INTEGRATING
LAW,
ETHICS AND
REGULATION

Dedication

A debt of gratitude for the reflections of many generations,
which continue to enrich current thinking.

INTEGRATING
LAW,
ETHICS AND
REGULATION

A GUIDE FOR NURSING AND HEALTH CARE STUDENTS

CATHERINE BERGLUND

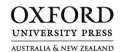

OXFORD
UNIVERSITY PRESS
AUSTRALIA & NEW ZEALAND

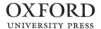

OXFORD
UNIVERSITY PRESS

Oxford University Press is a department of the University of Oxford.

It furthers the University's objective of excellence in research, scholarship, and education by publishing worldwide. Oxford is a registered trademark of Oxford University Press in the UK and in certain other countries. Published in Australia by
Oxford University Press
Level 8, 737 Bourke Street, Docklands, Victoria 3008, Australia

A catalogue record for this book is available from the National Library of Australia

ISBN 9780190311339

Edited by Philip Bryan
Typeset by Newgen KnowledgeWorks Pvt. Ltd., Chennai, India
Proofread by Naomi Saligari
Indexed by Jeanne Rudd
Printed in China by Leo Paper Products Ltd.

BRIEF CONTENTS

EXPANDED CONTENTS

LIST OF FIGURES AND TABLES

LIST OF PRACTICE EXAMPLES AND RESEARCH SKILLS

Practice examples

Research skills

ABBREVIATIONS

ACSQHC	Australian Council on Safety and Quality in Health Care
AHPRA	Australian Health Practitioner Regulation Agency
AHRC	Australian Human Rights Commission
AIN	Assistant in Nursing
ALRC	Australian Law Reform Commission
CLR	Commonwealth Law Reports
COAG	Coalition of Australian Governments
CPD	Continuing professional development
CTN	Clinical Trials Notification
CTX	Clinical Trials Exemption
EN	Enrolled Nurse
FDA	US Food and Drug Administration
GCP	good clinical practice
GDP	gross domestic product
GP	General Practitioner
HREC	human research ethics committees
ICH GCP	International Conference on Harmonisation Good Clinical Practice
IMS	Incident Management System
NDB	Notifiable Data Breaches
NDIS	National Disability Insurance Scheme
NNDSS	Australian National Notifiable Diseases Surveillance System
OAIC	Office of the Australian Information Commissioner
OECD	Organisation for Economic Co-operation and Development
ORI	Office of Research Integrity
QA	quality assurance
QI	quality improvement
RM	Registered Midwife
RN	Registered Nurse
S4D	Schedule 4D drugs
S8	Schedule 8 drugs
SOPs	standard operating procedures
TEQSA	Tertiary Education Quality and Standards Agency
TGA	Therapeutic Goods Administration
UNESCO	United Nations Educational, Scientific and Cultural Organization
WHO	World Health Organization

ABOUT THE AUTHOR

Catherine Berglund has worked in applied ethics and regulatory aspects of health care, standards and policy for close to 30 years. As well as completing a PhD on professional and community limits for medical research, Catherine taught health care ethics for over 20 years at undergraduate and postgraduate levels. She is legally qualified, and contributes to many regulatory and practical standards endeavours for registered health professionals and health care workers.

Contributors

Fiona Foxall has been a Registered Nurse for almost 35 years and has worked predominantly as an intensive care nurse in the UK and Australia. For over 20 years, she has worked in academia in the UK, Australia and Singapore and currently works as the Director of Undergraduate Nursing Studies in a West Australian University. Fiona is a qualified nurse teacher, has a Master of Arts degree in medical ethics and her PhD studies relate to the experiences of senior nurses and intensivists with the withdrawal of life-sustaining treatment from ICU patients and how those experiences shape decision making.

Jayne Hewitt has been a Registered Nurse for 30 years, working predominantly in critical care areas such as intensive care and coronary care. Having seen first-hand how the law impacts on the practice of nurses, Jayne undertook a Bachelor of Laws and Master of Health Law. This led her current role as an academic in the School of Nursing and Midwifery at Griffith University teaching health law and ethics to undergraduate health students. Continuing to combine her clinical experience and interest in law, Jayne is completing her PhD where she is exploring understandings of justice in health care. Jayne's current research focuses on patient safety and end of life issues.

Jennifer Haines is a Registered Nurse with an Intensive Care Certificate, Diploma of Law, Bachelor of Social Work, and a Graduate Certificate in Legal Practice. She is a Legal Practitioner in New South Wales, admitted to the Supreme Court in 2002. She has been a Registered Nurse for 40 years and spent most of those years practising in critical care areas, ICU, CCU, Neurosurgery ICU and Emergency Department. Jennifer trained at the Prince Henry Prince of Wales in the late 1970s, and worked in mixed wards after graduation at the Royal Prince Alfred Hospital. She was the General Secretary of the New South Wales Nurses Association from 1982 to 1987, and started teaching law and ethics to nurses in universities in 1991. Jennifer currently teaches at UTS and UWS.

Kath Weston is academic leader of Public Health in the School of Medicine, University of Wollongong (UOW) where she is passionate about engaging medical students in the science of public health and as public health advocates. Her research interests include historical aspects of outbreaks and public health, the history of prison medicine, and medical education. Kath leads the Research and Critical Analysis component of the UOW medical course, is a member of the UOW Human Research Ethics Committee, and a member of the Population Health and Ethics Assessment Panel of the Australian Medical Council.

Kay Tucker is the Law Library Manager at Monash University. She has extensive experience in designing and teaching legal research programs into undergraduate and postgraduate Faculty of Law courses. Prior to Monash, she worked in academic libraries in Sydney and Boston. Kay is co-author of Sue Milne and Kay Tucker, *A Practical Guide to Legal Research* (Thomson Reuters, 1st edn, 2008 and 2nd edn, 2010). She has also authored journal articles published in the *Australian Law Librarian* and the *Journal of Academic Language and Learning*, has been a member of the Editorial Board for the *Australian Law Librarian*, and has presented at numerous conferences on topics concerning students' research skills.

Narelle Biedermann is currently a Senior Lecturer at James Cook University. She is the course coordinator for the Master of Nursing program, and is also the Academic Lead–Blended Learning and Equity Contact Officer at the University. As a clinician, she served in the Australian Defence Force.

Susan Alexander has been a Registered Nurse for 12 years, working predominantly in palliative care and academia, but with a strong interest in professional issues. As well as clinical nursing, Susan has a background in managerial and administrative positions, experience that has contributed to the development of a nursing academic with a wide range of skills. After working in palliative care, Susan achieved her PhD in 2010, then continued with postgraduate studies in tertiary education, counselling and palliative care. During this time, Susan has continued teaching and researching as a lecturer in universities in Queensland, New South Wales and, currently, Western Australia. Topics taught include professional communication, ethics and law, palliative care and clinical skills.

PREFACE

An integrated understanding of law, regulation and ethics supports professionally responsible conduct. An integrated understanding helps professionals to be mindful of appropriate standards that support safe and competent practice, and to be able to recognise when a situation is potentially problematic and deserving of additional reflection and discussion—or expert advice. An integrated and practical understanding of law, regulation and ethics helps to ensure acceptable health care practice, and it is a professional competency.

In ***Integrating law, ethics and regulation: A guide for nursing and health care students***, fundamental concepts are defined and explained. Classic examples of principles or concepts in law and ethics are explored, and seminal discussions are included to illustrate the way these fields have contributed to contemporary practice standards. Regulatory examples are included to highlight regulation as a practical meeting point of ethics and law, supporting all health care professionals to act lawfully and ethically in their everyday practice. Examples of comment, research or reasoning exercises that have been published by people working in the health sector illustrate the active involvement of the health professions in integrated consideration of law, regulation and ethics issues. These references are drawn from a wide timeframe to highlight when complex issues have been considered within the health sector, and the reasoned ways forward that were suggested, which inform current and future practice. The text approach is compatible with the trend to teach ethics and law in an integrated way, within clinical streams, or in broad subject areas such as governance, professional identity or professional responsibility.

Integrating law, ethics and regulation: A guide for nursing and health care students is a practical text. The text is relevant for health care workers in all settings, from community health, public health, community support, disability and aged care, to small clinics and large organisation or tertiary hospital treatment delivery settings. As practice examples are drawn from diverse health care settings and health professions, readers will develop a deeper appreciation of their own professional role, as well as understanding the contribution others make to the health care endeavour.

When the knowledge drawn from law, ethics and regulation is understood in an integrated and practical way, the subject area remains interesting and relevant. The text approach is to encourage active reflective and critical reasoning and mindfulness for all routine and complex matters, so that the integrated analytical skills from law, ethics and regulation are developed, which can then be applied in an integrated and practical way across the whole scope of practice.

This text is a development of the earlier text *Ethics for health care*, originally published by Oxford University Press in 1998, and in its 4th edition in 2012.

GUIDED TOUR

Guided learning

Learning objectives are at the beginning of each chapter. These will help you focus on the chapter's key points and sharpen your skills in identifying potential problems you could face in the workforce.

Key terms help you pinpoint important concepts that you need to know to be an effective and competent health care professional. These terms are listed at the beginning of the chapter, defined in **margin notes** where they first appear, and collated in the **glossary** at the end of the book.

LEARNING OBJECTIVES

- To appreciate that law, regulation and ethics are all sources of standards and rules.
- To be able to find examples of laws, codes, policies and regulations.
- To be able to explain the importance of active reflection on conduct given expected standards.
- To understand the importance of shared objectives and specific roles in a health care team.
- To appreciate integrated standards in health care record keeping.

KEY TERMS

assault	law
autonomy	legislation
battery	medical ethics
beneficence	morals
bioethics	non-maleficence

Applying what you learn

Ethics and ethical dilemmas

PRACTICE EXAMPLE

Jennifer Haines

Jennifer has been a Registered Nurse for 40 years and spent most of those years practising in critical care areas, ICU, CCU, Neurosurgery ICU and Emergency Department.

When working through an ethical dilemma, we must ask the following:

- What is the ethical problem we are trying to solve?
- What are the facts?
- What ethical factors apply to the situation? What does our Code of Ethics say about the situation?
- What ethical factor takes priority in the situation?
- What does the law say about the situation?

Practice examples are provided by experienced health care professionals. These are potential 'real life' situations where you can put your learning into practice.

Reflections throughout the text encourage you to interact, explore and develop your legal, ethical and regulatory responsibilities that you may encounter as a health care professional.

REFLECTION POINT

On your marks, get set

How do you feel at the start of this learning on law, regulation and ethics and the standards and rules that will affect your professional practice? How familiar are you with any of these terms?

Make a note now in your portfolio, so that when you finish the course you will be able to look back to how you felt at the start of your reading and learning, and you will realise how much your own knowledge and understanding has grown. As you will read in this very first chapter, you should feel confident that you will have many experienced guides coming along with you on the journey.

CASE EXAMPLE

Five-minute overview

Nic is a nursing student who is lucky to have some work as an assistant in nursing, which makes for a busy schedule. As you read this chapter, keep a few notes that will help Nic develop an appreciation of professional practice responsibilities and fitness to ultimately register as a nurse. Imagine that Nic has a few minutes spare tomorrow and wants your five-minute overview of this chapter.

Case examples are scenarios or activities that will broaden your thinking on important topics and highlight the integrated nature of law, ethics and regulation. This will help you see the 'big picture' and how these issues impact the health care industry.

Pulling it all together

Integrated learning and practice boxes pose rhetorical questions that demonstrate the relevance of your learning to the working life of a health care professional.

INTEGRATED LEARNING AND PRACTICE

Is there a fundamental rule to consider before treating a patient?

Yes, there is a fundamental rule to consider. Before you can proceed with your part in any therapeutic encounter, consider the following:

- Law prompts you to consider if you have the person's agreement—in law, to touch without agreement can amount to **assault** or **battery**.
- Ethics reasoning frameworks prompt you to consider if you have the person's agreement to proceed, given the emphasis of respect for the person and their autonomy.
- Regulations support the application of these principles in practice. For instance, setting out what to do before proceeding with treatment, such as how to document the process of gaining informed agreement on a consent form.

Glossary **margin notes** make it easy to quickly identify and understand important concepts, which you need to be job-ready.

jurisdiction
Scope of authority and power to set and enforce laws and regulatory schemes.

Statute law

Statute law is legislation that has force because it has been passed into law by the government given a particular **jurisdiction**. Jurisdiction is a term for legal authority or power (Mann, 2013, p. 420). It represents the collected formally stated customary rules and principles that are used to regulate interaction within a community. The power is limited, as it can only be relied on to set rules and standards in a specific setting or context. Together, the power and the reach or scope of application of the power under that authority form the jurisdiction.

The **Summary** at the end of each chapter links the chapter's content back to the opening learning objectives. This enables you to make sure you are gaining the knowledge you need, for both your studies and future employment.

Summary

This chapter provides the foundation for understanding the integrated standards in health care. You have learnt that standards and rules are part of everyday life and also everyday work life, and that laws, regulations and ethics work together to provide that guidance on acceptable and appropriate standards. You have learnt a little about the structure and function of law and ethics from ancient and modern philosophers. When general principles are provided in law and ethics, the application of the principles is assisted by regulation. You have learnt that regulation contains the more precise details on how the standards are to be applied in practical contexts. The standards provide guidance for you. What is also needed is your active aspiration to act with integrity so that the relevant standards become part of your everyday practice.

STUDY QUESTIONS

1   Why is jurisdiction important in thinking about standards and rules?
2   What do law, ethics and regulations have in common?
3   Write the opening paragraph of an essay on 'The central importance of professional integrity in health care'.
4   Outline, in detail, with references, three significant regulatory requirements for record keeping in health care.
5   Have a glossary quiz. Turn to the glossary and select any glossary term that was covered in Chapter 1. (The numbers in brackets show you in which chapter the glossary term was defined.) See if you can define each term, and explain what it means when applied in a legal, ethical or regulatory context that you have read about in this book.

Study questions are provided for you at the end of each chapter to help you focus on the salient points of your learning.

Sample essay questions will help you think deeply about issues covered in the chapter to prepare you for assessment and practice.

SAMPLE ESSAY QUESTIONS

1   Identify the types of standards provided in a professional code of conduct or code of ethics. Describe the way the code was developed and the force of the rules or standards in it for the health profession.
2   Outline four examples of how the health care system is ready to identify mistakes and problems to better safeguard the public.
3   Research a contemporary safety and quality initiative at federal government level, and comment on why it is being undertaken, what it may achieve, and what progress has been made under the initiative so far.

References, legislation and cases are provided to help you identify further resources to support your learning.

REFERENCES

Australian Commission on Safety and Quality in Health Care (ACSQHS). (2012, 2017). *National Safety and Quality Health Service Standards* (1st edn 2012; 2nd edn 2017). Sydney: Australian Government. Available at http://safetyandquality.gov.au

Australian Commission on Safety and Quality in Health Care (ACSQHS). *Clinical Care Standards*, updated as necessary. Retrieved from http://safetyandquality.gov.au

LEGISLATION

Evidence Act 1995 (NSW)

Health Practitioner Regulation National Law No 86 (NSW)

Health Practitioner Regulation National Law Act 2009 (Qld)

CASES

Allinson v General Council of Medical Education and Registration [1894] 1 QB 755.

Briginshaw v Briginshaw [1938] HCA 34.

Council of the Law Society of New South Wales v Foreman (1994) 34 NSWLR 408.

GLOSSARY

A **Glossary** is provided at the end of the book. This provides a quick reference to help you grasp unfamiliar terms and concepts.

Note: Numbers in brackets refer to chapters where these terms are defined.

Absolutism
An ethics theory in which a rule or rules are identified as fundamentally important, and of unvarying significance. (4)

Accountability
Process of being open to scrutiny for assessment of conduct of responsibilities. (3)

ACKNOWLEDGMENTS

Family and friends continue to be my inspiration for taking time to enjoy life and adventure as well as the pursuit of a challenge. So with time to explore, the flicker of an idea begins. While the notion of a book is exciting in itself, it takes a team to nurture it to completion. Grateful thanks are due to Debra James, Publishing Manager at Oxford University Press, who was thoughtfully enthusiastic throughout, including at the early concept and proposal stages. Encouragement is always welcome, and when given generously yet in measured terms by eminent academic peer reviewers, it is heartening and invaluable. I am hopeful that I can one day assist other writing colleagues with such a generous spirit, and I extend my heartfelt and collegial best wishes to them and their role – the comments and queries prompted an integrated and revised structure of the text throughout, for a much better result. Reflections, practice examples, case material and exercises have been helpfully contributed by many academic colleagues. To freelance editor Philip Bryan, and Alex Chambers, Editor, Sarah Fay, Associate Publisher, the cover and layout team, and all those behind the scenes at Oxford University Press who make a real book possible, thank you.

The author and the publisher wish to thank the following copyright holders for reproduction of their material.

Extract from Health Insurance (Professional Services Review) Regulations 1999 (Cth), section 5 and Health Insurance Act 1973 (Cth), at sections 128A or 128B sourced from the Federal Register of Legislation at 19 February 2019. For the latest information on Australian Government law please go to www. legislation.gov.au.; Medical Board of Australia. (2014). Good medical practice: a code of conduct for doctors in Australia, March 2014. Accessed from www.medicalboard.gov.au, © Medical Board of Australia; Extracts from Health Records and Information Privacy Act 2002 (NSW) and New South Wales Government. (2018). Budget Paper 3. Budget Estimates 2018–19. NSW Budget 2018–19. Accessed from www.budget.nsw.gov. au, © State of New South Wales through the Information and Privacy Commission NSW 2015; Quotes from the New South Wales Ministry of Health, © State of New South Wales NSW Ministry of Health. For current information go to www.health.nsw.gov.au for New South Wales Government, Ministry of Health. (2012). Health Care Records Documentation and Management and Information. Sydney: New South Wales Ministry of Health, PD2012_069. Accessed from http://www1.health.nsw.gov.au/pds/ActivePDSDocuments/PD2012_069.pdf; Extracts from Mental Health Act 2014 (Vic), State Government of Victoria, Department of Health. (2011). Guidelines for Victorian public health services on community detention, as at September 2011. Accessed from www2.health.vic.gov.au and State Government of Victoria, Department of Health. (2011), © State of Victoria; Quote from Thomson, J.J. (1971) *A Defense of Abortion, Philosophy & Public Affairs* by Blackwell Publishing, Inc. Reproduced with permission of Blackwell Publishing, Inc. in the format Book via Copyright Clearance Center; Quotes from the Western Australian Administrative Tribunal © State of Western Australia 2006. This information is the property of the State of Western Australia represented by the State Administrative Tribunal. It is intended for your general use and information. The information provided is correct to the best of our knowledge, but no warranty as to accuracy is given and each person or organisation should not act on the basis of its contents without taking appropriate advice. To the fullest extent permissible at law the State of Western Australia and its officers, employees, agents and others acting under its control are irrevocably and unconditionally released from any and all liability to each person or organisation using this site as a result of any information being incorrect. The material is made available on the understanding it does not constitute professional or expert advice. It may include views of third parties and does not necessarily reflect the views of the State Administrative Tribunal.

Every effort has been made to trace the original source of copyright material contained in this book. The publisher will be pleased to hear from copyright holders to rectify any errors or omissions.

CHAPTER 1

Beginning to understand the sources of standards and rules

LEARNING OBJECTIVES

- To appreciate that law, regulation and ethics are all sources of standards and rules.
- To be able to find examples of laws, codes, policies and regulations.
- To be able to explain the importance of active reflection on conduct given expected standards.
- To understand the importance of shared objectives and specific roles in a health care team.
- To appreciate integrated standards in health care record keeping.

KEY TERMS

assault	law
autonomy	legislation
battery	medical ethics
beneficence	morals
bioethics	non-maleficence
code of conduct	norms
ethics	professional
false imprisonment	professional code of ethics
good	regulation
health care worker	responsibility
health practitioner	rules
human rights	skill
ideals	standards
integrity	values
jurisdiction	virtue
justice	

Aiming for an integrated understanding from the start

The approach in this text in explaining the standards that underpin working within health settings is user-friendly, pragmatic and practical. As you work through the chapters and companion readings and exercises, you will start to feel that law, ethics and regulation are not as complex and unwieldy as they seemed at first, and you will be equipped with a conceptual framework to understand more about standards and rules as you train and work in the health sector.

REFLECTION POINT

On your marks, get set

How do you feel at the start of this learning on law, regulation and ethics and the standards and rules that will affect your professional practice? How familiar are you with any of these terms?

Make a note now in your portfolio, so that when you finish the course you will be able to look back to how you felt at the start of your reading and learning, and you will realise how much your own knowledge and understanding has grown. As you will read in this very first chapter, you should feel confident that you will have many experienced guides coming along with you on the journey.

---

standards
Accepted benchmarks that are defined and available.

law
Body of formal and customary rules and principles, used to regulate interactions in a community.

regulation
Standards, rules, restriction and procedures for social control and management in specific contexts.

ethics
Reflective process of analysing and examining moral issues and problems.

Your responsibilities as a health care professional are partly defined and informed by law, regulation and ethics. Some of your responsibilities are **standards** to uphold that are expressed in rules, codes, guidelines, policies and legislation. We begin by exploring how such standards were derived. Many examples and excerpts appear in this text; as you work your way through the text, you will become more comfortable with the diverse sources and styles of those standards. Examples of restrictions, standards and rules are sourced from a variety of legal, ethics, administrative, regulatory and policy arenas.

Law and **ethics** have quite a lot in common. As scholarly and intellectual endeavours with practical application, their common purpose is to facilitate fair and reasonable ways to live with others in a society. The principles in law and ethics are intended to be applied in practical contexts. Law and ethics inform and shape **regulation**.

The purpose of regulation is to set out operational restrictions, standards and rules to be applied in practice, in specific contexts. Regulation provides the bulk of practical day-to-day guidance for health care settings, for both institutions and the health care workers. Regulation also guides the way departures from acceptable standards are assessed. Discussion of the expected standards—and departures from those standards—highlights what society expects of both institutions and persons engaged in health care when the standards are applied in practical contexts, in real life.

Our philosophical great-grandparents left us forms of reasoning as their legacy, as well as the benefit of their discussion about how to live in a society in a peaceful and orderly way.

Ethics and law are their children, who in turn gave us the practical codes and laws in each nation-state. The youngest in the family tree, the next and current generation, are the lively and dynamic regulation-setters, who try to make living together fair and workable in the current day. Remembering the vast history and deep thought that has gone into setting standards will help you to understand how important it is to live up to the expected standards in your work.

INTEGRATED LEARNING AND PRACTICE

Is there a fundamental rule to consider before treating a patient?

Yes, there is a fundamental rule to consider. Before you can proceed with your part in any therapeutic encounter, consider the following:

- Law prompts you to consider if you have the person's agreement—in law, to touch without agreement can amount to **assault** or **battery**.
- Ethics reasoning frameworks prompt you to consider if you have the person's agreement to proceed, given the emphasis of respect for the person and their autonomy.
- Regulations support the application of these principles in practice. For instance, setting out what to do before proceeding with treatment, such as how to document the process of gaining informed agreement on a consent form.

assault
Physical interference or causing fear of physical interference to a person.

battery
An act of physical interference or force applied to a victim's body without consent. Battery is an old term. Many modern laws combine battery in the broader concept of assault, which includes the threat as well as actual force or touching.

It would be a good idea to reread Chapter 1 every now and then, when you want to look back over the general explanations of law, regulation and ethics.

Jurisdiction and laws

Law is an authoritative system of norms that can be written or unwritten, and which govern a society and can be enforced with sanctions (Mann, 2013, p. 432). It represents the basic duties of citizens and the accepted lower limits of their conduct. The law is a contemporary statement of the standards that you are expected to maintain in your dealings with the social institutions of your state and country, and in your dealings with others in personal interactions. Different countries and states define and expect different basic responsibilities from their people. In addition to the basic responsibilities owed to others under law, there are also special responsibilities for professionals under law.

Understanding a little about the legal system in your state and country will help you to more fully appreciate the legal requirements that apply to you. Our legal system is made up of:

- legislative instruments—which includes Statute law and related regulations
- case law—which includes civil or common law and criminal law court decisions.

Statute law

jurisdiction
Scope of authority and power to set and enforce laws and regulatory schemes.

Statute law is legislation that has force because it has been passed into law by the government given a particular **jurisdiction**. Jurisdiction is a term for legal authority or power (Mann, 2013, p. 420). It represents the collected formally stated customary rules and principles that are used to regulate interaction within a community. The power is limited, as it can only be relied on to set rules and standards in a specific setting or context. Together, the power and the reach or scope of application of the power under that authority form the jurisdiction.

Statute laws evolve when elected government representatives pass new pieces of **legislation**—or amend existing legislation—to try and correct an issue that has been brought to their attention. The head of state (e.g. the monarch or representative) then approves the legislation so that it is in force. These statutes and related regulations are meant to guide everyone's conduct as they live within the society.

legislation
Statutes and other rules in related instruments that are formally approved by parliament.

Case law

A tradition from English law dating back to 1584 that is in place in our legal system is that legislation also provides structure to a law court's considerations (*Heydon's Case* (1584), as cited in Cook, Creyke, Geddes & Hamer, 2009, p. 233). So statute law and case law work together in a practical way to set and maintain standards within society. Statutes guide individuals in their conduct and they also guide the courts when resolving disputes or redressing wrongs that have been committed. Judges' wisdom on fair dealings with each other in society is available in their judgments, which collectively forms the case law. In turn, case law principles in important judgments inform the further development of statute law.

Jurisdiction

Sovereign states have a specific geographic territory and a permanent population. This is their jurisdiction. They can make their own laws to 'rule' over their own people and also all the people present in their own geographic territory (Crawford, 2012, p. 452). The same principle applies to areas within a country, if the areas are recognised as being able to set their own laws.

So, the state and territory governments of Western Australia, South Australia, Victoria, Tasmania, New South Wales, Queensland, the Australian Capital Territory and the Northern Territory are able to pass laws on many matters that apply within their boundaries.

For instance, the state and territory governments pass laws that help them to run public hospitals and implement service standards. The states existed before Federation in 1901—it was was the decision of the states to form a Commonwealth Government so that they could collaborate on practical matters, trade and foreign dealings. Given the agreed powers under the Constitution as a Federation, the Commonwealth Government then assumed the right to pass laws over certain matters, such as taxation and immigration. It can also rely on these constitutional powers to pass laws on related or incidental matters (*Commonwealth of Australia Constitution Act 1900* (Cth) (the Constitution), section 51). You can look up the full list of matters that the Commonwealth can pass laws on by reading section 51 when you look up the Constitution: <www.legislation.gov.au>.

As stated in section 5 of the Constitution:

> This Act, and all laws made by the Parliament of the Commonwealth under the Constitution, shall be binding on the courts, judges, and people of every State and of every part of the Commonwealth, notwithstanding anything in the laws of any State; and the laws of the Commonwealth shall be in force on all British ships, the Queen's ships of war excepted, whose first port of clearance and whose port of destination are in the Commonwealth.

The Federal Government funds and regulates Medicare, a universal health system, through a series of statutes including the:

- *Medicare Levy Act 1986* (Cth)
- *Human Services (Medicare) Act 1973* (Cth)
- *Human Services (Medicare) Regulations 1975* (Cth).

The Commonwealth is able to pass laws on the funding of medical services because the Constitution provides, in section 51(xxiiiA) that the Commonwealth can pass laws for the peace, order and good government of the Commonwealth with respect to:

> The provision of maternity allowances, widows pensions, child endowment, unemployment, pharmaceutical, sickness and hospital benefits, medical and dental services (but not so as to authorize any form of civil conscription), benefits to students and family allowances.

This power was added by amendment in 1946, well after Federation. This shows that the Constitution is a live document that can be amended from time to time so that our society is governed appropriately for its contemporary context. Medical services may include 'healing by drugs, surgery and manipulation'. Further laws and regulations on the way services are delivered by institutions such as public hospitals is a matter for the states and territories, unless additional powers under the Constitution are relied on (see McMillan, 1993, p. 34).

INTEGRATED LEARNING AND PRACTICE

How do providers get Medicare Provider Numbers?

A Medicare Provider Number is the mechanism for the partial reimbursement or contribution by the community to the cost of medical services that individuals receive through the Commonwealth Medicare scheme.

Medical practitioners apply to a Commonwealth government department (Human Services, Health) for a provider number for the location of their medical practice or service provision. Practitioners need to be able to show that they are eligible—that they have the correct qualifications and the required public hospital training. Practitioners are then able to bill certain item numbers in their own right, if the services are within the scope of their practice.

Other providers can also apply for provider numbers. For instance, registered psychologists and accredited mental health social workers can apply for provider

+ continued

numbers, if they have evidence from their own assessing authority that they are competent to provide certain services.

The Health Insurance scheme, including the *Health Insurance (Allied Health Services) Determination 2011* (Cth), supports the consideration of an individual's training and competence by a recognised assessing authority. This regulatory scheme provides public protection and enhances quality and safety—because only those who are appropriately trained and assessed by a recognised authority as being sufficiently skilled are then able to bill patients or Medicare directly for those item number services.

REFLECTION: LEGISLATION DISCOVERY

Understanding which governments' laws may be applied to you is important as a first step before you look for derived regulations and standards and rules.

You can get some idea of the vast number of legislative instruments that regulate interactions in health and health care by searching 'health' as a key term in your own jurisdiction. You can look at the listed legislative instruments by searching the Federal Register of Legislation for the Commonwealth legislation (legislation.gov.au) and then your state or territory jurisdiction legislation:

* legislation.act.gov.au
* legislation.nsw.gov.au
* legislation.nt.gov.au
* legislation.qld.gov.au
* legislation.sa.gov.au
* legislation.tas.gov.au
* legislation.vic.gov.au
* legislation.wa.gov.au.

1 Browse your lists to see the wide range of topic areas that have been considered in your jurisdictions as part of setting standards for health and health care.

2 Note your reaction to the list you have identified. Understanding your responsibilities starts with an appreciation of the vast scope and detail of legislation that could be relevant to your field of professional work.

3 Choose one statute, an Act, and look at the 'object' or purpose section of your Act. This is in an early section of every instrument, and reading it first is essential—it guides the proper interpretation of the following detailed sections of the Act.

Research skills: Legislation

Kay Tucker, Law Library Manager, Monash University

As a law librarian in a large university, I see many students from Law and other faculties who need to find the law applying to a particular topic. I usually recommend that they start by reading a text, legal commentary service or journal article that summarises the law and identifies the relevant Acts and cases. Reading the work of an expert who has done this initial work for you could save you a lot of wasted research time. One such legal commentary service in the Health Law area is the *CCH Australian Health and Medical Reporter*. Find other texts via your library catalogue and databases.

If you know the title of the Act that regulates the issue you're researching, then you can easily find it on the official government website. However, these sites are not easy to search deeply. For example, if you are trying to find the Victorian Act that includes the Health Privacy Principles, searching for the occurrence of these words in the current Acts contained in the 'Victorian Law Today' section of the official site results in a number of Acts. You may need to go to a few of them to read the terms in context, before looking at the *Health Records Act 2001* (Vic) where the Principles are included as Schedule 1.

Rather than search each government website separately, you can use a subscription-based database to help you find legislation from all Australian jurisdictions. The main databases are LawNow (LexisNexis), LawOne (TimeBase) and Lawlex (SAI Global). Lawlex provides a freely available browse facility to help find legislation related to particular topics. Selecting the topic 'Health' initiates a number of subcategories such as Aged Care, Medical Practice and Treatment, Mental Health, Privacy, and Regulatory Bodies. From there, you will see a list of the relevant Acts and Regulations for the selected jurisdictions. For example, if you're interested in the privacy of medical records, and you select the Privacy category, you may need to look at a few Acts, including the *My Health Record Act 2012* (Cth) and the *Privacy Act 1988* (Cth).

Once you have an Act, how do you know which provisions (or sections) of an Act apply to your problem? You can look through the Table of Provisions at the start of the Act—but you will often need to read a number of sections to place them in context. You can also use the search facility in AustLII <www.austlii.edu.au>, a free web database that provides access to Australian legislation, where search results are listed at the section level. For example, if you select to search Consolidated Commonwealth Acts and type in Privacy NEAR Protection NEAR Health, a top result is the *Privacy Act 1988—section 95A Guidelines for Australian Privacy Principles about health information*. You can link through to read the section. However, if you use or reference the Act, always go back to the official government website as the authoritative source.

More tips for researching:

+ Make sure that you are looking at the most current version of the Act. At the top of the Act under the Short Title, you will see wording such 'includes amendments up to …' or 'Authorised Version incorporating amendments as at'. One of the hazards of googling an Act is that you may link through to an older version.

+ continued

+ If you want to see what the amendments to an Act have been over time, look at the Endnotes of the Act, where you will find the Table of Amendments or Amendment History. You may then need to look at the Amending Act to understand the change. For example, the *Privacy Act 1988* (Cth) was amended by the *Privacy Amendment (Notifiable Data Breaches) Act 2017* (Cth). Lawlex can also help you identify changes to Acts and the dates the changes commence.

+ Look at the Explanatory Memorandum (published along with the Bill) to understand the meaning of an Act. Read the Second Reading Speech for the Bill to learn more about the context and intent of the Bill. These 'Extrinsic Materials' are valuable research sources, available on the Parliamentary websites and legislation databases.

References

Australasian Legal Information Institute: <http://www.austlii.edu.au/>.

Bates, Philip, *Australian Health and Medical Reporter* (CCH Australia, 2007).

Victorian Legislation and Parliamentary Documents: <http://www.legislation.vic.gov.au/>.

Jeremy Bentham, one of the famous scholars in law and philosophy, is an example of a jurist, philosopher and social reformer who promoted a particular view of how law and ethics are related. An early utilitarian, Bentham espoused the principle of achieving the greatest good for the greatest number. The utility he concentrated on was felicity, or happiness. The means to pursue felicity, Bentham thought, were reason and law. He thought that the stability of law would provide the structure to achieve happiness. He felt that this fundamental aim should be recognised in law, and he set about suggesting legal and societal constructions that would achieve it. His concern was at a societal and governmental level (Honderich, 1995, p. 85). Bentham's utilitarianism was a grand plan to express societal goals and limits in a legal system.

REFLECTION: LAW AS A BASIC STANDARD

You have already thought about the law on assault, the ethical importance of autonomy, and the regulations about gaining permission to treat—which applies to all therapeutic interactions. The standard is that you should always ask for permission before touching a patient.

To begin examining what the law could mean for you in a practical sense, and identifying basic standards you should be mindful of in your interactions in your community, try the following exercise.

1 Look up a statute in your jurisdiction, and read a section that sets out a legal rule about required action or unacceptable conduct. You could look up tax evasion, or

the definition of assault in a state or territory Criminal Code or Crimes Act, or perhaps check on whether driving without a licence is illegal, or another issue you choose.

2   Consider if that legal rule promotes stability for the jurisdiction and felicity in the people who live within the jurisdiction.

The law is an empowering force in health care. Society uses laws to give professions authority and power to define standards of knowledge and skill in their profession. Laws can be relied on to constrain professionals if the appropriate standard is not met.

The state and territory governments can seek Commonwealth Government assistance or co-ordination at times. States have sought Commonwealth assistance to coordinate nationally consistent regulations in relation to registration for registered health professionals, who may use the title 'practitioner'. The Australian Health Practitioner Regulation Agency (AHPRA) is a national agency that holds the registers of health practitioners on behalf of national boards. States and territories agreed to pass state laws that are broadly consistent to enable this coordination, the *Health Practitioner Regulation National Law 2009* (Cth), so that the law has force in their own jurisdictions (AHPRA, 2017). There are some minor variations between the state and territory legislative instruments, which collectively put in place the practical objectives agreed between all the governments.

Currently in Australia practitioners in the following professions are subject to specific registration requirements, which is set out in legislation:

- Aboriginal and Torres Strait Islander health
- Chinese medicine
- chiropractic
- dental
- medical
- medical radiation practice
- nursing and midwifery
- occupational therapy
- optometry
- osteopathy
- paramedicine
- pharmacy
- physiotherapy
- podiatry
- psychology.

The standards expected of those registered health care practitioners is also partly defined by legislation. The National Boards of those professions can set codes of conduct and ethics for their members and, under the National Law, these codes have legal force as appropriate standards for professional conduct or practice. (For instance, see *Health Practitioner Regulation National Law 2009* (Vic), sections 38–41.) The legislation also sets out the process for investigating and considering potentially unsatisfactory professional conduct. Some provisions in the National Law also apply to health services provided by unregistered providers—for instance, prohibition orders that prevent persons who have lost their registered status from working in certain health care service roles.

health care worker
Person working in health service delivery who is not registered as a health practitioner.

health practitioner
Health care professional who is registered under the Health Practitioner Regulation National Law.

Some uniform conduct standards are also being developed for **health care workers** who are not regulated as 'registered **health practitioners**', as they are not registered under the AHPRA regulatory scheme. However, some professionals may be referred to as 'unregistered health practitioners' in some states. A *National Code of Conduct for health care workers (NCC)* (Coalition of Australian Governments, 2015) is available for states and territories to formalise through their own laws. In addition, abiding by the NCC may be set as a requirement of working in certain settings, such as under nationally funded schemes. Endorsed by the Coalition of Australian Governments (COAG), the purpose of the National Code is to encourage consistent minimum requirements, so that all unregistered health care workers who provide a health service can be held accountable to those standards. A prohibition order could be issued if a serious risk to public health and safety would be posed if that worker continued to work in health service care roles (Coalition of Australian Governments, 2015).

Also, all the normal municipal civil and criminal laws on acceptable conduct apply to all health care workers and registered health practitioners, just as they do to all other unregistered health care professionals and support workers in the health care sector. This includes social workers, counsellors, assistants in nursing, disability and aged care support workers, infection control and cleaning staff, reception staff, information management and information technology workers, public health unit staff, dieticians, food preparation staff, and many more.

International agreements

There are many international commitments that are relevant to health and health care. These are most commonly expressed in treaties, declarations and conventions as agreements to uphold fundamental rights and principles.

human rights
Basic rights, thought to be due to all human beings.

The United Nations has issued numerous **human rights**, civil and political rights and economic, social and cultural rights documents on behalf of its member states, which together are known as the International Bill of Human Rights. You could go to the United Nations website <www.un.org> for documents such as the:

- *Universal Declaration of Human Rights, 1948*
- *International Covenant on Civil and Political Rights, 1966*
- *International Covenant on Economic, Social and Cultural Rights, 1966.*

There are optional protocols that support these documents, and these are publicly available through the United National Office of the High Commissioner for Human Rights <www.ochr.org>.

Some of the rights to be protected as human rights are:

- rights to life
- right to freedom from fear
- right to self-determination
- right to be able to pursue one's own economic, social and cultural development
- right not to be detained unreasonably.

There is a proviso that the rights should be protected unless infringement of the rights is protected by law and restriction of the right is reasonable and necessary and proportionate to the purpose of the restrictive law (Australian Human Rights Commission, 2017).

In international law, countries are referred to as member states. Each member state can choose to make agreements with other states. They must be able to demonstrate the stability of their government, so that others can rely on them to have the capacity to enter into such international agreements—and also to live up to those agreements (Crawford, 2012, p. 115). This is a broader commitment than specific trade agreements that are negotiated and made between states, so that fair trading can be conducted between those two states.

If a member state chooses to be party to an international agreement, a representative signs the agreement, and the agreement is then ratified, which carries with it an obligation to explain to the whole international community how the commitment is being put into action. Each state translates the principles of the agreement into practice in its own geographic territory as it sees fit, because each state has the exclusive jurisdiction—or right—to legislate and regulate within its territory (Crawford, 2012, p. 452).

The absolute right not to be subjected to cruel, inhuman or degrading treatment is set out in the *International Covenant on Civil and Political Rights* (ICCPR): 'No one shall be subjected to torture or to cruel, inhuman or degrading treatment or punishment. In particular, no one shall be subjected without his free consent to medical or scientific experimentation' (United Nations, 1966a, Article 7). The ICCPR was ratified by Australia in 1975.

As you will read in Chapter 7 'The limits of care', our ethics approval requirements and local institution governance processes for health and medical research safeguard the commitment that Australia has made to the international community.

In 2017, the Australian Government also recommitted to ratification of the United Nations *Optional Protocol to the Convention Against Torture and Other Cruel and Degrading Treatment or Punishment* (United Nations, 2002; Australian Human Rights Commission, 2017). This Optional Protocol obliges member states to monitor places of detention in order to prevent violence and abuse. This will arguably include mental health facilities and other secure residential facilities where people with disabilities may be living.

INTEGRATED LEARNING AND PRACTICE

Why is the restraint or restriction of patients problematic?

Promoting human dignity and human rights and freedom is expressed as an international commitment in the *Universal Declaration on Bioethics and Human Rights*. The Declaration refers to collective responsibility to promote health and social development; respect and integrity of individuals; and protection of the vulnerable in health care and research contexts (United Nations Educational, Scientific and Cultural Organization, 2005).

Keeping someone in an environment, either directly or negligently, without their consent, or without lawful or reasonable reason to act without their consent, can

+ continued

false imprisonment
Unlawful physical
or psychological
restraint of
freedom, including
detention.

amount to **false imprisonment**, if the person reasonably feels they have no reasonable means of escaping from that environment.

The area of law called torts law provides the case law principles on false imprisonment, as torts law protects the freedom of movement of a person (Balkin & Davis, 2013, p. 49). You will read more about torts law in Chapter 3. Knowing you have lost the freedom of movement is the injury that is the subject of the tort, but knowing the freedom has been lost is not always required—for instance, if someone is locked into an environment while they are asleep, the containment has still occurred.

So as not to cause injury to this freedom, consent to retaining someone in an environment is presumed to be essential, and there are only rare instances when authorised consent is not required. Following the legal and regulatory provisions before retaining a person in an environment are crucial to acting lawfully. For instance, if you think someone is a danger to themselves or others, a person can be 'scheduled' to remain in the care environment.

Society sets out what a reasonable infringement of a person's freedom is, and the type of circumstances that justify the curtailing of rights, and provides an authority with the power to provide that consent. The term 'schedule' means that the provisions of the regulation or 'schedule' have been properly applied to make detaining the person lawful. You will read more about this in Chapter 7.

If any restriction of a patient is to be used against their will, for their own safety or the safety of others, then only the least restrictive option reasonably available is lawful. Policies support the prevention of disturbed behaviour, or minimising the disturbed behaviour episode, and rarely using restrictive practices—for instance in mental health and aged care. While the use of restrictive practices has declined, a recent report states that more work is needed in the disability sector (Melbourne Social Equity Institute, 2014). Quarantine restrictions of liberty are not false imprisonment of a person provided the proper procedures are followed so that the detention is lawful.

International agreements underpin many other more routine aspects of safeguarding basic rights and promoting the best health possible for all people. A practical example of joint action to enhance health is the current multilateral *Agreement to Ban Smoking on International Passenger Flights* (Multilateral agreement, 1994), which Australia implemented soon afterwards in its own legislation through the *Transport Legislation Amendment Act (No 2) 1995* (Cth) and *Air Navigation Regulations (Amendment) 1996* (Cth) (SR No 113).

To understand the obligations that are derived from international treaties, declarations or conventions in your jurisdiction, you can check whether a member state has:

- become a signatory to the agreement
- ratified the agreement in specific terms, or varied some terms
- put in place any regulation or legislation that gives legal effect within its jurisdiction to the commitment.

REFLECTION: INTERNATIONAL OBLIGATIONS

Look up the Australian Treaties Database, which is hosted by the Australian Government Department of Foreign Affairs and Trade (DFAT) at <www.info.dfat.gov.au/treaties>.

1   Find out when Australia signed, and if and when Australia has ratified some of the other international Declarations and Conventions and Agreements.

2   Also on <www.info.dfat.gov.au>, see which legislation is listed as giving effect to the agreements, and find up-to-date information on the ongoing policy work towards ratification or implementation of Australia's obligations under these agreements.

3   Note your reaction to the list you have identified. Did you notice any of these legislative instruments in your earlier search?

Ethics reasoning traditions

Ethics is a shorthand term for the process of analysis and derivation of basic values and objectives, norms or standards, and reasoning to identify optimum aims or objectives of thoughts and actions, standards, and behaviour. The essence of ethics lies in a process of debate and thought and reflection, either on an individual or group basis. It is the process of analysis as much as the position that is argued, and that is the subject of ethics writings and discussions.

Ethics helps you to decide what to do in routine and complex or difficult situations. It acts as a guide, and a reasoned 'voice'. Thinking and reflecting is the hallmark of ethics—as it is an active process. It is a tool that is meant to be used in practical situations. It helps you to reflect on real-life issues, and it is a process that can be applied to real concerns and situations as they unfold.

Ethics in health contexts is sometimes simply called 'ethics'; at other times it is called 'bioethics', or 'medical ethics'. You may like to choose a definition of ethics that you understand best from the following options, which were crafted by experts:

- ethics—'ways of understanding and examining the moral life' (Gillon, 1986, p. 2)
- **bioethics**—'a popular contraction for "biomedical ethics", which is the study of moral value in the life sciences and in their clinical application' (Moreno, 1995, p. 4)
- **medical ethics**—'the analytical activity in which the concepts, assumptions, beliefs, attitudes, emotion, reasons, and arguments underlying medico-moral decision making are examined critically' (Gillon, 1986, p. 2).

There is an impetus in ethics to aim higher than the basic minimum of social responsibilities. The common process of the reflection is that **moral** issues are identified and examined. To some people, moral reflection means to reflect on a lesson that has been handed down in significant religious texts, to strive to distinguish between right and wrong, and act

bioethics
Reflective ethics process applied to the health care context and life sciences.

medical ethics
Specific term for ethics in the medical and biomedical context.

morals
Significant lessons prompting reflection to identify virtuous, right, or acceptable course of conduct.

accordingly, given that lesson. It can also be a practical lesson learnt from past experience and reflection, again reflected on in terms of significance and importance. In this text, the word *moral* is used in a broad sense to mean a reflective examination of values and objectives, including reference to lessons, with an examination of the implications of thought and action for oneself and others.

For centuries, philosophers have been motivated to understand and explain the process of judgment and reflection in a moral being. Some philosophers have concentrated on a categorical imperative (or law) that must be followed, and autonomy of the will, while recognising that judgment illustrates the purposiveness of nature. Reasoning and judgment are explained as part of personal agency, responsibility and moral law—for example, in Kant's seminal work, the *Critique of Judgment* (Honderich, 1995, pp. 435–9).

REFLECTION POINT

Everyday ethics

Take a minute to think about how you live your life. In your own words, try to identify whether there is one fundamental value or principle in the way you live your life, and in the way you live alongside others.

---

norms
Accepted standards, which can be used to guide conduct.

Many of the philosophers whose work we draw upon in professional ethics wrote about individual ethics—the ethics of decisions made by individuals—such as in virtue ethics traditions. Other philosophers concentrated on group standards or **norms**—such as in descriptive ethics or normative ethics—to search for expressions of acceptable standards. Some ethicists in meta-ethics traditions considered the significance of defining some value or rule or norm identified as right or wrong.

Early philosophers thought about how we should live our lives and relate to others. They thought about the structure of our society; about what we, as individuals, owe to our society; and about what we can, and should, expect in return. They also thought also about our higher duties to God. Today, religion is often separated from professional ethics, but if it is a part of how you live your life, it would be artificial for you to ignore it. You will see comments and exercises from many early philosophers dotted throughout this book.

virtue
Worth or quality of particular moral excellence.

Socrates was an important early philosopher. The key feature of his discussions was the way in which participants were encouraged to elicit and question beliefs. Some of the central values that Socrates espoused were justice, courage and pity (Borchert, 2006, pp. 105–6). He tried to define the values through reflection and discussion, like the Reflection you have just completed. This reflection process is also appropriate for your professional life. As nurses advance their clients' interests and strive to maximise the autonomy of their clients, justice and courage have been identified as **virtues** espoused in modern nursing (Beauchamp & Childress, 1994, p. 465).

values
Concepts given worth or importance in life and interactions, making up a value system.

Our **values** form our ethics standards—and they determine what we expect from others. In some ethics frameworks, virtue and the formation of central values is paramount in moral self-development. We probably apply this notion of moral self-development in our own lives without thinking about it. For instance, we do not expect children to be rational and moral in the way that they relate to others and the world because we know that some of this is learnt. We gradually teach them what is expected, what we value, and what we hope that they will value. As they grow older, children begin to recognise that it is not just because these values are advocated by their parents and guardians that makes them desirable as guides for life—they come to value the virtues themselves.

In ancient Greece and Rome, there were forums that were used for debating what was right and virtuous. Learned people were trained to reflect and to hold monologues or debates challenging others to refine their thoughts, actions and reasoning. Socrates and Plato led this tradition, and there was an expectation that people who rose to prominence in society would learn to reflect and debate personal and social ethics. Plato was Socrates' student and Aristotle's teacher. Plato espoused the work on systematic techniques of argument, and emphasised that winning a debate was not the purpose of the discussion. The purpose was to search for the truth. The dialogue between Socrates and Plato became famous, and can be the basis of philosophy exercises to this day (Borchert, 2006, pp. 105–14).

REFLECTION POINT
Virtue and ideals

1　When you think about how you try to live, think about the virtue you aspire to.
2　What is that virtue? How would you define it, and how do you know if you have achieved it?

When you are applying for a job, you should consider the values and objectives of the institution and the aims it pursues; in other words, the way the institutional services are delivered. What service is offered is only part of the information that you need. Values may be expressed in mission statements and visions as they relate to the institution's strategic objectives (Gillon, 1986, p. 2). Even though health care institutions all aim to provide goods and deliver health care, how they define goods, and how they deliver health care can vary subtly. Sometimes this is because of the underlying ethic or morality system of the institution, such as in Catholic and Seventh Day Adventist hospitals.

REFLECTION POINT
Shared goals

Make a note of the goals or mission statement of a health centre, community health service or hospital near you, and of your own prospective or current place of employment.
　Once you discover these values, you need to decide whether they are compatible with your ethics and belief system—as the values will affect the way your work is defined and carried out in that institution.

Ethics in health care is really about three things:

* individual ethics and values
* group ethics and values
* professional ethics and values.

Writers on health care ethics who favour different ethics theories and frameworks vary in their approach. Some concentrate on individual virtue, others on group notions of ethics, or on philosophical analysis of ethical stances and values.

You will read more about ethics reflection and the reasoning frameworks that you can choose from for ethics analysis in Chapter 4.

Integrating ethics and skill

Individual reflection on standards, skill and ethics is vital, yet individual reflection alone is problematic. It is difficult to act responsibly without some guidance. Some of that guidance is found in discussion with fellow professionals, and some is found in written form in professional codes. A modern well accepted definition (Barker, 1992), is that a profession is an occupation that:

* is skilled
* requires training to a high level (to which considerable time is devoted, leading to the expectation of relatively high remuneration)
* gives rise to expectations of a high standard of proficiency
* is bound by a code of ethics of ideals of service to society.

INTEGRATED LEARNING AND PRACTICE

Isn't being technically proficient the main objective for any professional?

Technical proficiency is important, of course, but a professional should also recognise that the broader aspects of making the skill available and then delivering the service—and also representing the profession well at all times—are integral to being a **professional**. A professional is a person who has become skilled to a level judged by the profession to be adequate to hold themselves to be competent, and who applies their competencies in keeping with the values and ethics that are acceptable to their body of professional peers.

professional
Skilled person with high standards of skill and ethics, which they offer in the service of the community.

code of conduct
Comprehensive listing of rules or principles to guide members of a group in their thought and considered action.

Codes of conduct are a form of self-regulation by the group that makes up the profession, stating required and important principles to guide professional practice. Increasingly, professions and health registration boards include performance standards and ethics in the one professional code. Codes of conduct include competencies, and contain detail about what properly equips professionals to deliver services. A code provides practical guidance on acceptable professional standards—and how these should be upheld.

Learning to be a professional is partly about understanding tasks and becoming skilled in them, and partly about becoming able to put those **skills** into action. The skills aspect of professional work is inextricably linked to professional ethics. As Pellegrino has stated, the ethics of a profession are not 'the norms actually followed by professionals, or the professional codes they espouse, but rather the moral obligations deductible from the kinds of activity in which they are engaged' (Pellegrino, 1989, p. 56). So your individual ideals and values—and the skills you learn—are bound together in your sense of professional ethics.

> **skill**
> Level of competence in a specific tasks or series of tasks.

Philosophically, the principles that professions seek to uphold translate into moral rules that guide behaviour (Reich, 1978, p. 410). Many different ethical frameworks support, to some extent, the notion of practical rules. Moral rules are especially important in rule forms of deontology and utilitarianism, which regard rules as ethically necessary (Beauchamp & Childress, 1994, p. 45). **Rules** can be formed and adopted so that moral goals may be achieved. While the rules can be formed by individuals, according to Kant, the collective notion of shared rationality implies that rules formed by rational individuals will be shared and will have commonalities (Sullivan, 1989, p. 214).

> **rules**
> Derived and specific expression of fundamental principles or ideals that are agreed by a group to have force, in a moral obligation of members of the group to abide by them.

As a professional working in a community of other member professionals, you are expected to:

- share some common 'professional ethics' rules
- have a sense of purpose in expressing those rules
- strive to abide by those rules.

Your strict professional duties can be defined with reference to the rules that your profession adopts. Your goals go further than that: you have a general duty to aspire to the optimal goals—in other words, to go beyond minimum duties. Thus, goals and duties go hand in hand.

In professional and personal life you will encounter the setting of moral rules and the expression of moral ideals. Moral rules may not be left to individual discretion as much as moral ideals. A moral rule is something that must be obeyed, and can therefore form the basis of a list of prohibitions—such as 'Thou shalt not kill'. In contrast, a moral ideal is something that should be strived for; it requires some positive action (Gert, 1992, p. 19).

So, there is a sense that 'lower' limits of behaviour exist and that we should strive for 'upper' ideals. If we should abide by moral rules, we would regard behaviour that breaks these rules with disfavour. We might be forgiving when ideals are not upheld, as long as the person strives for them in the future with a moral imperative to strive towards the aspirational goods (Freckleton, 1996, p. 134). A written code makes this more explicit, and provides members—as well as outsiders—with clear expectations of the rules and ideals that are central to the profession.

It seems appropriate that the group of people who best understand the professional skill and actions involved are ethically active—in effect setting their own goals and limits. It is worrying if outsiders have too much control over the ethics of a profession. As one commentator has stated, 'a morality of those whose hands are clean only because they have the position of an observer, charging others with the responsibility, seems doubtful' (Tomaszewski, 1979, p. 131).

professional code of ethics
Expression of principles, rules, ideals and values of specific professional group, creating responsibility to strive for states, ideals and goals, and to uphold certain rules, in each member professional's conduct.

responsibility
Obligation and duty to fulfil certain tasks or series of tasks.

As **professional codes of ethics** provide guidance on the values and aspirations of a profession, there is little doubt that codes are looked to by the profession and public as a measure of professional approach and standards. The formation of the code is a valuable ethical process and, as explained by Stephen Cohen and Damian Grace, the process of reflection is perhaps ethically more important than eventually enshrining a code (Cohen & Grace, 2005, p. 179). The process of reflecting on professional caring, identifying important aspects of caring, and debating what professionals should aim for continues the tradition of ancient debates, albeit in a different guise. In professional debates, try to remember to keep discussion constructive, as is urged in Plato's tradition. The reflection process is more important than keeping score.

Codes of ethics can be thought of as 'general action guides' for professionals (Reich, 1978, p. 407). In a general sense, they are a form of regulation. As a health care professional, you have a **responsibility** to abide by your association's code of ethics in carrying out your work.

Your code is a potential influence on your conduct, because it can define how you should act, and mould you to conform with your profession's standards. The code expresses a collective responsibility in the ethical conduct of health care by you and your fellow member professionals (Tomaszewski, 1979).

The codes may be evidence of existing ethics standards, rather than creating obligations in themselves. According to Knultgen, the purpose of a professional code is to promote a sense of community among members, to discipline the behaviour of members, and to ensure public trust in professional actions (Knultgen, 1988, pp. 212, 213, 215).

The existence of a code should not replace individual conscience and reflection; we need to distinguish between the teaching of custom (or group norms) and what is moral. Continual assessment of the existing standards in the codes of ethics is needed as part of ethical reflection. This proposition seems simple but many philosophers have pondered why continued reflection on defined principles or rules is still needed.

Joseph Butler wrote extensively on the importance of individual conscience in all matters, emphasising that when conscience was exercised, virtue would be expressed, as he argued that human nature was positive rather than evil (Collinson, 1987, p. 79; Borchert, 2006, pp. 780–4). The philosopher John Rawls thought that principles of conduct, such as those we find in some codes of ethics, were important. He also thought that we need more than principles to bring ethics into action. Rawls distinguished between the principles and the subsequent judgments of value in relation to those principles (Rawls, 1971, pp. 20, 48, 120, 579). Individual and collective judgments are needed before principles are put into practice. So shared contribution to standards will remain important.

You might apply principles slightly differently from another health care worker, or someone else in your own profession. Part of that difference may be the values that you use when you interpret and apply the principle. One of Rawls's points is that the judgments we make may depend on the contractual situation to which the principles and values are applied (the word *contractual* refers to any agreement between people, whether implied or explicit).

We can expect some differences in 'ethical behaviour'. Just because someone behaves differently does not necessarily mean that they are unethical. But it does give us pause for reflection and discussion. The next time you see something quite different in the application of a principle, think about the values that may have influenced that professional's behaviour, and the contractual situation in which it was applied. You may be witness to extreme values or a contractual situation that puts considerable constraints on professional behaviour.

From time to time, guidelines are updated. As a profession develops and the context in which it operates is required to practise changes, so codes become increasingly defined. You should be ready to be part of the discussion and be alert to changes in context and professional bounds. It is preferable that all professional members actively consider their ethical stance and their stance on standards, and be ready to explain it or pursue further discussion on it.

So, when a person becomes a member of a profession, they become one of the people who help define the **ideals** of the profession. They bring their own ethics to the profession, and their ethics are influenced by what others have defined as appropriate ethical standards for that profession. It is a fluid process of sharing thoughts, and of learning to work together towards a common **good**. (Note: The word 'good' is used as a noun here—it is a thing or a concept, not an adjective.)

All codes of ethics for health care professionals include statements on respecting the integrity and autonomy of each individual. This is a reminder that gaining consent for any therapeutic process is vital. Nursing codes emphasise autonomy, with nursing roles aligned more explicitly with patient advocacy (Seal, 2007, pp. 29–36). The Australian Association of Social Workers emphasise respect for persons, social justice and professional **integrity** in their Code of Ethics (Australian Association of Social Workers, 2010). The subtle differences in codes and the different professional roles that are undertaken can mean that different professionals apply their own particular codes and make different assessments of their responsibilities in the same shared care or interprofessional situation.

ideals
A standard of excellence, which is aimed to be met.

good
A desirable end or object.

integrity
Willingness to actively reflect upon and uphold the highest principles and standards of conduct consistent with roles, responsibilities and duties.

beneficence
The principle of doing good and providing care for others.

non-maleficence
The principle of not harming others, and of minimising harm to them.

autonomy
The principle of allowing and promoting self-rule, of people making decisions about their lives.

justice
The principle of fair allocation of community resources and burdens.

REFLECTION: GENERAL PRINCIPLES IN CODES OF CONDUCT AND ETHICS

You should have at hand your relevant Code of Conduct or Code of Ethics. If you do not already have it, you could try looking up the association website or the relevant registration authority websites. The latest codes outline duties to patients, the community and the profession. Make sure you always obtain updates whenever your code is altered.

Using your own code, summarise the principles and comments of guidance in your code of ethics under the broad headings listed below of **beneficence**, **non-maleficence**, **autonomy** and **justice**.

Beneficence encompasses the obligation to do good, to care for people; non-maleficence is the paired obligation to do no harm to them.

Autonomy is the principle of self-rule, of clients making decisions about their own lives.

Justice is about fair distribution of resources, particularly when the pool of resources is limited. These were chosen by Beauchamp and Childress, as they are principles that can be applied within the different ethics theories and frameworks (Beauchamp & Childress, 1994, pp. 38, 45).

INTEGRATED LEARNING AND PRACTICE

Rules and aspirations in codes

This is an extension question, and can be tackled as a group or individually if you are ready for more complex considerations.

Identify principles that are mandatory, and expressed as a 'rule'—these principles will form a list of things you must do if you accept this role as a professional. Then use your law research skills to identify a parallel law that is the equivalent of this in society.

Next, identify an aspirational principle, such as striving to deliver the best available care. This is not a 'rule', but a guiding principle. Professionals won't be judged as harshly if circumstances prevent them from achieving the aim. Do search—but you are unlikely to find a parallel law for this.

Remember that some responsibilities are specific to each profession. They can include both legal responsibilities and professional responsibilities that professionals are obliged to fulfil—or try to live up to. There is more discussion about professional assessment of standards in Chapter 2.

REFLECTION: GUIDANCE IN CODES

1   Think about one of the basic principles that you, as a registered health practitioner, might find in your board's code of conduct or code of ethics, or your relevant code as a health care worker. (Alternatively, you might like to look at another profession's code.)

2   Think of situations in which you have applied this principle. Make a note of how you have seen others apply it.

Community trust in health care professions and their professional standards is based on the expectation that the community as a whole will ultimately be served by the profession. If this trust is shaken, society may judge that more outside regulation is needed, effectively limiting the power and discretion of professionals. Professions have sometimes refined and discussed their standards precisely because of the threat of such an external imposition of standards.

Interprofessional teamwork

Throughout your health care career you will work alongside different professions and health care workers. This is termed *multidisciplinary*, *interprofessional* or *interdisciplinary* teamwork. When tasks and responsibilities are shared in a health care team, the team as a whole is also responsible for the comprehensiveness of care of the individual patient. You can expect that different professionals are equipped to deliver different specific aspects of care. One step towards professionals working well together is to understand each other's different skills and objectives in providing care.

It is important that a team ethic of caring is acknowledged, and that teams discuss and define team goals. The discussion should extend to values and ethics, as well as to technical skill and tasks, so that minimum rules and optimal ideals are identified, compatibilities in acceptable aims are recognised, and potential problem areas are identified before they occur in practice. It is a natural extension of professional standards to broaden the discussion to others who are engaged in a similar endeavour.

Because of your shared objectives—and despite your differences—you must learn to work together, because you need each other's skills to provide comprehensive health care. The basic aim of all health professions is to care for clients or patients, to be beneficent, and to serve and protect the health of the community. Health care is a system, partly because that is the most efficient and effective way that our society has available to share the skills of the health care workforce. Society needs you to work well together.

Working as a team does not mean always working 'under' another profession. It means being aware of and working towards goals, and on occasions being 'guided by others who possess greater knowledge and expertise' (Alexandra & Woodruff, 1996, p. 242). Of course, establishing team leadership will depend on the team goals and objectives, and on who has the skills to lead the team towards that goal. Junior residents find themselves learning a great deal from senior unit nurses. Experienced nurses and their favourite doctors appear to work effortlessly. Perhaps they have come to a common understanding of the goals of care in their own context and appreciate each other's skills so much that there is true team harmony in providing that care. You could apply the same assessment of successful teamwork to other professional combinations.

Bear in mind that full discussion is as valuable in reflection as the ultimate decision that you reach. There is a danger that aiming for consensus too early—and sacrificing differences of opinion to achieve that consensus—can hide the difficulty of an issue, or even hide divergent views on an issue (Moreno, 1995). It is a reminder that challenging issues warrant detailed reflection and discussion.

In ethics education at a university health centre in the United States, the complexity of issues that students training in different health professions brought to the ethics discussion was noticed and valued as a benefit to all students. The lecturers felt that when students understood each of the team members' roles and responsibilities, they also further developed their understanding of discharging their ethical obligations to their patients in an appropriate manner (Yarborough et al., 2000, p. 794). So, ethics discussion and decisions cannot be made in isolation from other interdisciplinary team members for them to be realistic and practical.

It's crucial to have guidance on proper behaviour by those with relevant expertise. As Hans Jonas has said, it is especially difficult to define ethical conduct in a technologically complex situation—which modern health care inevitably is. People who have the relevant technological expertise can help to predict the consequences of actions. Without their help, actions—even if done with good intentions—could easily result in harm to others (Jonas, 1984, pp. 5–6). This has particular relevance for health care teams that combine different sorts of expertise. You should get used to checking matters of professional conduct and professional ethics with the whole team. The minimum is to check with your own professional peers.

The importance of relying on others for guidance is evident even in Kant's otherwise individualist writings, which stress virtue in relation to one's own moral laws. According to Kant, the acceptability of actions to others is important because the praise of others is essential in reinforcing virtuous actions (Sullivan, 1989, p. 29). It is a practical safeguard that you check and discuss matters with your colleagues to see if you have acted properly or if your planned action is acceptable and ethical. It is appropriate that the diverse group of people who together can comprehensively understand the scope of professional skill and actions in health care settings contribute to the reflection.

Learning about how your institution, ward, department or clinic has approached a range of practical issues in the past is a privilege, as you then share in some of the corporate memory. An 'acceptable' course of action may already be defined by other experienced team members. If the legal, regulatory and ethical reasons remain unarticulated, take the time to draw people out so that you understand how issues have been solved in the past. This provides you with a toolkit for approaching challenges in the future.

Checking all perspectives does not mean you lose the capacity to form your own position, even though some reasoning frameworks may minimise the moral authority of any one position. The theory of relativism suggests that there are no hard and fast rules in ethics. Rather, ethics can change depending on the perspectives of key participants in a dilemma and the stance of the group to which they belong. To adopt an extreme relativist position on all matters is quite controversial, but the basic process of searching for perspectives is less controversial. Finding and comparing different possible perspectives on what might be best or right is helpful in identifying if a practical agreement is possible. Harman, a philosopher who has defended relativism, claims that a judgment of proper conduct by one party towards another depends on the agreement between the two parties (Harman, 1975, p. 3). In a professional–client relationship, both parties should agree that what is being undertaken is proper. In the context of a health care team, the team should also agree that it is proper. Remember that they might agree for different reasons. Reaching this agreement does not necessarily mean minimal standards. In any contractual situation, an upper level, beyond a bare minimum, can be negotiated. Teams may choose to strive to go beyond the minimum and aim for an outcome that will raise and uphold standards.

Ethics and ethical dilemmas

Jennifer Haines

Jennifer has been a Registered Nurse for 40 years and spent most of those years practising in critical care areas, ICU, CCU, Neurosurgery ICU and Emergency Department.

When working through an ethical dilemma, we must ask the following:

- What is the ethical problem we are trying to solve?
- What are the facts?
- What ethical factors apply to the situation? What does our Code of Ethics say about the situation?
- What ethical factor takes priority in the situation?
- What does the law say about the situation?
- What course of action should an ethical nurse take?

An ethical dilemma

Doctors have been working all day on a patient, reviving them after repeated cardiac arrests. They meet and decide that continuing to resuscitate the patient is not helping the patient and may well be causing harm. They approach the family, who want every measure of treatment continued. The doctors advise against it, but the family insist. The doctors decide that the next time the patient arrests, they will pretend to resuscitate the patient, and that will fail, and the patient will die. The doctors did this, and the patient died.

- Did the doctors behave ethically? Why, or why not?

Practical local regulation

Standards and rules are part of everyday life. For instance, when you go to a local park, you want to relax and have fun. As a law-abiding citizen, you also try to use the public area safely and in a way that does not damage the property or cause harm to other people.

You might see a sign at the park that lists the things you can do in that park—and perhaps lists activities that are prohibited. At the bottom of the sign you will probably find the name of an Act, which is the legislation that gives the general authority for the rules, or the name of a Regulation, which is relied on by the local area to implement specific rules that make the park enjoyable for everyone.

You might find that you are able to walk a dog, but not allowed to let the dog off the leash. There is nothing to suggest you are prohibited from an ordinary, well accepted use, such as a picnic on the grass, but if you see an image of a tent with a cross through it you know that you would not be allowed to camp in the park overnight. These rules are partly about public safety, and partly about sharing the use of the public facility in a fair and reasonable way. You can decide whether to use that park, based on the rules and local regulations. There may be warnings, or advice given on particular risks, such as the grading of a bush walk as 'very steep' or difficult and uneven, meant for experienced walkers, and that you should carry plenty of water. You can then decide whether to embark on the walk given the risks involved.

Regulations are the applied legal and administrative requirements that are made as part of a process of social control and management of a particular process or setting in a specific context. So finding out what the regulations are in that setting is an important first step. Then, your integrity and commitment to upholding standards that are expected of you and behaving ethically—even if other people can't see you—will help you to decide if your plans were fine, or whether you need to rethink what you will do while you are in the park.

Let's look at another everyday example. Before you drive a vehicle, you will have applied for a licence to drive, or a provisional permit to learn to drive. You will have passed a test of some sort to show that you are competent and safe enough for the licence to be issued to you. The licence issued to you will have restrictions: you may be entitled to drive a motorbike or car but not a large truck, or you may be licensed to drive an automatic but not a manual vehicle. When you drive on the road, road rules such as speed limits also apply. These standards, restrictions and rules are all provided to regulate driving so that it is as safe as possible. Parking restrictions also apply for safety reasons—and so that you do not park in a way that is inconvenient to others. The local area is best placed to decide what is acceptable for local conditions, and this is why the speed limits or parking rules applied can vary. Your driving is subject to the regulations of the area that you travel in. Also, it is subject to the type of licence that you have. You have a responsibility to inform the licensing authority if you become unfit to still hold your license, and you have an everyday responsibility to restrict yourself from being behind the wheel if you are temporarily unsafe to drive. Your reflection on the importance of acting within your agreed driving competence, being safe, and respecting road rules is most importantly upheld by you even when others are not monitoring or observing you.

Sanctions can apply when people do not abide by these standards and rules. This is to:

- redress the harm caused
- act as a deterrent for repeated transgressions
- encourage others to uphold the rules because they are important and meaningful standards for our communities.

When you choose to work in the health sector, you can expect that similar restrictions, standards and rules will apply. Health care is a heavily regulated sector as there is a need to protect the safety of the public, and the practical imperative to use public resources wisely. Health facilities are licensed and health care providers are trained to appropriate standards and may also be registered.

Care is taken to make health care delivery as safe as possible for workers, as well as for patients. The training and qualification you have allows you to work in certain roles, and always with some limits. It is your responsibility to find out what local rules and regulations apply to your work in the particular setting that you are working in. For instance, even if you have the necessary skill and qualifications, the scope of procedures that can be undertaken will be different in a small day clinic than a larger hospital. You can't drive at 110 km/h through a local town, and you also need to adjust in every setting so that you use your skills in the most appropriate, safe and effective manner.

Health service institutions always operate within a state or territory and national context, and some regulation is set as subordinate part of the legislative instruments in each jurisdiction. Each health-service setting and institution endeavours to ensure that laws and regulations are complied with and that employees and people presenting to the service are treated lawfully. If any person suffers harm on the premises or through the action of an employee or agent of the institution, institutions can be sued in law as an entity. You will read more about this in Chapter 3.

Following the precise requirements of all relevant regulations is an expected and routine part of the privilege you have accepted in becoming a health professional to serve the public. Each health care institution helps to set the culture of aiming for best practice and compliance with regulations.

Local institutional rules, such as standard operating procedures, prompt you to consider competent and ethical aspects of your practice, including:

- appropriate levels of training and skill for particular jobs
- what care to offer and how to deliver it
- social expectations of what would be a priority in particular situations.

For each health setting, remember that it is as if you are in a local park and on local roads. You should expect that some local standards, regulations and rules will apply, as well as the general laws and codes that guide your conduct. The regulations aim to support the safe, effective and fair delivery of health care in each of our local communities.

Some regulations are like basic road rules, and they will become second nature to you as you build your career in the health sector. Special responsibilities as a health care worker are set out in a practical way in regulations, such as what makes up an adequate health care record.

Shared responsibilities in record keeping

Health care professionals share in the responsibility to keep a health record of the assessment and care that each patient receives. Health records should be accurate and complete; they can be initiated or added to by any health care worker; and they become the basis of noting and assessing progress as the client is engaged in treatment.

An adequate record was defined in the *Health Insurance (Professional Services Review) Regulations 1999* (Cth), under section 5, as follows:

5 An adequate record

For the definition of adequate and contemporaneous records in section 81 of the Act, the standard to be met in order that a record of service rendered or initiated be adequate is that:

(a) the record clearly identify the name of the patient; and

(b) the record contain a separate entry for each attendance by the patient for a service and the date on which the service was rendered or initiated; and

(c) each entry provide clinical information adequate to explain the type of service rendered or initiated; and

(d) each entry be sufficiently comprehensible that another practitioner, relying on the record, can effectively undertake the patient's ongoing care.

Under section 6, it must be contemporaneous—that is, 'completed at the time the practitioner rendered or initiated the service', or as soon as practicable.

Health departments recognise the importance of health records, and issue guidelines like these:

The main purpose of a health care record is to provide a means of communication to facilitate the safe care and treatment of a patient/client. A health care record is the primary repository of information including medical and therapeutic treatment and intervention for the health and well being of the patient/client during an episode of care and informs care in future episodes. The health care record is a documented account of a patient/client's history of illness; health care plan/s; health investigation and evaluation; diagnosis; care; treatment; progress and health outcome for each health service intervention or interaction.

(New South Wales Government, 2012, p. 2)

Making health records or medical records is not just the responsibility of medical practitioners. It is a responsibility shared by different care providers in different clinical settings. The basic requirements are that records:

• have entries that are legible and non-erasable
• are identified as relating to a particular person
• are organised chronologically
• are made available to authorised persons.

The accuracy and completeness of the records you make is relied upon by others, and is an essential supplement—but not a replacement—for a full verbal handover between staff (O'Brien, 2002).

Taking notes and making records is one of the key skills of health professionals. It is vital in terms of effective teamwork. Other health practitioners and workers who care for the same client need be able to refer to detailed information about the client without asking for the same information all over again. They also need to know the exact nature of care that has already been delivered so that future care is safe, informed and effective.

Inadequate, inaccurate or misleading documentation by a nurse in any health record or report can be found to amount to unsatisfactory professional performance/conduct,

---

REFLECTION: ACCURACY AND RECORDS

Think about the following example, which is from a Masters course in clinical ethics:

> A nurse makes a mistake with the amount of medicine he dispenses to a patient. He realises the mistake, as does a fellow nurse. The patient's records show that the correct amount has been given. Neither corrects the records, nor reports the mistake to the charge nurse or the attending doctor.
>
> *(Berglund, Mitchell & Cox, 1993, pp. 195–6)*

1 What do you think could be the effect of the mistake?

2 What ethics responsibility is being degraded by not rectifying the records?

---

and may be considered by a tribunal, panel or committee to be unprofessional conduct. In one case, a caution to mark the disapproval of the conduct was ordered, and conditions to safeguard the public in the future were put in place for the nurse practitioner (AHPRA, 2016).

All health care workers need to be vigilant in upholding responsibilities in their roles. Team work and accountability to others is regulated in some aspects of record keeping.

For instance, drug regulations have a practical impact on many routine aspects of health care, including making accurate records of the handling and administration of them. Rigorous prescribing and supply restrictions apply to S4D and S8 drugs and these restrictions have particular significance for the health professionals handling and administering them. The *Standard for the Uniform Scheduling of Medicines and Poisons* (SUSMP), is given effect through each state or territory's legislation (Australian Government, 2018).

These drugs are called Schedule 4D (S4D) and Schedule 8 (S8) drugs because they are listed in regulation in the schedules, which are then read with the relevant legislation. Schedule 4 covers prescription-only medicines, and particular further restrictions apply to those listed in Schedule 4D, such as benzodiazepines and amphetamines. Schedule 8 drugs are controlled drugs, and include opiates. The restrictions are because of the dangers associated with the drugs: they have addictive qualities, and cause harmful effects if used in excessive quantities or over lengthy timeframes.

When doctors prescribe these drugs, which nurses then administer, the combined regulatory framework is made up by the Commonwealth schedules, as well as Therapeutic Goods Administration (TGA) requirements, the state legislation, and the local health facility standard operating procedures, which clearly set out staff members' responsibilities and practical procedures to comply with these requirements.

One example of local procedures is that of the Royal Hospital for Women in Sydney, which sets out principles for the storage, supply and administration of the drugs. For instance, the nurse in charge of a ward is responsible for the storage of the S4D and S8 drugs, which are stored in a locked dangerous drugs cupboard, except if needed on a designated trolley for anaesthetic purposes. A nurse employed in a permanent capacity carries the key, and recording and checking requirements apply. Two members of staff, including one registered nurse or registered midwife, must check out and witness administration of all S4D and S8 drugs. Requirements for recording drugs in a register, and documenting and witnessing wastage or spillage are also strict (Royal Hospital for Women, 2016).

The further significance of the records, including the drug register, and the records of administration, is that they are legal documents. When you sign off any step in the storage, supply or administration of these drugs, you are declaring that the step you document and place your signature or initials next to has actually occurred. This is a matter of significant professional integrity and responsibility. You are entrusted with this responsibility given the trust that the community places in you as a health professional. There are potentially serious legal consequences for making a false record. The community trusts that the integrity of the professional will provide the motivation to ensure that regulatory requirements are carried out.

REFLECTION: CAN YOU SIGN OFF PLEASE?

Imagine that you are part of the nursing team working in a particular institution. Find out more about the rules that would apply in the place you work. Look up that institution's regulations on the handling and administration of S4D and S8 drugs to refresh your understanding of what your responsibilities would be if you were asked to witness the administration of these drugs to a patient.

1   Share what you have found out with your colleague, so that they are up to date with the regulations and know that you are fully aware of your regulatory responsibilities. How would you approach this in your team setting? What level of formality do you feel comfortable with? The context will make a difference to the type of language you would use to summarise what you know.

2   Think about what you would say if you are asked to sign off on a process in order to satisfy the regulatory requirements—but you had not actually witnessed each step of the process that you should have seen.

Consistent with all administrative law and application of administrative regulations, if the regulations are too onerous, or impose too great a burden on any one person or organisation, it is possible to rebalance the burden imposed. (You will read more about this in Chapter 3 'How the law shapes health care'.) Checking each other's decisions in more routine procedural issues is part of normal and expected practice. At the moment, the regulation of having two personnel sign off S4D and S8 administration is not thought to be too onerous. It is clear what each person is responsible for. The requirements are clear and protect the public interest.

Legislation and regulatory mechanisms to weigh competing public interests in safeguarding and allowing or limiting access and use of personal health information are discussed in Chapter 6 'Personal information privacy and public interests'. Chapter 10 'Regulation and availability of health and community services' includes a discussion of national funding and billing regulations, and of local resource allocation discretionary policy.

Continual reflection and development of standards

It is part of being a professional to use the skills available to you in both the technical and procedural and reflective spheres, and to identify a responsible way forward. A commitment to the further refinement of standards or rules is also central to being a health professional. This is because, together with others, you form the health care profession.

Standards are also continually reflected on and developed, partly due to the dynamic nature of law and ethics and the complementary relationship between the two. Lower limits are defined and debated, and optimal standards are more readily defined as a result. The interplay is a social process, and to treat law and ethics as totally separate would be artificial. Broader societal expectations and standards are applied by law. Such laws are expressions of the lower limits of behaviour that society will tolerate.

Professional guidelines and regulations—although derived from groups' mores and ethics—sometimes have force as important standards because of statute law and common law principles and doctrines. These limits are constantly debated by politicians, and can change. The process of debating new laws exposes the reasoning behind the laws. There is an opportunity to view this in parliamentary debates or law reform discussion documents. Throughout this book, you will notice examples of discussions from law reform processes.

You need to stay up to date, because abiding by standards and undertaking ongoing reflection on responsible practice is part of your professional obligation.

Summary

This chapter provides the foundation for understanding the integrated standards in health care. You have learnt that standards and rules are part of everyday life and also everyday work life, and that laws, regulations and ethics work together to provide that guidance on acceptable and appropriate standards. You have learnt a little about the structure and function of law and ethics from ancient and modern philosophers. When general principles are provided in law and ethics, the application of the principles is assisted by regulation. You have learnt that regulation contains the more precise details on how the standards are to be applied in practical contexts. The standards provide guidance for you. What is also needed is your active aspiration to act with integrity so that the relevant standards become part of your everyday practice.

STUDY QUESTIONS

1 Why is jurisdiction important in thinking about standards and rules?

2 What do law, ethics and regulations have in common?

3 Write the opening paragraph of an essay on 'The central importance of professional integrity in health care'.

4 Outline, in detail, with references, three significant regulatory requirements for record keeping in health care.

5 Have a glossary quiz. Turn to the glossary and select any glossary term that was covered in Chapter 1. (The numbers in brackets show you in which chapter the glossary term was defined.) See if you can define each term, and explain what it means when applied in a legal, ethical or regulatory context that you have read about in this book.

REFERENCES

Alexandra, A., & Woodruff, A. (1996). A Code of Ethics for the Nursing Profession. In M. Coady & S. Bloch (Eds). *Codes of Ethics and the Professions*. Melbourne: Melbourne University Press.

Australian Association of Social Workers [AASW]. (2010). *Code of ethics*. Retrieved from www.aasw.asn.au

Australian Government, Department of Foreign Affairs and Trade. (n.d.). *The Australian Treaties Database*. Retrieved from www.info.dfat.gov.au/treaties

Australian Government, Department of Health. (2018). Therapeutic Goods Administration, Scheduling Basics. Retrieved from http://tga.gov.au

Australian Human Rights Commission [AHRC]. (2017). *Consultations on OPCAT*, 2017. Australian Government. Retrieved from www.humanrights.gov.au

Australian Health Practitioner Regulation Agency [AHPRA]. (2016). *Panel decisions*, Case 2016.0761, decision dated 1/9/16, Qld Nursing and Midwifery. Retrieved from www.ahpra.gov.au

Australian Health Practitioner Regulation Agency [AHPRA]. (2017). *Regulatory principles for the National Scheme*. Retrieved from www.ahpra.gov.au

Australian Human Rights Commission. (2017). *Permissible limitation on rights*. Retrieved from www.humanrights.gov.au

Balkin, R.P., & Davis, J.L.R. (2013). *Law of torts* (5th edn). Australia: LexisNexis Butterworths.

Barker, S.F. (1992). What is a profession? *Professional Ethics: A Multidisciplinary Journal, 1(1–2)*, 73–99.

Beauchamp, T.L., & Childress, J.F. (1994). *Principles of biomedical ethics* (4th edn). London: Oxford University Press.

Berglund, C.A., Mitchell, K., & Cox. K. (1993). *Exploring clinical ethics* (2nd edn). Distance module in a Masters of Clinical Education program. Sydney: University of New South Wales.

Borchert, D.M. (Ed.). (2006). *Encyclopedia of philosophy* (2nd edn). Farmington Hills MI: Thomson Gale.

Coalition of Australian Governments Health Council. (2015). *A National Code of Conduct for health care workers*. Australian Health Ministers' Advisory Council 2014, Australian Government. Retrieved from www.coaghealthcouncil.gov.au

Cohen, S., & Grace, D. (2005). *Business ethics* (3rd edn). Melbourne: Oxford University Press.

Collinson, D. (1987). *Fifty major philosophers: A reference guide*. London: Routledge.

Cook, C., Creyke, R., Geddes, R., & Hamer, D. (2009). *Laying down the law* (7th edn). Australia: LexisNexis Butterworths.

Crawford, J. (2012). *Brownlie's principles of public international law* (8th edn). Oxford: Oxford University Press.

Freckelton, I. (1996). Enforcement of ethics. In M. Coady & Bloch, S. (Eds), *Codes of ethics and the professions*. Melbourne: Melbourne University Press.

Gert, B. (1992). Morality, moral theory, and applied and professional ethics. *Professional Ethics: A Multidisciplinary Journal*, 1(1–2), 5–24.

Gillon, R. (1986). *Philosophical medical ethics*. Chichester, United Kingdom: John Wiley & Sons.

Harman, G. (1975). Moral relativism defended. *Philosophical Review*, 84, 3–22.

Honderich, T. (Ed.). (1995). *The Oxford companion to philosophy*. New York: Oxford University Press.

Jonas, H. (1984). The imperative of responsibility: In search of an ethics for the technological age. Chicago: University of Chicago Press.

Knultgen, J. (1988). *Ethics and professionalism*. Philadelphia: University of Pennsylvania Press.

Mann, T. (2013). *Australian law dictionary* (2nd edn). South Melbourne, Australia: Oxford University Press.

McMillan, J. (1993). Commonwealth constitutional power over health. *Consumers Health Forum of Australia*, as cited in *Does the Commonwealth have Constitutional power to take over the administration of public hospitals?* Research Paper 2008–09 (36), Canberra: Parliament of Australia. Retrieved from www.aph.gov.au

Moreno, J.D. (1995). *Deciding together: Bioethics and moral consensus*. New York: Oxford University Press.

Melbourne Social Equity Institute. (2014). *Seclusion and Restraint Project Report*. Melbourne: University of Melbourne, for the National Mental Health Commission. Retrieved from http://socialequity.unimelb.edu.au

[Multilateral agreement.] (1994). *Agreement to Ban Smoking on International Passenger Flights*. ATS 5 Multilateral, 1 November 1994.

New South Wales Government, Ministry of Health. (2012). *Health care records documentation and management and information*. Sydney: New South Wales Ministry of Health, PD2012_069. Retrieved from http://www1.health.nsw.gov.au/pds/ActivePDSDocuments/PD2012_069.pdf

O'Brien, E. 2002. Making a note and handover. In C. Berglund & D. Saltman, *Communication for health care* (pp. 113–34). Melbourne: Oxford University Press.

Pellegrino, E.D. (1989). Character, virtue and self-interest in the ethics of the professions. *Journal of Contemporary Health Law and Policy*, 5, 53–73.

Rawls, J.A. (1971). *A theory of justice*. Harvard: Belknap Press.

Reich, W.T. (Ed.). (1978). *Encyclopedia of bioethics* (Vol. 1). New York: The Free Press.

Royal Hospital for Women. (2016). *Local Operating Procedure, Clinical Policies, Procedures & Guidelines, Medication—Schedule 4(d) and Schedule 8*. Sydney, New South Wales: Ministry of Health. Retrieved from http://seslhd.health.nsw.gov.au

Seal, M. (2007). Patient advocacy and advance care planning in the acute hospital setting. *Australian Journal of Advanced Nursing, 24*(4), 29–36.

Sullivan, R.J. (1989). *Immanuel Kant's moral theory*. Cambridge, United Kingdom: Cambridge University Press.

Tomaszewski, T. (1979). Ethical issues from an international perspective. *International Journal of Psychology, 124*, 131–5.

United Nations. (2002). *Optional Protocol to the Convention Against Torture and Other Cruel and Degrading Treatment or Punishment*. Entered into force 22 June 2006. Geneva: Office of the High Commissioner for Human Rights. Retrieved from http://ohchr.org

United Nations. (1948). *Universal Declaration of Human Rights*. United National Office of the High Commissioner for Human Rights. Retrieved from www.un.org

United Nations. (1966a). *International Covenant on Civil and Political Rights*. Retrieved from www.un.org

United Nations. (1966b). *International Covenant on Economic, Social and Cultural Rights*. Retrieved from www.un.org

United Nations Educational, Scientific and Cultural Organization. (2005). *Universal Declaration on Bioethics and Human Rights*. Retrieved from www.unesco.org

Yarborough, M., Jones, T., Cyr, T.A., Phillips, S., & Stelzner, D. (2000). Interprofessional education in ethics at an academic health sciences center. *Academic Medicine, 75*(8), 793–800.

LEGISLATION

Air Navigation Regulations (Amendment) 1996 (Cth) *(SR No 113)*

Commonwealth of Australia Constitution Act 1900 (Cth) (the Constitution), compilation prepared 4 September 2013

Health Practitioner Regulation National Law Act 2009 (Cth)

Health Practitioner Regulation National Law 2009 (Vic)

Health Insurance (Allied Health Services) Determination 2011 (Cth)

Health Insurance (Professional Services Review) Regulations 1999 (Cth)

Human Services (Medicare) Act 1973 (Cth)

Human Services (Medicare) Regulations 1975 (Cth)

Medicare Levy Act 1986 (Cth)

Transport Legislation Amendment Act (No 2) 1995 (Cth)

CASES

Heydon's Case (1584) 76 ER 637

CHAPTER 2

Standards for professional training and practice

LEARNING OBJECTIVES

- To appreciate the central importance of trust and professional integrity in health care.
- To appreciate the need to continually develop skills and knowledge and ensure fitness to practise.
- To appreciate the regulatory governance systems that ensure quality and safety in health service settings.
- To understand the importance of applying knowledge, skills and judgment in a proper and ethical manner.
- To explore the value of peer opinion on performance within acceptable and satisfactory standards.
- To understand how powers can be used to protect the public from departures from reasonable and acceptable standards.

KEY TERMS

belief	governance
character	health care
client	health care professionals
communitarianism	impairment
community	impropriety
competence	libertarianism
competencies	mandatory notification
consultation	obligation
cultural safety	patient
culture	principlism
deon	professional misconduct
deontology	propriety
duties	reflection
fit and proper person	unsatisfactory professional conduct
goals	

CASE EXAMPLE

Five-minute overview

Nic is a nursing student who is lucky to have some work as an assistant in nursing, which makes for a busy schedule. As you read this chapter, keep a few notes that will help Nic develop an appreciation of professional practice responsibilities and fitness to ultimately register as a nurse. Imagine that Nic has a few minutes spare tomorrow and wants your five-minute overview of this chapter.

---

health care
The provision of care with the objective of maintaining, restoring, or improving health or comfort.

health care professionals
Those trained in recognised professions to be providers of health care.

patient
Person receiving care.

Training and working as a health care professional

Choosing to become a health professional is a significant decision. Historically, people entered the equivalent of holy orders to receive the depth of training that was required in professions, and they often pledged themselves to the ideals of learning and service. To have a profession was, literally, to have professed oaths, such as obedience to church values, honesty and high standards of service (Barker, 1992, p. 86). This is similar to the intensity of devotion and long apprenticeship that a successful professional still needs today.

There is more to being a successful and productive professional **health care** worker than demonstrated aptitude for remembering facts and performing certain procedural skills. Selection panels search for those with the willingness to work with others, the preparedness to reflect on difficult problems, and the virtue of wanting to care, to serve, and to meet the needs of others. They are interested in why people want to become **health care professionals**, to contribute to furthering the health and wellbeing of each **patient**.

REFLECTION: STARTING OUT

Think back to when you started your training. Why did you choose to train in your health profession? Did you believe you had an aptitude for the type of work in a particular field? Did you hold certain values and ideals of caring, or was it something else that prompted you to choose your field of health care work?

1   Write down what type of work you thought you would be trained for, and any specific procedural skills that you thought you would be trained in.

2   Describe the person you were then, and your ideals and values as a beginning clinical student.

3   Have any of your initial expectations changed?

4   Describe your current ideals and values further.

(Adapted from an exercise by Professor Ken Cox (Berglund, Mitchell & Cox, 1993, p. 4).)

Your own **beliefs** remain important in your professional practice. A training program in systematic personal ethics consideration for trainee physicians, called CARE, acknowledged the personal beliefs of the carer as well as the practical context in which that care is applied. The initials CARE stand for:

C—the physician's *core* beliefs

A—*action* in similar situations in the past

R—*reasoned* opinions of others

E—the *experience* of others in similar situations in the past.

Each item is critiqued as part of the ethics reflection, so the model is shorthand to prompt reflection on reasonable and acceptable directions in care (Schneider & Snell, 2000).

belief
Firmly held opinion or accepted understanding.

Continuing professional development

The process of learning, and the awareness of the culture of caring starts early and continues throughout professional life. Your own early learning should be recognised, even if it appears to be less glamorous than 'real' health care or 'real' professional work. Many students take on part-time work in health contexts, and this exposes them to a variety of health care work, and to the reality of the day-to-day aspects of health care. It provides a unique opportunity to learn to respond to the needs and wishes of others, behave with respect and courtesy, and work smoothly as a team to contribute to the ethic of caring.

Professional training is necessarily a slow process. It takes time to accumulate knowledge and skill, and to develop insight into proper standards. Society acknowledges that it is necessary to fund training through public taxes. Public training institutions are eligible for funding if they are accredited, demonstrating appropriate curriculum and assessment of their students. Graduates are eligible for registration if they have attended accredited training programs in their chosen health profession, and approved programs of study are approved by each health profession. For instance, the Nursing and Midwifery Board of Australia lists the various approved programs for enrolled nurses (EN), registered nurses (RN) and registered midwives (RM), which make graduates eligible for endorsement.

Teaching hospitals work in partnership with colleges and universities to train a skilled and experienced workforce. Our system of teaching hospitals lets students and juniors observe and gradually contribute to health work under supervision, in the presence of a trained person to support, supervise, and step in as needed. As their skill and knowledge level increases, students undertake increasingly difficult tasks under decreasing supervision. The professional skill and 'right' manner in carrying out that work is slowly transferred from supervisor to student. Through mentoring, academic instruction, role modelling, group discussion, and other systems, we gradually form the new generation of trained professionals in a safe, publicly accountable system. Higher Education Providers meet accreditation standards through the federal government's Tertiary Education Quality and Standards Agency (TEQSA), as well as the standards set by the relevant accreditation authorities for each professional course offered. This is to ensure that graduates have received training through a curriculum that meets appropriate standards.

You will be assigned a clinical supervisor for each placement. When you perform tasks in a clinical setting, you will be very closely supervised, and even though you may be allowed opportunities to practise taking observations such as blood pressure, your observations will be supervised, and necessary observations for each patient will also be made by another trained person who records and signs their own observations. (See both your clinical placement scope of practice in your training institution and the local health facility policies on training placements or pracs.)

You will already be aware of some regulations for you as a health care student, which affect your clearance to take part in that training. For instance, if you are training to be a registered health professional, before you enter hospitals or clinic settings, you will have given personal details to your training institution, which lodges those details with the national board for your health profession, which in turn informs the Australian Health Practitioner Regulation Agency (AHPRA) that you are registered, so that you can enter the clinical teaching setting. You then have an obligation under the relevant jurisdiction's National Law to inform the National Board or AHPRA if you have been convicted of an offence punishable by imprisonment, or if you are charged with an offence for which a 12 month or longer sentence of imprisonment could apply, or if your student registration is suspended or cancelled in another country. You likely had a police check before being issued with security identification and access to a health facility. Your immunisation status will have been checked. (See your local health training institution governance provisions.)

REFLECTION POINT

Reading legislation

Look up the Health Practitioner Regulation National Law Acts in each jurisdiction, and read the relevant sections on student registration requirements. For instance, in the Queensland legislation, *Health Practitioner Regulation National Law Act 2009* (Qld), look to sections 87, 89 and 130.

Make a note in your portfolio on what you noticed about the language used in the legislation.

Ethics and professional integrity are a core part of every assessment you undertake in your training. When you submit your university or college assignments, you will be aware that your honesty and integrity is essential. There are significant academic penalties—such as suspension or loss of your training place—which can be applied if you are found to have plagiarised or copied another student's work and presented it as your own. (See your training institution policies on student misconduct and plagiarism, and look at the declaration you make at the top of your assignment submission form.) You could find the wording of the actual law, standard, or rule for each of these in your own context—that is, in Australia; in your state or territory for your health service; in the training health institution; and in your academic institution.

REFLECTION POINT

Identifying standards for your context

You now know that standards can be found in many sources, and are derived from law, ethics and regulation. Think about one further standard for professionals or students in training and make a note of how and when you learnt about it.

You may have chosen a level of knowledge (or practical skill), or you may have chosen a standard that is more about the way that skill is delivered. Learning increasingly difficult and finely tuned professional standards is part of becoming a professional carer. You learn, in fine detail, what the job is, and how you are expected to do it.

When you complete your basic training at college or university, you will have started to acquire the privileged knowledge of your chosen profession. Part of being a professional is to commit to keep learning and improving, constantly updating or extending your knowledge and skill base, so you can deliver the best possible care for your clients. The flip side is that there are always limits to your knowledge and skill.

REFLECTION POINT

Learning and limits

Find somewhere you can sit quietly without interruption. Think about each of the following statements and how you would complete each sentence, based on your own safe limits. Think of a skill that you are still learning, and try the following reflection.

My safe limits in performing the skill are …

My judgment of my safe limit is based on …

The consequences of exceeding this limit for the client and the public is …

Recognising your limits in skill is very helpful, because it starts you on a process of self-reflection. You need to have **insight** into how knowledgeable and capable you are. There is a danger for others if you think that you are much more skilled than you actually are, and you go beyond your safe limits in dealing with people. **Reflection** is a key part of responsible practice. When you work on your reflective portfolio, you are learning the reflective skills that will stay with you throughout your professional life.

You are already encountering some very challenging issues. For instance, there is a heightened practice risk that has ethical significance when you perform a procedure for the first time.

Thinking about what you would say is important because it is a part of training that there simply has to be a first time for every procedure that is learnt. Ensuring adequate supervision for your level of skill and experience is in place is an essential safeguard of patient safety and trust, and of the derived principle of veracity.

insight
A reflective process of examining own behavior and motivations, and recognising deficiencies.

reflection
A process of thought and analysis on past, present or future issues, applying deep and serious consideration.

> **REFLECTION POINT**
>
> ## Learning skills
>
> Think about a non-invasive procedure that you can undertake, such as taking observations, taking blood pressure (BP), or recording a pulse. Try to remember the first time you carried out such a procedure on a patient or a fellow student.
>
> Did you disclose to them that you hadn't carried out that procedure ever before? Practise stating aloud, in your own words, your level of skill and experience, and that some supervision would be beneficial as you start to learn to undertake the procedure.

Also, being open and honest about your skill and limits is sensible and protective for you as well. The standards expected of health care professionals takes into account their level of training and experience.

Professional associations and boards are responsible for defining:

- the profession's collective goals
- the expected role, and corresponding duties of professionals
- the limits of the service that the profession and member professionals can be expected to provide.

The associations and national boards of health professions discuss these issues regularly, and you can find their statements on professional responsibilities on their websites. The expected skill set of individual professionals is expressed in competencies or standards, and scope of practice statements.

For instance, the Nursing and Midwifery Board of Australia sets the expected requirements for Enrolled Nurses (ENs) in 'Enrolled nurse standards for practice'. For instance, an enrolled nurse: 'interprets information from a range of sources in order to contribute to planning appropriate care', and 'collaborates with the RN, the person receiving care and the healthcare team when developing plans of care' (Nursing and Midwifery Board of Australia, 2016a, p. 5).

As can be found in course information for Assistants in Nursing (AIN) training, AINs are assistants to nurses and also to doctors and other health professionals who are treating patients. They can assist the patient to be more comfortable, and help with activities such as eating, dressing and changing clothes, and showering, as well as performing duties such as cleaning patients' rooms, and carrying out routine sterilization. AINs communicate with nurses and doctors about their observations of a patient, such as improvement or other reaction to treatment that has been given.

obligation
Something one is bound to fulfill or perform.

Basic duties can translate into lists of duties, or **obligations**, and prohibitions, all of which are outlined for you before you start working in your profession. The first documentation you might see when starting a new job is a 'statement of duties', or a general job description that implies 'duties'. These vary widely between professions because of the different skills and corresponding responsibilities involved in that profession or sub-specialty. They also vary between different health care institutions and units as different services need to be provided in different settings.

The following position descriptions were adapted from advertised jobs. Notice how different the basic duties of each health care role is, and how different the day-to-day aspect of the work would be. The skill aspect of the job is defined, given the level of training and experience that is needed.

- A qualified speech pathologist is sought to provide speech pathology assessment, discharge planning and therapeutic intervention to clients known to the community and rehabilitation service. The role involves consultation and coordination with the client, their carer, other members of the community health and rehabilitation service team and other key stakeholders. There is scope to be involved in planning, implementation, evaluation and reporting on clinical services for the service, and quality improvement projects, as well as education for staff and students.
- A physiotherapist with at least two years post-qualifying experience is sought for a rehabilitation and aged care role in a busy public outpatient program. Drivers licence and registration with AHPRA essential.

Try to look at a few more position descriptions in real advertisements, and you may also notice how roles can vary depending on the seniority of the position, commensurate with higher level training or experience.

In any field there are further differences in job roles and duties—for instance, in different divisions of registration. A registered midwife is a partner in a process of childbirth, so the focus is on wellbeing and the natural health changes, with the added skills to recognise when additional support is needed, and an awareness of the challenges of health issues and of social disadvantage:

> The midwife, as registered by the Nursing and Midwifery Board of Australia (NMBA) and defined by the International Confederation of Midwives (2017), is educated, competent and authorised to provide safe, effective delivery of quality services that promote health and wellbeing for pregnancy, birth, the postnatal period and transition to parenting.
>
> (Nursing and Midwifery Board of Australia, 2018a)

These recent competency standards also recognise a broader role for the use of midwifery skills, now regarded as part of midwifery practice:

> This practice includes working in clinical and non-clinical relationships with the woman and other clients as well as working in management, administration, education, research, advisory, regulatory, and policy development roles.
>
> (Nursing and Midwifery Board of Australia, 2018a)

A nurse practitioner is endorsed for a specific scope of practice, as a nurse practitioner who has practised three years full-time at the clinical advanced nursing practice level. Scope of practice as an endorsed nurse practitioner is determined by the nurse and their employer. Each nurse practitioner must ensure that they have the necessary skills and training for the scope of practice that they offer in a particular context (Nursing and Midwifery Board of Australia, 2016b, 2016c).

Medical graduates can apply to work in supervised, accredited intern positions, and may not work as medical practitioners outside their allocated internship position, as their registration is provisional. The terms they complete as an intern are varied, so that they have experience in emergency medical care, medicine, surgery—as well as other approved terms—before they are able to apply for general registration (Medical Board of Australia, 2018). The job description of an intern is defined by the state and training institution they are allocated to.

Language proficiency is defined as part of professional competence, along with sufficient physical and mental capacity and professional skill. See for instance the *Health Practitioner Regulation National Law No 86* (NSW) at section 55(1)(d). Assessment of competence in English is a routine part of the screening process for suitability for registration of overseas medical practitioners, as a safeguard for safe and effective teamwork and communication with patients.

REFLECTION POINT

On the job

Find a few job descriptions of different health care workers. Notice the unique contribution that each worker will make to the health care setting, given their skill set, and how they will be expected to use those skills.

The core competencies and scope of practice for registered professionals can be quite different in different jurisdictions, so if you plan to work in another country at any time, remember to check the scope of practice and consider whether you can meet the list of duties in the job description.

Duties are something you are obliged to fulfil. In an ethics sense, it is a minimal position to only fulfil strict duties without also considering higher goals. **Goals** are something to aspire to—they are the ethically optimal position.

The distinction between duties and goals is often expressed in codes of ethics. For instance, the Code of Ethics for occupational therapists states: 'all members of the occupational therapist profession have an individual responsibility to maintain their own level of professional competence and each of them must strive to improve and update knowledge and skills' (Occupational Therapy Australia, 2014, p. 6).

One of the legacies of Aristotle's work is that the process of striving for ideals—and considering why the virtue of striving for optimal goals is adopted—is ethically significant. This is an important area of reflection for health care professionals who, given their special roles, assume higher responsibilities than others. These responsibilities include the expectation to exceed normal moral requirements towards what would be regarded as moral ideals and excellence in others (Beauchamp & Childress, 2001, p. 45).

Reflective practice depends on an awareness of current research evidence and professional clinical knowledge, so sharing in the transfer of that knowledge is essential.

duties
Obligations and specific tasks that you are bound to fulfil, or actions from which you are bound to refrain.

goals
Ideals and objectives aimed towards.

Reflective practice depends on your willingness to source current expected standards for your profession and role—for your level of training and experience—so that you can meet the expected competency standards. Reflective practice depends on your willingness to strive to learn your craft and offer it competently, safely, effectively and ethically. The community gives you the privilege of working in health care, and depends on you to remain an active learner and take responsibility for actively reflecting on appropriate and optimal practice in all of the roles you will hold throughout your career as a health care professional.

INTEGRATED LEARNING AND PRACTICE

Why do I need to do CPD?

Continuing professional development (CPD) is part of the registration requirements for every registered health practitioner, as a way of demonstrating that they are staying up to date for routine accreditation or credentialing purposes. CPD is part of maintaining quality standards for all professions.

The CPD requirements are set by your health profession board or association. Accurately documenting that you have completed a range of activities, and being ready to lodge further information to demonstrate your compliance, will become a routine aspect of your professional life. This is an example of regulation driven by your own profession, so that professional standards are maintained in a transparent and accountable way. Your professional integrity in this endeavour is vital.

CPD is often documented on an honesty basis, with individual professionals lodging summaries of the activities they have undertaken, or a signed statement that they have achieved at least the minimum required CPD. Monitoring can be undertaken—a bit like the tax audit system—with some random or targeted subsection of professional members being asked to provide further evidence supporting their compliance. You will need to keep records for your CPD in case you are asked to provide it.

Many professionals exceed the requirements, and active learners appreciate the opportunity to attend in-service training to reinforce and extend their skill base and competency, and to maintain their capacity for learning so that they can look forward to a long and enjoyable career. Remember that the profession you enter will change over time, and you will need to be ready to be part of the developing knowledge base of your field. You will become used to actively seeking out lectures and conferences, online modules and in-service sessions, and you may one day even contribute to their delivery to share your knowledge and expertise.

Mentoring and supervision is routine in health care teams, so that more junior members are supported in their roles to provide quality care. The supervision you can expect to have available to you is in keeping with the scope of your practice and position description. Discussion with colleagues becomes a routine part of work for fully trained professionals, and many continue to seek mentoring as part of their own professional development, as well as contributing to the profession by in turn mentoring or supervising more junior colleagues.

Ethics, character and propriety

propriety
In keeping with prudent and supported conventional standards.

character
Moral qualities of a person.

Satisfactory professional conduct depends on skill and competence, and the fitness, **propriety** and **character** of the professional, as well as the ethical way that professional provides their health service. The intertwining of professional skill and proper and ethical conduct is recognised at law.

Ethical conduct is partly defined in professional codes of conduct or professional codes of ethics. A common law concept is that a professional should not fall significantly below the standards expected by a peer of good repute, so improper behaviour is unethical for a professional as well. 'Improper or unethical conduct relating to the practice or purported practice of the practitioner's profession' is also listed as other conduct that could amount to unsatisfactory professional conduct in the *Health Practitioner Regulation National Law No 86* (NSW), at section 139B(1)(l).

Legal practitioners and medical practitioners feature in many of the classic cases on character and ethics and fitness to practise—that's because these professions have long established professional standards and membership or registration procedures. When registration is challenged, formal court hearings can follow. If an applicant is judged by a registration body to be an 'unsuitable person', that may prevent registration. Being found to be unfit on character grounds can justify a finding of professional misconduct, and can lead to deregistration of a registered practitioner, if they are deemed not suitable to be a member of the registered profession.

AHPRA lists some conduct that would be inconsistent with a practitioner being fit and proper to be a registered health practitioner:

- abusing a professional position—for instance, engaging in a sexual or personal relationship with a patient or someone close to the patient
- inappropriate patient examinations
- acts of indecency, sexual assault or violence
- fraud or dishonesty
- serious criminal acts (Australian Health Practitioner Regulation Agency, 2018).

Case law reasoning, the judgment and reasons in cases that have been decided by the courts, provide a way of thinking about character as the acceptance of high standards, and then also acting in accordance with those standards under pressure (*Council of the Law Society of New South Wales v Foreman* (1994), per Mahoney JA, at paragraph 449). If a person needs to prove they are fit and of good character, their moral standards, attitudes and qualities are weighed, as 'good character' is not the summation of acts alone (*Ex Parte Tziniolis* [1967], at paragraph 377).

The circumstances of such conduct should be considered before assuming they indicate unfitness to be a registered health practitioner, as explained in the following seminal case. A legal practitioner was hit on the head and face repeatedly in an altercation at a bar. He had intervened to stop a drunk seaman approaching two young women but was then attacked by the seaman. After police attended and the drunk seaman was arrested, the injured practitioner drove off in his car. Unfortunately, he had an accident in which someone else died, and was struck off the roll of medical practitioners, as he had been convicted of manslaughter. The majority of the High Court judges who sat on the appeal case found that the mere fact of a conviction does not necessarily demonstrate conclusively that someone is unfit to practise (*Ziems v The Prothonotary of the Supreme Court of New South Wales* (1957)). There has been considerable comment on this case in the professions, because it sets the precedent for the process of deciding if someone is fit and proper. In Ziems' case, he was not found to have a tendency to violence or lack of probity, and the conviction was not connected with his professional function. However, the High Court emphasised that some personal misconduct could show that a person was not a **fit and proper person** to practise (DalPont, 2014, p. 8). This means that conduct outside a professional context can be considered to determine whether a person is a fit and proper person to practise.

Related issues of **impropriety** have also been considered, and historical precedents are found in cases on the conduct of legal and medical practitioners, as well as cases about other people in responsible positions—such as company directors. Impropriety does not need to be intentional. As an objective standard, the onus is on each person to know the limits of their authority. This means that if you act knowingly or recklessly outside the scope of your role, this could be viewed as improper. The take-home message is that you should always find out the scope of your role and of your delegated authority to make decisions and act on behalf of the organisation in which you are working.

In a High Court case involving commercial company directors, an explanation of impropriety was provided (*R v Byrnes* [1995]). The explanation is now relied on in professional standards considerations for other professions:

> Impropriety does not depend on an alleged offender's consciousness of impropriety. Impropriety consists in a breach of the standards of conduct that would be expected of a person in the position of the alleged offender by reasonable persons with knowledge of the duties, powers and authority of the position and the circumstances of the case. When impropriety is said to consist in an abuse of power, the state of mind of the alleged offender is important (*R v Yuill* (1994) 34 NSWLR 179 at 193–194; see also *R v Donald; Ex parte Attorney-General (Q)* [1993] 2 Qd R 680.): the alleged offender's knowledge or means of knowledge of the circumstances in which the power is exercised and his purpose or intention in exercising the power are important factors in determining the question whether the power has been abused. But impropriety is not restricted to abuse of power. It may consist in the doing of an act which a director or officer knows or ought to know that he has no authority to do.

Look up the case on the High Court website if you want to read the full judgment: <http://hcourt.gov.au>.

A professional is of good character, fit to practise, appropriately trained and skilled for the role they undertake, committed to upholding acceptable practice standards in their professional responsibilities, and further striving for best practice standards.

fit and proper person
A suitable person deserving of the trust of others to exercise certain privileges in an ethical manner.

impropriety
Imprudence; stark and distasteful contravention to conventional standards.

There is provision for finding someone is 'unsuitable' to be registered under the *Health Practitioner Regulation National Law* (see section 55), so if there is sufficient information in the view of the registering authority to indicate someone is not suitable, they could be precluded from being registered when they first apply.

Governance and safety and acceptable practice settings

The practice setting enables every health care worker to be able to bring their skills into action in the service of the public. You can expect your credentials to be checked thoroughly before you start every new job.

INTEGRATED LEARNING AND PRACTICE

Why is there so much paperwork when starting a new job?

As a way of minimising risks undertaken under the umbrella of the service, the administration will routinely conduct checks on prospective staff as a condition of employment, with their agreement. Local sector regulation and employer standards are both additional and important protective features of the health care system. Different aspects of regulation will cover all staff, as the whole team combines to deliver health, community services and health care effectively, safely and efficiently to the community.

The curriculum vitae, qualifications and experience of each prospective employee will be double-checked to ensure that people with appropriate skills and qualifications and experience are hired.

Criminal checks of each prospective employee are routine—this is to ensure reasonable confidence in the honesty and integrity of staff. The appropriate authority carries out the check, with the applicant's agreement, and the results are made available to the institution. In keeping with Child Protection Laws, employers are required to make sure employees are regarded as safe to work with children prior to commencing, and these administrative conduct and criminal background checks may take into account allegations as well as proven offences. The laws prompt institutions and the appropriate authorities to carry out the checks because they are required and empowered to do so. Checks may be repeated and employees may be required to notify if they are charged with a serious offence.

Asking prospective staff to sign their agreement to abide by codes of conduct—and to uphold the values of the organisation—provides further reassurance that people who agree to work alongside others in the institution have an understanding about how they are to carry out their role.

Paperwork and rigorous checking applies for every institution as well before it offers services on an ongoing basis. Public hospitals and other health service organisations are accredited after meeting the national standards for quality and safety, with good systems in place to improve health services and minimise the risk of harm to patients. The emphasis is on safe clinical practice that meet the expectation of the health care public, who are the consumers of health care services. Health ministers of the Australian governments have endorsed both the standards and a national accreditation scheme. The initiative is ongoing, and current standards are available on the Australian Commission on Safety and Quality in Health Care's website (ACSQHS, 2012, 2017).

The standards apply to all hospital and day procedure services in Australia, and the majority of public dental services. In readiness for assessment, services gather their own evidence of improvement in quality and safety.

If an institution is accredited, the public and the staff can rely on that rigorous assessment that it is properly staffed and equipped, and that it is aiming for further improvement in quality and safety. However, the practice setting is only safe and acceptable if properly staffed and every health worker in that setting is aware of their part in the collective objective to deliver safe and acceptable care.

Potential employees and contractors would be prudent to check that the facility they may work in is licensed for the services offered, including being properly equipped and adequately staffed. Professionals should be aware of the licensing limitations of every setting. You could be responsible for harm to patients if you work in an unlicensed setting, because working there as a professional lends credibility to the institution, as patients will expect that acceptable services will be provided.

The local institution accepts a responsibility as a licensed provider to ensure that relevant regulations are applied. This is so that services are as safe as possible, and delivered to expected standards.

In an overseas jurisdiction, the District of Columbia Health Department of Health (DOH) (2016) has set out an informative policy on the development of standard operating procedures (SOPs) for use within its institutions, which reflects the shared wisdom of the field of health care **governance**.

governance
Controlling, directing or regulating activities.

The purposes of SOPs for specific DOH tasks and responsibilities are to:

- improve efficiency and effectiveness
- provide clear guidance on and requirements for implementing DOH processes
- aid in training all persons working for or assigned to DOH
- promote consistent and uniform results
- document how to comply with applicable laws, rules and regulations governing DOH's operations
- document best practices within the relevant subject matter
- provide managers with the tools necessary to ensure that DOH tasks and responsibilities are being uniformly and consistently performed.

In general, each SOP should document all operating processes and work expectations for the particular tasks enumerated in that SOP. Each SOP should articulate all tasks within the process flow and identify the office or bureau that is accountable for the processes.

Guidance documents from reputable councils and specialist colleges are plentiful, representing the best advice of the health professions, and academic, government and non-government organisations. Some internationally sourced documents are relevant to health settings worldwide. For instance, the UK Nuffield Council on Bioethics, which is highly regarded internationally, aims to stimulate debate and assist policy makers and professionals with general guidance as they explore issues in biology and medicine. The UK Clinical Ethics Network advises on reflective processes in clinical ethics committees and as they arise in clinical practice. The US Office of Research Integrity can assist institutions if they are considering best practice issues, or potential misconduct, by their research staff or affiliates. As these organisations provide their advisory documents free on public access websites, institutions can use them wherever they are situated in the world:

- http://www.nuffieldbioethics.org
- http://www.ukcen.net
- http://www.ori.hhs.gov.

The guidance found in these documents can be very helpful but won't ordinarily be enforceable, unless there is a local commitment for them to be strictly applied, or a contractual obligation arising out of an agreement between people or companies in different countries that a particular set of guidelines or protocols must be followed.

Best practice standards are routinely considered as part of providing comprehensive standard operating procedures at local state and territory government health department level. Jurisdictions often share resources when they develop new policies and procedures. The benefit of this wisdom and jurisdiction and local laws are integrated into the local policies and procedures, and updated as required.

Each institution is legally responsible for taking proper care to ensure they have complied with legal requirements that apply to health care. Managers actively seek advice and information on the different aspects of law to identify acceptable and required standards and limits. The governance department of a large institution such as a health department is a busy place. The people there are checking quality and acceptability of services, and generating policies and procedures that are informed by the current law so that risks for patients, staff and the institution are managed as much as possible. They are using the principles of law and generating the policies and SOPs that will keep health care professionals safely within their lawful scope of practice.

Some governance policies provide crucial guidance for lawful and documented consent processes, as you will read in Chapter 8 'Lifelong practice in decision making'. You will also notice practical judgment positions within some standard procedures, which have been resolved as a matter of policy. For instance, guidelines and limits in relation to the prioritisation of patients for admission into public hospitals are discussed in Chapter 10 'Regulation and availability of health and community services'.

> ### REFLECTION POINT
>
> ## A job in governance
>
> Read a role description of a job in governance. The description should outline what would be expected as part of this role, showing the nature of the work and the unit, or the scope of the role of the governance unit in a health service setting—what regulatory and institutional standards they are considering and applying.
>
> - Imagine working in that role in an institution, as part of the team to 'govern' and manage the risk in employment and maintaining safe and acceptable standards. Describe one of their roles.

Striving for quality care and improvement

Discussions on quality and care help to ensure that appropriate standards are achieved in the care that is offered. Case conferences or grand rounds are a formal way of hearing a comprehensive professional assessment of a current case, but many informal opportunities also present themselves. A system of mentorship and supervision is in place in health professions, so that more experienced professionals pass on their opinions and advice to more junior professionals. At team meetings or at handovers, you are called on to provide your opinion on current situations to your colleagues. What you say is informed by training and experience, and you will be relied on to have accessed relevant professional literature, if that is necessary to give your considered professional opinion.

Those directly involved in care are in a unique position to observe potential problems, and reporting potential issues to those who can manage them is part of normal practice, so that individual patients receive the best possible care. Institutions can also require staff to report incidents and adverse events—partly so that the potential for problems to arise again is managed.

Adverse events

Adverse events—also called 'sentinel events'—are reported, such as in annual reports to the Australian Commission on Safety and Quality in Health Care (ACSQHC). This is to enable system-wide consideration of improvements in management of risks in health care settings. Serious adverse drug reactions are reported under Therapeutic Goods Administration (TGA) regulation requirements (Therapeutic Goods Administration, 2016), so that information on anything that potentially poses a risk to the public is made known to the relevant authorities. Adverse events experienced as part of a research trial are additionally reported to the ethics committee, as it may mean that a research trial should be monitored more closely or halted. Responsibilities to report and also take action in response to the event are shared by the principal investigator, the sponsor of the trial, the human research ethics committee, the institution hosting the research work and the TGA.

Incident management

At institution level, incidents are reported which any person feels are outside current policies and procedures—particularly if they have impacted or could potentially impact on patient or workplace safety. Then the local administration can consider whether further steps are needed. The Incident Management System (IMS) or incident report is a familiar term in large public health services institutions (New South Wales Government Ministry of Health, 2018). Public hospital staff are now accustomed to documenting an issue on the relevant form, and lodging the form in a timely manner. Then information is available so that the risks can be mitigated or managed more effectively.

These are institutional level responses to safeguard each person—and the institution—from excessive risk. The institutional responses rely on individuals with the relevant information to report that concern of actual or heightened possibility of risk. A capacity for reflection and a commitment to the identification or standards that should be applied is part of the effective management of the institutions.

Performance management

Managers actively manage performance and undertake performance improvement plans appropriately with team members. Care needs to be taken to act reasonably, as bullying is experienced when a person or group of people act unreasonably in repeated conduct towards another person or group and that conduct creates a risk to health and safety for a person or group.

Unreasonable work demands can constitute bullying, as can teasing and other conduct. Government authorities and agencies such as Fair Work Australia and Safe Work Australia provide guidance on how to actively manage performance and improvement so that a person does not feel bullied in the workplace (Safe Work Australia, 2018). Staged and supportive performance improvement plans protect workers' health—as well as the health of the **clients** that they ultimately serve.

client
Person investigating or receiving service.

Formal institutional review processes of quality improvement (QI) or quality assurance (QA) aim to maintain and improve the quality and safety of care that is offered within the institution. These processes provide an opportunity to consider patterns of care and outcomes at an institutional or clinic level, and to identify potential problems in standards of practice. The aim is to ensure that high standards of care are maintained. Sometimes guidelines are developed from patterns of care that seem appropriate for particular conditions or types of clients.

Each healthy institution maintains a continual process of reflection on the quality and safety of its services, independent of any formal audit or accreditation round. Hospitals actively encourage QA assessments and initiatives within service units. Essentially, these QA activities are research, as they collect personal information from patients or health records, such as health services received and outcomes of those services. A review of the ethics of the research activity is required before they proceed. You will find more about research ethics consideration in Chapter 6 and Chapter 7.

QA processes promise a public benefit, as they provide opportunities for institutions and services to check that appropriate standards of quality and safety are being met, and to refine their systems for service delivery.

For instance, improved QA in wound management protocols has been credited with improvements in wound infection rates. Even small decreases in infection rates have a large impact on reducing patient complication rates because of infection, and reducing the funding needed for patient care required because of the complications of surgery (Goldstone, 1998).

Continual improvement in wound management and infection control remains a consistent theme in health care, and being informed of the latest protocols will become a routine feature of your own CPD as you stay up to date with the latest clinical knowledge.

At government level, quality and safety initiatives—such as Royal Commission inquiries—can be prompted when there is need to consider if large scale or systemic issues exist and, if so, how to address them. The Royal Commission into Aged Care Quality and Safety, announced by the Australian Government in 2018, attracted immediate comment from health professionals, concerned that there was already considerable information on what was needed to address the crisis in aged care, so that addressing systemic issues of funding and planning for adequate staff ratios should not be further delayed (Bastian 2018).

Community expectations and cultural safety

The process of defining acceptable health care and delivery is a joint responsibility of government, administrators, professionals and the **community**.

When policy on service delivery and legislative reform of laws is considered, it is an established and routine requirement to undertake public engagement and community **consultation** (Peel, 1999; Australian Law Reform Commission, 2017).

Have a look at the composition of the governing board of a local health care institution. You will find that there are some community representatives there. These representatives have a say in setting the operating objectives and priorities, as well as the policy and regulation within that institution. They also help to ensure accountability and transparency, in considering the extent to which the institution meets its stated purpose and objectives—including its stated values.

Under specified **principlism**, principles can be identified, but their meaning and application should be defined with reference to cultural norms or standards (De Grazia, 1992, p. 525). Under **communitarianism**, issues of social moral import are emphasised. A strong sense of community limits—self-defined by the community—is essential to communitarianism (Zwart, 1993).

community
Group of people defined by shared social engagement.

consultation
Active process of facilitating the expression of opinions, taking advice and cooperative deliberation.

principlism
An ethics framework in which issues are understood and analysed with the assistance of broad descriptive principles.

communitarianism
An ethics theory in which the relationship of a person to a specific community is identified, and the interests and needs of that community as a whole take priority over individual interests and needs.

REFLECTION: SCAN THE LOCAL NEWS

Have a look in a local or regional newspaper to see what has made the news in your community.

1 Which issues are causing concern or generating discussion? Do these concerns raise ethical or legal issues that you have heard about elsewhere?

2 Note what you learn about community concerns, and if this is the first time you were aware of the concerns.

3 Write in your own words why it is important to consult and gauge community views and concerns, if you agree that it is important in principle, or if you agree it is important for the topics you have found.

Community consultation is compatible with many ethics frameworks, because they implicitly rely on a collective community view to identify best practice and the limits of acceptability. You will learn more about these frameworks in Chapter 4.

libertarianism
An ethics theory that aims for the greatest good for the greatest number, with good defined by each person pursuing their own defined wishes and liberties.

deontology
An ethics theory in which the process and components of actual or proposed action is the focus, with reference to agreed values and rules.

deon
Established morally fundamental rule.

In liberalism, in which there is little role for cohesive community control over individual actions, there is still a sense of a general community consensus on the limits to autonomy. **Libertarianism** assumes that there is some kind of community agreement on reasonable limits to liberty that can be expressed, and that there are obligations to endure certain burdens for the good of the society to which we belong. Within the framework of libertarianism, only a majority community view—the general will—would be the acceptable basis of a limitation placed on liberty (Mill, 1975).

In **deontology**, there is an ethical standard expressed in a rule, or **deon**, that one would expect to be shared among members of the community, below which these community members should not go. In Kant's work, there is a sense that we should respect others, and that there should be a limit to how much we interfere or harm them, so that each person can develop his or her own moral self, and identify the categorical imperative (Sullivan, 1989).

At a minimum, the diversity of values in the community should be recognised when offering health care, as has been consistently promoted by the World Health Organization (WHO):

> To be ethical, our responses must be both honest and humane: first, they must be applicable to people's concrete circumstances and meaningful to them; and second, they must be respectful of their rights, values, and personal dilemmas, as lived within their own communities. In other words, ethical issues must be worked out with the people concerned.

(Nakajima, 1996, p. 3)

Health professionals are drawn from diverse cultural backgrounds and are trained to work in different local settings and contexts, and to serve different cultures. You have the benefit of a more comprehensive knowledge of cultures other than your own. This is partly because you have the opportunity to travel, live and work in different countries, and partly because of the culturally and linguistically diverse community that we live in. So, you are partly prepared for the fact that people are often culturally different to you.

Culture shapes expectations and understanding of illness, health and care. Anticipating that clients' expectations and understandings may be different from yours is part of respecting diversity.

Cultural safety takes into account the environment and the personal experience of the person (Victorian Aboriginal Child Care Agency, 2010).

If a health care service is not viewed as culturally safe by prospective clients, they might delay seeking effective health care. Health care workers contribute to cultural safety and cultural security by seeking training so that they are culturally competent. Diversity must be valued by professionals and the health system before a true partnership can be achieved in a spirit of respect.

culture
Social expectations and norms of a particular community or civilisation.

cultural safety
Safety for a person given their culture, environment and personal experience.

PRACTICE EXAMPLE

Departing from standards

Susan Alexander

Susan has been a Registered Nurse for 12 years, working predominantly in palliative care and academia, and has a strong interest in professional issues.

Jocelyn is a nurse in a mental health care facility. She is caring for Ronald, who has been admitted following an episode of psychosis thought to be related to substance abuse over a long period of time.

Jocelyn is married with four children, but is currently experiencing difficulties at home. Ronald is fifteen years younger than Jocelyn. Although he has had some episodes of psychosis, Jocelyn finds Ronald exciting because he has travelled widely and has participated in activities that she considers to be risky—but attractive. Jocelyn starts to spend more time with Ronald, to the extent that her other patients are neglected.

When Ronald is released from the facility, Jocelyn drives him home and gives him her personal contact details. She tells Ronald not to tell anybody that she has done so because her employer does not allow staff to provide personal contact details to patients.

A few days later, Jocelyn calls on Ronald to see how he is progressing. She continues to visit him on a regular basis and starts discussing her difficulties at home. Although not intimate, Ronald suggests to Jocelyn that they have a close friendship. He tells Jocelyn how much he requires medication but cannot afford to visit his GP to obtain a prescription. He asks Jocelyn to obtain the medication for him. When Jocelyn refuses, Ronald threatens to tell her employer and the nursing regulatory authority about their relationship.

1 What should Jocelyn do in this situation?

2 Which NMBA standards has Jocelyn breached?

3 Why is it not appropriate for a health professional to have a relationship with a patient other than the health-care provider–patient relationship?

4 Patients are typically considered to be vulnerable. What additional characteristics does Ronald have that exacerbate his vulnerability in this scenario?

If a context is culturally secure, policies and practices are in place so that 'interactions adequately meet cultural needs'. That is, each person feels culturally safe. This has been explored by the Australian Human Rights Commission (2011), noting Māori nurses in New Zealand have described this as:

> an environment that is safe for people: where there is no assault, challenge or denial of their identity, of who they are and what they need. It is about shared respect, shared meaning, shared knowledge and experience of learning, living and working together with dignity and truly listening.
>
> (AHRC 2011; also citing Williams, 1999, p. 213)

The peak body Victorian Aboriginal Child Care Agency (VACCA) offered participants' views of cultural safety to the Commission to explain the concept, including one participant's view: 'Feeling safe in the knowledge that you're listened to, that your contribution to the community is important, just as much as anyone else's'. Particular attention was given in the Social Justice Report to cultural safety and security as tools to address lateral violence (Australian Human Rights Commission, 2011; also citing Frankland et al., 2010, p. 63).

Professional integrity and accountability

The professional upholds their responsibilities by ensuring they are ready to practise their skills. Safe and acceptable practice includes having adequate training, knowledge and judgment, and exercising care so that skill and knowledge is put into practice in an acceptable way. Individuals must also act with integrity, and in a way that is accountable to their profession, institution and the community.

competence
Capacity to perform a specified task, and readiness to do so.

competencies
Skills that have been assessed and demonstrated by a person as able to be performed to an acceptable standard.

You are able to practise if you are competent. Professional **competence** is a readiness to use your knowledge, skills and judgment in the practice of your profession and role. Competence or mental capacity also applies to patients, who need to have a readiness to consider their choices and decide on what they consent to for their care. You will read more about this in Chapter 8 'Lifelong practice in decision making'. Some of the earlier writers use the term *competence*, but *capacity* is the current term for the decision-making readiness of patients.

Precise skills are often referred to as **competencies**.

Part of your professional integrity is to actively reflect on your competence, competencies and readiness to practise at all times. You are the primary safeguard that safe and effective care can be delivered by you at the time you perform each task and role. The hallmark of a professional is in maintaining a strong commitment to high standards and optimal principles—a commitment to professional integrity. Professionals also have a shared responsibility to their profession, to notice if standards are not adequate due to the actions of their fellow professionals, and to bring this to the attention of those who could remedy the situation.

Remedial action can be taken at institutional level if any individual worker is not performing to expected standards. If the work of an employee is falling short of existing standards, an institution could try and remedy the deficits in that employee's approach to their work—for example, by arranging an education program or closer supervision.

Performance plans prompt education and periodic assessment of a person's performance. If this approach is not successful, the institution may prefer to dismiss that employee, rather than allowing them to risk either the work of the institution or the public's trust that the institution will provide safe and effective care. The process followed and the decision made can be challenged, and unions or professional associations or insurers can assist their members in bringing proceedings of unfair dismissal, so that the matter can be reviewed.

Counselling, performance assessments and performance reviews can also be carried out by professional councils, responding to complaints or concerns—see, for instance, under the *Health Practitioner Regulation National Law No 86* (NSW), section 145B—to consider if conditions need to be placed on a practitioner's registration, such as further education and working under formal supervision. This is in addition to any education or supervision an employer may require.

The public places significant trust in the health care system, the care setting, and their carers. The general public should be able to trust that safe and acceptable care will be available. Maintaining public confidence in professions and practice settings is essential because it goes to the heart of health care. When people need health care, they are potentially vulnerable. If their trust in the system, practice setting, a profession or their carer is damaged, they may even feel unable to seek further health care.

A central part of the protective regulatory scheme for the maintenance of acceptable practice standards in Australia is that many health professions in the health workforce are registered. A national register of those who are suitably qualified to be registered health practitioners is held by AHPRA on behalf of each of the health profession boards. An acceptable standard of practice is initially safeguarded by only registering those who are properly trained and fit to practise. This is combined with inquiry powers at state level into performance and conduct matters to provide a national system of professional practice regulation. The privilege of being registered can be withdrawn, and conditions can be placed on a registered professional's practice if it is necessary to protect the public.

Health review commissioners, complaints commissions, health services commissioners, health care complaints commissioners, and health ombudsmen systems exist in each state and territory, so that matters of concern with any aspect of health services or conduct by health workers that affects patients can be inquired into by the relevant public authority, to minimise further risk to person or persons, if any is found, and so that the public is protected.

REFLECTION: PROTECTIVE SCHEMES

Look up the relevant complaints body and commissioner in your jurisdiction:

- Health Complaints Commissioner (Tas)
- Health Care Complaints Commission (NSW)
- Health Services Complaints Commissioner (Vic)
- Health and Community Services Complaints Commissioner (SA, NT)
- Health Services Commissioner (ACT)

+ continued

- Office of the Health Ombudsman (Qld)
- Health and Disability Services Complaints Officer (WA).

1   Look at the website for your jurisdiction to find out what the protective purpose of that body is, and describe it in your own words.

2   Make a note of what happens when someone makes a complaint, and how the protective scheme in your jurisdiction works in practice. Complaints can be made about any registered or unregistered health service provider or worker in the health sector and the health organisation.

Deciding if knowledge, skill, judgment and care are exercised within reasonable standards

Conduct and performance can be assessed formally if a concern is raised by any person, professional, patient or other member of the public. Any concerned person can make complaints, including other health care workers and members of the public. Notifications of concerns can be made to AHPRA, to individual health councils and to the complaints bodies in each jurisdiction. Health councils, boards and the complaints investigating authorities share responsibility for appropriately handling complaints and making sure a process is in place for the assessment of any potential ongoing risks to the public, against the relevant reasonable and acceptable professional standards. Complaints can also be made about health service providers who are not registered. Their conduct is potentially judged against the *National Code of Conduct for health care workers* as the relevant standard as you read in Chapter 1.

Professionals have a duty to speak up if they hold a reasonable belief that a practitioner poses a potential risk to the public. Australian-registered practitioners are subject to legislated notification provisions if they form a reasonable belief of risk posed by a registered practitioner. Mandatory notification provisions vary between jurisdictions.

Legislative notification obligations are in place for health professionals to alert their registering authority if they hold a reasonable belief that any health professional poses a significant risk to the public or any person or persons.

Under the *Health Practitioner Regulation National Law* (the National Law), registered health practitioners, employers and education providers must make a **mandatory notification** of a complaint or concern if a reasonable belief is held that a practitioner:

mandatory notification
Required alert to relevant authorities.

- is placing the public at risk
- is practising in an unsafe way
- has an impairment that could lead to making unsafe judgments about their own patients.

See, for instance, *Health Practitioner Regulation National Law No 86* (NSW), at sections 140–143. Some of the National Law rules about notifying another health practitioner do not apply in Western Australia, but similar principles supporting notification of a serious concern are found in the health professions' Codes of Conduct or Codes of Ethics.

The Health Complaints Commissioner in Victoria has noted an increase in complaints— possibly because more information about the complaints processes is now available to the public. Health service complaints made up the majority of complaints to the Commission, and an increase in complaints about certain services and providers was noted—such as prison health service providers. When a practitioner provider's type was considered, by far the largest number of complaints were received about medical practitioners. Complaints about non-registered providers such as massage therapists, counsellors, alternative therapists and speech therapists have also increased (Health Complaints Commissioner, 2017).

Each complaint needs to be assessed, and investigations can be undertaken by a complaints commission or health ombudsman, or the board or council of a health profession, after a consultation process between their agencies. Investigation into the complaint is then coordinated, and the concerns may be able to be addressed by interviewing or counselling the practitioner or worker concerned. Performance reviews can be held at Council level, and the practitioner or worker could be asked to submit to a formal independent assessment of their competencies in a clinical context. The focus is on protecting the public, rather than offering redress for any harm that has befallen a particular patient.

If the matter is potentially a significant departure from expected professional standards, a more formal inquiry may be undertaken. An independent panel of health professional members, a legal member, and another member who is not a registered health professional undertakes the inquiry. The panel makes findings and considers the next best step, bearing in mind the protective nature of the jurisdiction and that the priority is to act in the interests of the public.

The most up-to-date Code of Conduct guides a health practitioner's current conduct, but as a matter of fairness, when a complaint is made about past conduct, the Code that was in place at that time is used to consider if there was departure from acceptable standards. For instance, the standards of the time would apply to the conduct of a nurse or midwife, even though the new 2018 *Code of Conduct for nurses* and the *Code of Conduct for midwives* have been issued to guide current conduct (Nursing and Midwifery Board of Australia, 2018b and 2018c).

Legislative provisions and case law from New South Wales is used to explain the inquiry into complaints of departure from accepted standards. The principles of assessing potentially **unsatisfactory professional conduct** are provided in the definition of the departure in the National Law:

> Conduct that demonstrates the knowledge, skill or judgment possessed, or care exercised, by the practitioner in the practice of the practitioner's profession is significantly below the standard reasonably expected of a practitioner of an equivalent level of training or experience.
>
> *(Health Practitioner Regulation National Law No 86* (NSW), *section 139B(1)(a))*

unsatisfactory professional conduct
Conduct that is judged by peers of good repute to be significantly below acceptable standards.

professional misconduct
Unsatisfactory professional conduct that is so serious it could warrant suspension from practice or deregistration.

Professional misconduct is conduct that is unsatisfactory, of a type that is so serious that it could result in suspension or loss of registration. The extent to which the conduct departs from acceptable or 'proper' standards is central to this consideration. The conduct can be a single instance of **unsatisfactory professional conduct** that is serious, or multiple instances of unsatisfactory professional conduct that together make up **professional misconduct** (*Health Practitioner Regulation National Law No 86* (NSW), section 139E).

Note that the definitions are found in the relevant legislation. The terms 'unsatisfactory professional performance' and 'unprofessional conduct' can also be used to refer to conduct that is below the standards reasonably expected (*Health Practitioner Regulation National Law (Queensland) 2009*).

A traditional case from the United Kingdom is often cited to define professional misconduct as 'deliberate departure from accepted standards or such serious negligence as, although not deliberate, to portray indifference and an abuse of the privileges which accompany registration as a medical practitioner' (*Allinson v General Council of Medical Education and Registration [1894]*, at paragraphs 760–761).

So, for instance, if a relatively minor problem was repeated, and the public could no longer trust that a practitioner would apply proper standards, the instances of repeated departure together could amount to professional misconduct.

The character of a professional, as demonstrated in conduct, is also open to scrutiny in inquiries of departure from acceptable practice standards, as it can form a complaint that an inquiry then considers. Being of good character is a key part of being fit to be registered and to practise in that registered profession. If a person is judged unsuitable, they would not then become registered. A lack of good character could amount to professional misconduct.

> ### REFLECTION POINT
>
> ## Protection of the public
>
> 1   Express the section 139B(1) and section 139E National Law elements in your own words.
>
> 2   If you are after more of a challenge, use statutory interpretation principles to consider the purposive interpretation of section 139E, to protect the public and deter other practitioners, and check how this protection is achieved by first reading *HCCC v Do* [2014], at paragraph 35.

Expert peer reviewers interpret the expected standards, and give an opinion on whether certain conduct represents a departure from the expected professional standards. This role is undertaken by experienced practitioners. The importance of their assessment is supported in case law. If a departure from standards is shown in the conduct, and the departure reasonably incurs strong disapproval of peers of good repute and competence, then it could be judged to be professional misconduct (*Qidwai v Brown* [1984], at paragraph 105). So, the level of criticism that peers feel is warranted carries weight in an inquiry into the practitioner's conduct.

Findings are made, and reasons are provided for those findings, which explain the evidence relied on by the inquiry panel. The *Briginshaw v Briginshaw* standard of proof applies, as it does in all civil proceedings. This means inquiries consider the evidence on the balance of probabilities, in a way that also is proportional to the seriousness of the consequences of the findings and consequential orders that are made (*Briginshaw v Briginshaw* [1938]).

Any protective orders that are made must be relevant to the findings, and should also achieve protection of the public in the least restrictive way feasible—that is, in a way that is proportional to the risk posed, and the need to protect the public, and maintain their trust, and uphold the reputation of the profession.

Orders can include a reprimand, or suspension or deregistration, if the matter has been heard by the upper level tribunal, or judicial hearing, and removal from the register is necessary to protect the public. Alternatively—and more routinely—protective conditions can be imposed. These include:

- educational programs—to remedy defined deficits in knowledge and skill
- mentoring—for continued professional development
- audits
- monitoring mechanisms for any aspect of practice
- restrictions on practice.

Sometimes a practitioner may have already undertaken protective steps for themself, such as:

- attending a relevant course
- reflecting on their errors and developed insight into their seriousness
- seeking help for any health or medical issues they have that have impacted on their professional work or fitness to practise.

In these cases, checking the sufficiency and protective effect of those steps may be all that is needed in terms of protecting the public into the future.

Under the National Law in New South Wales, 'the protection of the health and safety of the public must be the paramount consideration', as in the *Health Practitioner Regulation National Law No 86* (NSW), section 3A, Objective and guiding principle (NSW).

The purpose of any investigation or inquiry is to protect the public—and to maintain public trust in professional services. The safety of the public is paramount. Protection of the reputation of the profession is part of this purpose. While a punitive effect on the practitioner is not the objective, a punitive effect can be the result of proper and sufficient steps to protect the public (*HCCC v Litchfield* (1997)). A deterrent effect is also part of protecting the public. Protection of the public includes sending a message of deterrence to the practitioner, and also to other practitioners from similar conduct (*HCCC v Do* [2014], at [35]).

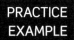

Mandatory reporting

Jayne Hewitt

Jayne has been a Registered Nurse for 30 years, working predominantly in critical care areas such as intensive care and coronary care.

Terry is an experienced and competent Registered Nurse (RN) who works on the medical ward in a small community hospital. A senior member of staff, Terry is frequently in charge of the ward, and responsible for supervising and supporting new or less experienced nurses. Terry's professional, gentle and caring approach to his work means that he is highly regarded by his colleagues and by the patients he cares for.

Lucy recently started work on the same medical ward as Terry. As a relatively inexperienced RN, she is grateful for the mentoring and support that she receives from Terry. After dinner on an afternoon shift, Terry tells Lucy that he is working his seventh shift in a row and that his 'back was killing him'. He asks Lucy whether any of the patients she is looking after are prescribed Valium. Terry indicates that, in the past, his back felt much better after he'd taken something to 'help relax'. Lucy is aware that Valium is prescribed for two of her patients and, when Terry inquires, she tells him who they are. Shortly afterwards, she sees Terry walk into one of the patient's rooms with a key to the medication drawer.

At the end of the shift, Terry and Lucy sit down to finalise their patients' documentation and prepare to hand over to the night staff. Lucy notices that Terry is having difficulty with his paperwork and is drifting off mid-sentence. She asks Terry whether he's okay. 'Yeah, feeling much better now,' he replies.

1 What is the ethical conflict that Lucy faces in this situation?
2 What information could Lucy rely on to form a 'reasonable belief' that Terry may have taken the patient's Valium?
3 What legal obligation does Lucy have in these circumstances?
4 How will Lucy satisfy her legal obligation?

The way registered professionals' potential departures from acceptable practice are assessed is informed by principles of reasoned inquiry and administrative decision making, including procedural fairness and natural justice. The same principles routinely apply in assessments of conduct for registered and non-registered health carers—for instance, at a hospital or area health board level. The process is as follows:

• A complaint is made, and the respondent has the right to be aware of the complaint and to respond.
• A person's training and role—or scope of practice—is explored.
• The acceptable standards for practising in that role are documented.

- A complaint is investigated, and then formally stated and inquired into, with a focus on the facts of what happened, and whether the conduct departed from acceptable and reasonable conduct in the circumstances.
- The authority bringing the complaint and the practitioner responding to the complaint can bring their own evidence; they can also make submissions before findings are made—these submissions can be about the facts, circumstances, standards, departure, and other relevant circumstances.
- Protective steps are also considered, sometimes as a separate stage in an inquiry. Parties can make submissions on protective orders.

If a complaint is made, or a concern is noted in a service unit, an employer is likely to first consider if it is safe to keep a person in their exact role, or whether it is better to reassign them—or even suspend them on pay—while further investigation of the facts is undertaken. An employer may have the resources to:

- offer training or supervision to a person while deficiencies in their practise are rectified
- offer ongoing education.

If a breach has been significant or if, after educative steps have been taken, a practitioner has not been able to demonstrate the capacity to practise safely and to the necessary standard in their role, the employer will consider whether an employment contract can continue.

In a case of an enrolled nurse in Western Australia, a number of findings and protective orders were made, which illustrate the range of orders that were thought necessary and sufficient to protect the public. In this case, the parties put forward what they thought were reasonable findings and protective orders, which were then considered further by the hearing member. This case also highlights the way an employing institution and the public registering authorities work together to protect the public.

The respondent practitioner admitted professional misconduct. These orders were made publicly available on the Western Australian State Administrative Tribunal website (Nursing and Midwifery Board of Australia, 2017). Although hearings are held in public, just like regular courts and public administrative inquiries, and the decisions are published, the name of the practitioner and institution has been deleted. The intended focus of citing the detail of the orders is education, so that you can appreciate in a practical way the range of orders that can be made.

> On application before Member David Maclean and upon a Minute of Consent Orders, signed on 29 August 2017, it is ordered:
>
> The Tribunal notes:
>
> 1 The Nursing and Midwifery Board of Australia (Applicant) alleged that there is proper cause for disciplinary action against XX (Respondent) pursuant to section 196 of the Health Practitioner Regulation National Law (National Law) because the Respondent has behaved in a way that constitutes professional misconduct as defined in section 5 of the National Law.
>
> 2 The Respondent has admitted that she has behaved in a way that constitutes professional misconduct contrary to the National Law and the parties have

agreed the terms upon which the proceedings could be settled pursuant to section 54(8) of the *State Administrative Tribunal Act 2004* (WA).

3   By written agreement between the parties dated XXXX the parties agreed the terms upon which the proceedings could be settled.

4   The Parties have agreed the relevant facts set out in Schedule 'A'.

The Tribunal orders:

5   Being satisfied by reason of the Respondent's admissions that proper cause exists for disciplinary action against the Respondent, and in order to give effect to the agreed terms of settlement of the proceeding, on date XXXX it is ordered, pursuant to s 54(8) of the *State Administrative Tribunal Act 2004* (WA) that:

6   The Respondent has behaved in a way that constitutes professional misconduct in terms of s 196(1)(b)(iii) of the National Law, in that she:

(a) misled Patient A to believe that the medication to be given by intramuscular injection was Olanzapine;

(b) administered an injection of 3mls of H2O to Patient A's left buttock in circumstances where:

(i)   it was not ordered by a Medical Officer or delegated or checked by a Registered Nurse;

(ii) it was not preceded by the 6 rights of medication administration checks;

(iii) there was no therapeutic basis to do so and it exposed Patient A to increased risk of haematoma, infection, irritation and lysis, in breach of THE HOSPITAL's Medications: Administration policy (C13.58) and the OVERARCHING HEALTH CARE ORGANISATION Health Care Code of Conduct (July 2014).

(c) by virtue of the conduct alleged at paragraphs a. and b. above, breached the Code of Professional Conduct for Nurses (May 2013), by failing to:

(i)   practise in a safe and competent manner;

(ii) practise in accordance with the standards of the profession and broader health system;

(iii) provide honest and accurate information in relation to nursing care;

(iv) support the informed decision making of a person requiring and receiving health care; and

(v)   practise nursing reflectively and ethically, in accordance with the Code of Ethics for Nurses in Australia (May 2013).

7   The Respondent is reprimanded;

8   The following conditions be imposed on the Respondent's registration:

Supervised practise

9   The Respondent must be supervised by another registered nurse (the supervisor) when undertaking medication management and medication administration.

10 For the purposes of this condition, 'supervised' is defined as: The Respondent must consult and follow the directions of the supervisor about the medication management of patients before medication is administered and must be directly observed by the supervisor who is physically present when attending to medication administration.

11 Within 14 days of the notice of imposition of this condition, the Respondent must, on the approved form (HPN10), nominate a primary supervisor and at least one alternate supervisor to be approved by the Chair of the Applicant. The Respondent must ensure that each nomination is accompanied by an acknowledgement, on the approved form (HPNA10), from each nominated supervisor that they are willing to undertake the role of supervisor and are aware that AHPRA will seek reports from them.

12 In the event that no approved supervisor is willing or able to provide the supervision required, the Respondent must cease practise immediately and must not resume practise until a new supervisor has been nominated by the Respondent and approved by the Chair of the Applicant.

13 Within 14 days of the notice of the imposition of these conditions, the Respondent is to provide to AHPRA, on the approved form (HP10) acknowledgement that AHPRA may:

   (a) obtain information from relevant authorities;

   (b) obtain information and/or a report from the senior person at each place of place of practise on a quarterly basis; and

   (c) obtain a report from the approved supervisor on a quarterly basis.

   14. Within 14 days of the notice of the imposition of these conditions, the Respondent is to provide to AHPRA, on the approved form (HPS10), acknowledgement from the senior person at each place of practise that AHPRA may seek reports from them.

Undertake education

15 The Respondent must undertake and successfully complete a program(s) of education, approved by the Chair of the Applicant, in relation to the following topics:

   (a) managing acute mental health related presentations;

   (b) medication management and administration; and

   (c) ethical decision making in clinical practice.

16 Within 1 month of the notice of the imposition of these conditions, the Respondent must, on the approved form (HPN24), nominate for approval by the Chair of the Applicant an education course(s), assessment(s) or program(s) (the education) addressing the topics required. The Respondent must ensure:

   (a) the nomination includes a copy of the curriculum of the education for each topic; and

   (b) the education consists of a minimum of 6 hours inclusive of all topics.

17 The Respondent must complete the education within 6 months of the notice of the Applicant's approval of the education.

18 Within 1 month of the completion of the education, the Respondent is to provide to AHPRA:

   (a) evidence of successful completion of the education; and

   (b) evidence of having undertaken and successfully completed the formal assessment component of the education.

19 Within 14 days notice of the imposition of these conditions the Respondent must provide to AHPRA, on the approved form (HPC), the contact details of a senior person, such as the Director of Nursing, Senior Practice Manager, Senior Manager, or equivalent (the senior person) at each a current place of practise. In providing this form, the Respondent acknowledges that:

   (a) AHPRA will contact the senior person and provide them with a copy of the conditions on the Respondent's registration or confirm that the senior person has received a copy of the conditions from the Respondent; and

   (b) the Respondent will be required to provide the same form:

      (i)   within 7 days of the commencement of practise at each and every subsequent place of practise; and

      (ii) within 7 days of each and every notice of any subsequent alteration of these conditions.

20 The review period for the above conditions is 3 months from the date of imposition.

21 All costs associated with compliance with the conditions on their registration are at the Respondent's own expense.

22 The Respondent pay the Applicant's costs of the Tribunal application, fixed in the sum of $2,000.

Mitigating factors which were put forward in the Schedule A were considered before the protective orders were imposed. The parties noted in Schedule A:

The Respondent contends that the following are mitigating factors in relation to penalty:

a   she was open and honest immediately following the event and admitted the conduct to her employer and to the Applicant;

b   she has apologised for her actions and confirmed that there was no malice or intent towards the patient. She has apologised for placing the patient, the patient's family and all staff concerned into the situation, and is extremely remorseful;

c   at the relevant time, she had been under an extreme amount of mental strain, which she had sought medical treatment for;

d   the acuity of the psychiatric intensive care unit was extremely high at the relevant time, she had been feeling very undervalued and alone, and was trying to do her job the best she could with heightened anxiety and an extreme amount of mental strain; and e she was suspended for one month following the incident, transferred to another department and placed on a two week super-numerary program.

She also received further education and close monitoring of her performance, with a 10 week period of being considered non-medication competent, and is undergoing a 12 month Clinical Enhancement Program; and

f she otherwise has a clean disciplinary history.

(Nursing and Midwifery Board of Australia, 2017)

A professional's registration and conditions of registration—and history of orders and conditions that have been made—are noted on a practitioner's registration history. Current practice conditions are listed on the AHPRA website register, and the decisions of standards committees and tribunals are generally also available to the public. Committees and tribunals can take the opportunity to pass their findings on to relevant professional associations, colleges, health departments and hospitals, so that the lowered professional standards can be rectified, guarding against further unsatisfactory practice.

The integrated responsibility of providing information and giving evidence

In formal settings, such as administrative and court proceedings, a variety of information is brought before decision makers so that a reasoned decision is made on the best available information.

Providing information

If you are asked to provide information to any authorised formal inquiry setting, you are obliged to do so to the best of your ability, in a way that is comprehensive, truthful and accurate. Expect to be periodically asked throughout your career about aspects of professional care that you have provided. The records that you keep about your part in health care are essential as a record of your involvement in each person's care.

A professional appreciates the importance of professional standards, and the importance for mechanisms that are in place to ensure standards are upheld, or deficits are rectified. One way of demonstrating fitness to continue practising is to respect and uphold the ability of the public and professional authorities to maintain standards and investigate potential risks to the public. It is a matter of professional integrity that any account given to your employer, professional association, registering authority, police, court, or administrative authority must be truthful, complete so as not to be misleading, and accurate.

Responsibilities and rights relating to legitimate investigations of a practitioner or a practice are addressed in codes—such as the following code for medical practitioners: 'Good medical practice involves ... cooperating with any legitimate inquiry into the treatment of a patient and with any complaints procedure that applies to your work' (Medical Board of Australia, 2014, p. 20). Similar statements appear in other codes, and case law supports the expectation that:

- a professional will assist in the public protective endeavour of an inquiry
- adverse inferences can be made if the professional does not give evidence and the evidence the practitioner could give is only within their knowledge.

If you are asked to provide information on factual events or circumstances as a witness of fact, you will be 'sworn in' and asked to promise to tell the truth in the same way as any other witness.

These examples of an oath and affirmation are drawn from the *Evidence Act 2008* (Vic), Schedule 1, at section 21(2) and section 22(2). Each is a solemn promise to tell the truth:

> I swear (or the person taking the oath may promise) by Almighty God (or the person may name a god recognised by his or her religion) that the evidence I shall give will be the truth, the whole truth and nothing but the truth.

> I solemnly and sincerely declare and affirm that the evidence I shall give will be the truth, the whole truth and nothing but the truth.

Take the time to think about the importance of this promise.

Giving evidence

If you are called as a witness of fact, you will need to think carefully about what you feel confident that you remember. You should be ready to explain how you support the information that you provide. You may have a clear recollection of the facts. Alternatively, you may rely on such earlier records that you made at the time or shortly afterwards as an accurate record of events.

For instance, a nurse manager was called to give evidence at a case about whether a person had capacity to make a will, as she was one of the witnesses of the making of a patient's final will. The nurses' notes were also called for, as they provided possible information on capacity during the patient's admission (*Loosely v Powell* [2018], at paragraphs 64–67). Any nurse who had made a relevant entry in the notes could also have been called as a witness of fact.

As well as being witnesses of fact, professionals can be asked to give evidence as experts. For instance, health professionals can be asked to assist an inquiry by providing a professional clinical assessment, such as:

- providing a diagnosis
- explaining the processes of illness
- explaining the likely effects of a particular injury
- explaining the process of rehabilitation.

When standards of professional practice are considered in administrative inquiry settings, senior and experienced members of the profession can be asked about the acceptable standards of practice that apply in particular practice settings, and also whether an individual's conduct represented a significant departure from acceptable standards.

It is well accepted legal principle that if you are giving expert opinion evidence, then you have a recognised area of expertise, and you can demonstrate your training and experience in that area of expertise. If you are asked to comment on any matter, first consider whether your expertise is well suited to the role you have been asked to fulfil. Your body of knowledge needs to be sufficiently sound and reliable, and you need to be suitably qualified in that field (Kumar, Odgers & Peden, 2012, p. 294). Your opinion as an expert can then be given on a mixture of observed facts and opinion, such as in observing and describing a wound and giving your opinion about what likely caused such an injury—but remember that the ultimate fact-finding is up to the tribunal if facts are in dispute.

To be qualified as an expert witness, this expertise is then placed on 'the record', with information about your expertise read onto the court record or transcript. You can expect to be asked preliminary questions about your background, training, study and experience, as this is what qualifies you to offer an opinion.

The decision makers will only be able to safely rely on your opinion if it is wholly or substantially based on your expertise, and you can demonstrate how you have formed your opinion, given the known facts or assumptions you are making.

A case excerpt that explains this is a case from the High Court of Australia: *Dasreef v Hawchar*. The personal injury case had examined, with the help of expert evidence, whether the plaintiff's employer could reasonably foresee that an employee exposed to silica dust could suffer a silica-related injury; what procedures an employer have taken to materially reduce the risk of injury; and, if those steps had been carried out, whether Mr Hawchar's risk of injury would have been minimised (*Dasreef v Hawchar* [2011], at paragraph 12).

The lower court's use of the expert's evidence was subsequently contested in the High Court. As it is the highest court in our nation, the High Court provides important precedent and guidance for all lower courts and administrative inquiry settings in Australian jurisdictions.

The High Court restated the *Evidence Act 1995* (NSW) provision at paragraphs 30–40:

> Section 79(1) of the Evidence Act must be understood in its statutory context. Section 76(1) of the Evidence Act provides that "[e]vidence of an opinion is not admissible to prove the existence of a fact about the existence of which the opinion was expressed". That exclusionary rule is referred to in the Evidence Act as "the opinion rule". Subsequent provisions of the Evidence Act provide a number of exceptions to the opinion rule. Section 79(1) provides that:
>
>> If a person has specialised knowledge based on the person's training, study or experience, the opinion rule does not apply to evidence of an opinion of that person that is wholly or substantially based on that knowledge.

The decision and reasons explained how this is applied, as set out by their Honours French CJ, Gummow J, Hayne J, Crennan J, Kiefel J and Bell J, from paragraph 34:

> ... it may greatly be doubted that Dr Basden sought to express an opinion about the numerical or quantitative level of respirable silica to which Mr Hawchar had been exposed. On the voir dire he denied that this was what he was trying to do. Read as a whole, Dr Basden's written report is better understood as offering an opinion

about what measures could have been taken to prevent Mr Hawchar contracting silicosis if he was exposed to respirable silica at levels as much as 1000 times greater than permissible levels. And in Dr Basden's evidence on the voir dire, that was what he said he was doing. But as also explained earlier in these reasons, that was not how the primary judge or the Court of Appeal used Dr Basden's evidence. Both the primary judge and the Court of Appeal took his evidence as expressing an opinion about the numerical or quantitative level of exposure encountered by Mr Hawchar. That is, his evidence was taken as expressing an opinion that could found the calculations made by the primary judge of the time weighted average level of respirable silica to which Mr Hawchar had been exposed. If that opinion was expressed, was it an opinion based on specialised knowledge Dr Basden had that was based on his training, study or experience?

In order for Dr Basden to proffer an admissible opinion about the numerical or quantitative level of Mr Hawchar's exposure to silica dust it would have been necessary for the party tendering his evidence to demonstrate first that Dr Basden had specialised knowledge based on his training, study or experience that permitted him to measure or estimate the amount of respirable silica to which a worker undertaking the relevant work would be exposed in the conditions in which the worker was undertaking the work. Secondly, it would have been necessary for the party tendering the evidence to demonstrate that the opinion which Dr Basden expressed about Mr Hawchar's exposure was wholly or substantially based on that knowledge.

In this case, demonstration of those matters could come only from evidence given by Dr Basden. That is why, in *HG v The Queen*, Gleeson CJ pointed out that, '[b]y directing attention to whether an opinion is wholly or substantially based on specialised knowledge based on training, study or experience, [s 79] requires that the opinion is presented in a form which makes it possible to answer that question'. (*HG v The Queen* (1999) 197 CLR 414 at 427 [39]; [1999] HCA 2.)

It should be unnecessary, but it is nonetheless important, to emphasise that what was said by Gleeson CJ in *HG* (and later by Heydon JA in the Court of Appeal in *Makita (Australia) Pty Ltd v Sprowles* (2001) 52 NSWLR 705 at 743–744 [85]) is to be read with one basic proposition at the forefront of consideration. The admissibility of opinion evidence is to be determined by application of the requirements of the Evidence Act rather than by any attempt to parse and analyse particular statements in decided cases divorced from the context in which those statements were made. Accepting that to be so, it remains useful to record that it is ordinarily the case, as Heydon JA said in *Makita*, that 'the expert's evidence must explain how the field of 'specialised knowledge' in which the witness is expert by reason of 'training, study or experience', and on which the opinion is 'wholly or substantially based', applies to the facts assumed or observed so as to produce the opinion propounded'. The way in which s 79(1) is drafted necessarily makes the description of these requirements very long. But that is not to say that the requirements cannot be met in many, perhaps most, cases very quickly and easily. That a specialist medical practitioner expressing a diagnostic opinion in his or her relevant field of specialisation is applying 'specialised knowledge' based on his or her 'training, study or experience', being an opinion 'wholly or substantially based' on that 'specialised knowledge', will require little explicit articulation or amplification once the witness has described his or her qualifications and experience, and has identified the subject matter about which the opinion is proffered.

But that was not this case.

Dr Basden gave evidence of his training, study and experience. He did not give evidence asserting that his training, his study or his experience permitted him to provide anything more than what he called a 'ballpark' figure estimating the amount of respirable silica dust to which a worker using an angle grinder would be exposed if that worker was using it in the manner depicted in the photograph of Mr Hawchar or in a video recording Dr Basden was shown. Indeed, in his written report, Dr Basden had pointed out that he had seen the use of an angle grinder in this way only once before. And he gave no evidence that he had then, or on any other occasion, measured directly, or sought to calculate inferentially, the amount of respirable dust to which such an operator was or would be exposed.

There was, in these circumstances, no footing on which the primary judge could conclude that a numerical or quantitative opinion expressed by Dr Basden was wholly or substantially based on specialised knowledge based on training, study or experience.

And at [42]:

A failure to demonstrate that an opinion expressed by a witness is based on the witness's specialised knowledge based on training, study or experience is a matter that goes to the admissibility of the evidence, not its weight. To observe, as the Court of Appeal did, that what Dr Basden said about the volume of respirable dust to which Mr Hawchar was exposed over time was 'an estimate' that was 'contestable and inexact' no doubt did direct attention to its worth and its weight. But more importantly, it directed attention to what exactly Dr Basden was saying in his evidence and to whether any numerical or quantitative assessment he proffered was admissible. And if, as the Court of Appeal observed ([2010] NSWCA 154 at [44].), his opinion on that matter lacked reasoning, the absence of reasoning pointed (in this case, inexorably) to the lack of any sufficient connection between a numerical or quantitative assessment or estimate and relevant specialised knowledge.

This means you should be careful that, if you agree to apply your knowledge and skill in that area of expertise to a set of agreed or assumed facts, and provide the formal inquiry panel with your opinion, to:

- stay within your area of recognised expertise as you offer your opinion
- base your opinion on clearly stated observed or assumed facts
- explain clearly how your opinion relies on your expert reasoning process.

If you are asked to provide evidence as an expert, as well as being 'sworn in' and taking an oath or affirmation, you will additionally be asked to formally agree to be bound by the Expert witness code of conduct.

These codes are now similar in all jurisdictions, given the harmonised national code for expert witnesses that was approved by the Council of Chief Justices in 2016. As set out in the Expert witness code of conduct—for instance, in the updated version of Schedule 7 of the *Uniform Civil Procedure Rules 2005* (NSW), and the *Supreme Court (Chapter 1 Expert Witness Code Amendment) Rules 2016* (Vic):

> An expert witness is not an advocate for a party and has a paramount duty, overriding any duty to the party to the proceedings or other person retaining the expert witness, to assist the court impartially on matters relevant to the area of expertise of the witness.

An expert may prepare a report, and prepares to be questioned further on the report during the hearing. The overriding duty is to the court, and each expert is to remain mindful of the strength and limitations of their report and evidence, and is able to make this active reflection on limitations available to the decision makers.

The code of conduct sets out the requirements for the Content at Schedule 7 of the *Uniform Civil Procedure Rules 2005* (NSW) secton 3:

> Every report prepared by an expert witness for use in court must clearly state the opinion or opinions of the expert and must state, specify or provide:
>
> (a) the name and address of the expert, and
>
> (b) an acknowledgement that the expert has read this code and agrees to be bound by it, and
>
> (c) the qualifications of the expert to prepare the report, and
>
> (d) the assumptions and material facts on which each opinion expressed in the report is based (a letter of instructions may be annexed), and
>
> (e) the reasons for and any literature or other materials utilised in support of each such opinion, and
>
> (f) (if applicable) that a particular question, issue or matter falls outside the expert's field of expertise, and
>
> (g) any examinations, tests or other investigations on which the expert has relied, identifying the person who carried them out and that person's qualifications, and
>
> (h) the extent to which any opinion which the expert has expressed involves the acceptance of another person's opinion, the identification of that other person and the opinion expressed by that other person, and
>
> (i) a declaration that the expert has made all the inquiries which the expert believes are desirable and appropriate (save for any matters identified explicitly in the report), and that no matters of significance which the expert regards as relevant have, to the knowledge of the expert, been withheld from the court, and
>
> (j) any qualification of an opinion expressed in the report without which the report is or may be incomplete or inaccurate, and
>
> (k) whether any opinion expressed in the report is not a concluded opinion because of insufficient research or insufficient data or for any other reason, and
>
> (l) where the report is lengthy or complex, a brief summary of the report at the beginning of the report.

Panel formats can be used in some court proceedings. Experts can confer and then are questioned together by legal representatives from both sides in a dispute, giving concurrent evidence. They can give their own opinion and also explain what they agree on and how their considered opinions differ, and give an opinion on the other expert's view. The Australian Law Reform Commission (ALRC) has encouraged the use of expert panels if two or more experts in the same field are to be called for evidence to be adduced (2000, Recommendation 67, p. 40), noting a supportive submission from the Federal Court:

> It has been the judges' experience that having both parties' experts present their views at the same time is very valuable. In contrast to the conventional approach, where an interval of up to several weeks may separate the experts' testimony, the panel approach enables the judge to compare and consider the competing opinions on a fair basis. In addition, the Court has found that experts themselves approve of the procedures and they welcome it as a better way of informing the Court. There is also symbolic and practical importance in removing the experts from their position in the camp of the party who called them.
>
> *(Australian Law Reform Commission, 2000, 6.117, p. 457)*

A change in the Federal Court Rules subsequently allowed the calling of the witnesses together, with the aim of reducing partisan and confrontational hearing processes, increasing court efficiency and facilitating greater accessibility of the decision maker to precise and accurate expert evidence, for appropriate cases. (See the Concurrent expert evidence practice Notes (GPN–EXPT), which are the guidelines for how expert evidence is given in the Federal Court.) Australian courts are leaders in this innovative practice (Rares, 2013).

Administrative tribunals have also supported concurrent evidence in practice, so that large volumes of detailed and technical expert evidence can be understood, and experts can be questioned in a timely, efficient and effective way.

Impairment and public safety

As part of standards maintenance and improvement, professional councils are involved in proactive education, increased peer discussion forums for information exchange, monitoring of performance, and support for higher risk practitioners, such as practitioners with an **impairment**. Health programs are offered by some professional councils to support impaired practitioners when they remain in practice. The programs necessarily include an element of periodic assessment, monitoring and treatment being provided as needed for the practitioner, and practice limits may be applied, so that the risk to the public is minimised. Such safeguards may be needed at any time in a professional's career, for reasons of physical or psychological impairment. They rely to a great extent on the insight of the practitioner that further help is needed, should a change in their condition or a crisis occur, and the practitioner's willingness to practise within safe limits.

impairment
Condition detrimentally impacting on competencies or capacity.

Under the National Law, section 5, impairment is defined as the 'physical or mental impairment, disability, condition or disorder (including substance abuse or dependence), that detrimentally affects or is likely to detrimentally affect' a registered health practitioner's capacity to safely practise the profession or a student's capacity to undertake clinical training.

If a health practitioner or student has a health impairment, conditions may be imposed on their registration to ensure safe practise limits are in place. AHPRA and the national boards and health councils work together so that drug and alcohol screening standards and policies are regularly reviewed—see, for instance, the Drummer (2014) review. Then best-practice drug and alcohol screening protocols and health monitoring standards are implemented to maintain safe standards for the protection of the public. Drug and alcohol testing can involve a combination of breathalyser, a urine screen, and hair sample testing, then implemented in accordance with screening protocols.

There may be an additional challenge in applying these conditions to students or professionals in periods of rapid learning and the application of new skills. Students are in a process of rapid skill acquisition rather than skill maintenance and routine professional development learning. The challenge is to support the individual practitioner or worker or student, and anticipate and manage periods of heightened risk, so that patients remain safe at all times. For all professionals, effective and alert mentors and supervisors are vital, and they can fill a special protective role for a potentially impaired professional and the public.

Care for self is also a routine professional responsibility: you should endeavour to stay safe and well, to pay attention to your health needs just like any member of the community, and to preserve your physical and cognitive fitness to practise, so that the public are protected each time you turn up for work.

CASE EXAMPLE

Clock on

Remember Nic who was pushed for time and is waiting for your quick summary of what you have learnt? Here is more about what Nic has been up to lately. Nic is an assistant in nursing, and he is also studying nursing. He is rostered on the Monday evening shift. Nic has been at university during the day, and will be again tomorrow. Oh, and Nic went out on the weekend and had a great time—but little sleep.

1   If Nic is already tired at the start of the shift, is he close to or beyond sensible or prudent personal physical and cognitive limits? What is threatened by breaching this limit?

2   Does your estimate vary if you consider 'safe' or 'optimal' work capacity?
    This exercise will lead you back to a consideration of skill and limits, duties and goals.

3   Draw up a new weekly schedule for work, uni, study and fun for Nic, including the weekends, perhaps with a 'pumpkin hour' or curfew to be home by. Draft a friendly

note listing some of the advantages of complying with the schedule. You could check sleep hygiene with a standard such as is used in mental health units. Then decide what your brief summary will be for Nic.

A person's current capacity is essential in carrying out expected responsibilities. The environment also needs to be conducive to safe and effective practice for your professional responsibilities to be met.

Now consider if your concern is further heightened if you have a reasonable belief that Nic has developed a 'habit' of using recreational drugs, which is possibly affecting his time at work or clinical uni placements.

4   What help is available? Look at a health board or council website, as well as a local health service and private health services to gather your ideas.

5   What mandatory notification and voluntary notification provisions apply? You may like to look at the guidelines accessible from the AHPRA website: Australian Health Practitioner Regulation Agency (2014). *National Board guidelines for registered health practitioners, Mandatory notifications guidelines, March 2014*. Retrieved from <http://ahpra.gov.au>.

6   Can you identify a supervisor or mentor who you could or should speak with to clarify your obligations? What notification provisions apply to training institutions?

Summary

You have learnt that integrated standards support the safe and systematic building of your knowledge and competencies throughout your training, and that standards derived from law, ethics and regulation will continue to guide your conduct when you offer your skills and training in health care work. You appreciate that this regulated system helps to define safe and acceptable standards of individuals who work in their chosen field as health carers, and to define the governance and safety of health care settings, and the quality and acceptability of the services provided. You now know that an ongoing appraisal of individual conduct extends far beyond your student years, and will be a feature of your professional life.

Looking back to integrated questions such as 'Why do I need to do CPD?' and 'Why is there so much paperwork to do when starting a new job?', you can revisit practical aspects of upholding standards and accountability. You will now appreciate the way society and each profession combine efforts to provide standards and mechanisms for addressing any departures from acceptable standards. An individual acting with integrity and striving for best practice standards is an essential part of the professional delivery of lawful and ethical health care delivery.

STUDY QUESTIONS

1   What is the significance of a professional's skill and limits in providing a professional opinion?
2   Why is reflection on skill and limits important for every person working in the health sector?
3   Describe (and reference) the legal, regulatory and ethics mechanism for encouraging safety and quality in practice.
4   Having read the example of orders made after a professional misconduct finding, explain how the orders safeguard the public from similar problematic conduct.
5   Using two practical examples, explain the professional importance of reflection on standards.

SAMPLE ESSAY QUESTIONS

1   Identify the types of standards provided in a professional code of conduct or code of ethics. Describe the way the code was developed and the force of the rules or standards in it for the health profession.
2   Outline four examples of how the health care system is ready to identify mistakes and problems to better safeguard the public.
3   Research a contemporary safety and quality initiative at federal government level, and comment on why it is being undertaken, what it may achieve, and what progress has been made under the initiative so far.

REFERENCES

Australian Commission on Safety and Quality in Health Care (ACSQHS). (2012, 2017). *National Safety and Quality Health Service Standards* (1st edn 2012; 2nd edn 2017). Sydney: Australian Government. Available at http://safetyandquality.gov.au

Australian Commission on Safety and Quality in Health Care (ACSQHS). *Clinical Care Standards*, updated as necessary. Retrieved from http://safetyandquality.gov.au

Australian Commission on Safety and Quality in Health Care (ACSQHS). *National Standards for Mental Health Services*. Retrieved from http://safetyandquality.gov.au

Australian Health Practitioner Regulation Agency (AHPRA). (2014). *National Board guidelines for registered health practitioners: Mandatory notifications guidelines*, March 2014. Retrieved from http://ahpra.gov.au

Australian Health Practitioner Regulation Agency (AHPRA). (2018). *What complaints or concerns can AHPRA consider?* Retrieved from http://ahpra.gov.au

Australian Human Rights Commission [AHRC]. (2011). *Social Justice Report*. Sydney: Australian Government. Retrieved from http://humanrights.gov.au

Australian Law Reform Commission (ALRC). (2000). *Managing justice: A review of the Federal Civil Justice System*. ALRC Report No. 89. Sydney: Australian Government.

Australian Law Reform Commission (ALRC). (2017). *Consultation*. Retrieved from www.alrc.gov.au

Barker, S.F. (1992). What is a profession? *Professional Ethics: A Multidisciplinary Journal*, 1(1–2), 73–99.

Bastian, D. (2018). Royal Commission into aged care sector: nurses react. *Nursing Review*, 17 September 2018. Retrieved from www.nursingreview.com.au

Beauchamp, T.L. & Childress, J.F. (2001). *Principles of biomedical ethics* (5th edn). New York: Oxford University Press.

Berglund, C.A., Mitchell, K., & Cox. K. (1993). *Exploring clinical ethics* (2nd edn). Distance module in a Masters of Clinical Education program. Sydney: University of New South Wales.

Dal Pont, G. (2014). When the personal becomes professional: Personal misbehavior is hardly immune from professional disciplinary consequences. *Ethics*, July. Retrieved from http://lawsocietywa.asn.au

De Grazia, D. (1992). Moving forward in bioethical theory: Theories, cases, and specified principlism. *Journal of Medicine and Philosophy, 17*, 511–39.

District of Columbia Department of Health. (2016). *Standard Operating Procedure Development 200.100* (Rev. edn August). Retrieved from http://dohc.dc.gov

Drummer, O. (2014). Professor Olaf Drummer, *Testing for impairing substances in health care professionals*. Australian Health Practitioner Regulation Agency and Victorian Institute of Forensic Medicine.

Frankland, R., Bamblett, M., Lewis, P., & Trotter, R. (2010). *This is 'forever business': A framework for maintaining and restoring cultural safety in Aboriginal Victoria*. Melbourne: Victorian Aboriginal Child Care Agency.

Goldstone, J. (1998). The role of quality assurance versus continuous quality improvement. *Journal of Vascular Surgery, 8*(2), 378–80.

Health Complaints Commissioner. (2017). *2017 Annual report: Supporting safe and ethical healthcare*. Melbourne: Victorian Government. Retrieved from http://hcc.vic.gov.au

Kumar, M., Odgers, S., & Peden, E. (2012). *Uniform evidence law* (4th edn). Pyrmont, Thomson Reuters (Professional) Australia Ltd / Lawbook Co.

Medical Board of Australia. (2014). *Good medical practice: a code of conduct for doctors in Australia*. March 2014. Retrieved from http://medicalboard.gov.au

Medical Board of Australia. (2018). *Registration*. Retrieved from http://medicalboard.gov.au

Mill, J.S. (1975). On Liberty. In *Three essays* (pp. 92–114). London: Oxford University Press.

Nakajima, H. (1996) *Health, ethics and human rights. World Health, 5*, September–October, 3.

New South Wales Government, Ministry of Health. (2018 and as updated). *Clinical programs: Incident management system*. Retrieved from http://ehealth.nsw.gov.au

Nursing and Midwifery Board of Australia. *Approved programs of study*. Retrieved from http://nursingmidwiferyboard.gov.au

Nursing and Midwifery Board of Australia. (2016a). *Standards for practice: Enrolled nurses*. Retrieved from http://nursingandmidwiferyboard.gov.au

Nursing and Midwifery Board of Australia. (2016b). *Safety and quality guidelines for nurse practitioners*. Retrieved from http://nursingandmidwiferyboard.gov.au

Nursing and Midwifery Board of Australia. (2016c). *Registration standard: Endorsement as a nurse practitioner.* Retrieved from http://nursingandmidwiferyboard.gov.au

Nursing and Midwifery Board of Australia. (2018a). *National competency standards for the midwife.* Retrieved from http://nursingandmidwiferyboard.gov.au

Nursing and Midwifery Board of Australia. (2018b). *Code of conduct for nurses.* Retrieved from http://nursingandmidwiferyboard.gov.au

Nursing and Midwifery Board of Australia. (2018c). *Code of conduct for midwives.* Retrieved from http://nursingandmidwiferyboard.gov.au

Occupational Therapy Australia. (2014). *Code of ethics.* Retrieved from http://otaus.com.au

Office of the Health Ombudsman. (2017). *Quarterly performance report: Quarter four 2016–17.* Brisbane: Queensland Government.

Peel, P. (1999). Community participation in decision-making and service delivery. *Canberra Bulletin of Public Administration, 94*, 34–51.

Rares, S. (2013). Using the 'hot tub': How concurrent evidence aids understanding issues. *Judges Speeches.* Canberra: Federal Court of Australia. Retrieved from http://fedcourt.gov.au

Safe Work Australia (2018). *Safe Work Australia guide for preventing and responding to workplace bullying.* Canberra: Australian Government. Retrieved from http://fairwork.gov.au

Schneider, G.W., & Snell, L. (2000). C.A.R.E.: An approach for teaching ethics in medicine. *Social Science & Medicine, 51*(10), 2000, 1563–7.

Sullivan, R.J. (1989). *Immanuel Kant's moral theory.* Cambridge: Cambridge University Press.

Therapeutic Goods Administration. (2016). *Safety monitoring and reporting in clinical trials involving therapeutic goods.* Department of Health, Canberra: Australian Government. Retrieved from http://nhmrc.gov.au

Victorian Aboriginal Child Care Agency [VACCA]. (2010). *Making your organisation culturally safe.* Melbourne: VACCA. 2010. Retrieved from www.vacca.org

Williams R. (1999). Cultural safety: What does it mean for our work practice? *Australian and New Zealand Journal of Public Health, 23*(2), 213, 213.

Zwart, H. (1993) Rationing in the Netherlands: The liberal and communitarian perspective. *Health Care Analysis, 1*, 53–6.

LEGISLATION

Evidence Act 1995 (NSW)

Health Practitioner Regulation National Law No 86 (NSW)

Health Practitioner Regulation National Law Act 2009 (Qld)

Supreme Court (Chapter 1 Expert Witness Code Amendment) Rules 2016 (Vic)

Uniform Civil Procedure Rules 2005 (NSW)

CASES

Allinson v General Council of Medical Education and Registration [1894] 1 QB 755.

Briginshaw v Briginshaw [1938] HCA 34.

Council of the Law Society of New South Wales v Foreman (1994) 34 NSWLR 408.

Dasreef v Hawchar [2011] HCA 21.

Ex Parte Tziniolis [1967] 1 NSWLR 357.

HCCC v Do [2014] NSWCA 307.

HG v The Queen (1999) 197 CLR 414; [1999] HCA 2.

Loosely v Powell [2018] NZCA 3.

Makita (Australia) Pty Ltd v Sprowles (2001) 52 NSWLR 705.

Nursing and Midwifery Board of Australia, File No. VR:130/2017. Retrieved from http://ahpra.gov.au and
     http://nursingmidwiferyboard.gov.au and http://decisions.justice.wa.gov.au

Qidwai v Brown [1984] 1 NSWLR 100.

R v Byrnes [1995] HCA 1.

Ziems v The Prothonotary of the Supreme Court of New South Wales (1957) 97 CLR 279, [1957] HCA 46.

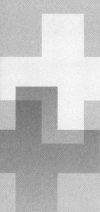

CHAPTER 3

How the law shapes health care

LEARNING OBJECTIVES

- To understand how the community relies on law to achieve peace and order in society.
- To appreciate some of the legal responsibilities of health care professionals in the delivery of services.
- To be able to recognise different aspects of law that are relied upon to identify standards and limits for conduct in health settings.

KEY TERMS

accountability	fiduciary duties
administrative law	judiciary
common law	prima facie
contract law	tort law
criminal law	utilitarianism

CASE EXAMPLE

A brand new society

Imagine this scenario. A new state has just been formed on an island, and new laws are to be drafted. The leaders ask the people for suggestions on guiding principles for the laws. One suggestion is for strict control. Another suggestion is for absolute freedom for all individuals who live there.

New laws need to be drafted to support these suggestions.

1   Work on a consultancy brief to advise on a preferable solution for the health care sector, taking into account the types of laws that will be needed.
2   Gather your ideas as you work through this chapter.

A system of reasonable limits in a community

Law is developed and applied within a community context. To refresh your memory, here are some of the key ethics terms you read about in earlier chapters. You can find definitions for them in the glossary.

assault	rules
battery	duties
jurisdiction	fit and proper person
legislation	mandatory notification
human rights	unsatisfactory professional conduct
false imprisonment	professional misconduct

When you keep reading, remember that you will be learning about other law terms, so this is just your starting list.

Legislative instruments

Elected representatives listen to their constituents and then sit in parliament with other elected representatives to debate proposed bills and amendments to existing legislative instruments—so creating the legislative structure on behalf of the community. The members of parliament consider statutes or 'Acts', and subordinate legislation (or regulation) that provides the administrative backing to statute law already passed, are all tabled for parliament's approval.

This legislative structure applies to many activities, including health care. For instance, laws support the use of land for public hospital and community health facilities, and laws support the building of facilities to appropriate standards. Public funding for some aspects of health care flows from taxation provisions in legislation. Further legislation and regulation supports the appropriate staffing and equipment of the health care facilities. Consultations and services—including choices of procedures, medications and therapeutic devices—are delivered by trained professional and support staff, because those activities are supported and regulated by legislative instruments. Education and training of health care workers and research and development of health care processes are also facilitated and supported by legislation. Safe workplaces are supported by laws, and statutes or criminal codes define conduct that would be criminal or otherwise unacceptable—including in health care settings.

REFLECTION: DEBATING LEGISLATIVE INSTRUMENTS

1 Recap what you learnt in Chapter 1 about statute law. Then have a look at a parliament website and share with your colleagues what you find out about how bills are debated in one jurisdiction. Relevant websites include:

- www.aph.gov.au
- www.parliament.act.gov.au
- www.parliament.nsw.gov.au
- www.parliament.qld.gov.au
- www.parliament.nt.gov.au

- www.parliament.sa.gov.au
- www.parliament.tas.gov.au
- www.parliament.vic.gov.au
- www.parliament.wa.gov.au.

2 Look on the website you have selected to see where you can read draft bills, and the research and discussion papers that have informed the debate about the wording of Acts.

3 Note your initial reaction to the forums for debating bills (draft laws) and explain the importance of those forums in your own words.

INTEGRATED LEARNING AND PRACTICE

How are community concerns translated into action in laws and regulations?

Laws that affect health care and health services constantly change.

After Parliaments pass laws, another part of the government (the Executive) shapes and implements the practical administrative aspects of the laws as part of running the state and regulating dealings by institutions or between its people. This includes formulating policy for efficient administration and checking on the safe and effective health care service delivery by institutions and individuals working in health care.

With a renewed public emphasis on privacy, recent amendments to the *Privacy Act 1988* (Cth), in the *Privacy Amendment (Notifiable Data Breaches) Act 2017* (Cth), established the Notifiable Data Breaches (NDB) scheme in Australia. From 22 February 2018, certain data breaches must be self-reported by agencies and organisations that have existing personal information security obligations under the Act. The mandatory data breach notification requirements are explained in supporting documents issued by the Office of the Australian Information Commissioner (OAIC) (2018).

With increasing concern about the treatment of people in vulnerable circumstances, such as people with disability and the elderly, who depend on others for their basic care needs, certain reporting frameworks about alleged abuse are being strengthened. The National Disability Insurance Scheme provides funds for people with disability. The providers of services are required to comply with a Quality and Safeguarding Framework, to be overseen by a Commission established in 2018, and given authority through the passing of the *National Disability Insurance Scheme Amendment (Quality and Safeguards Commission and Other Measures) Bill 2017* (Cth) by the Australian Parliament on 4 December 2017. The regulatory scheme was anticipated to be in place in all jurisdictions by 2020.

These are just two examples of initiatives in law or law reform and the corresponding regulations that have recently come into effect, which further support the recognition of the integrity of each person. The *Privacy Act* focuses on the integrity of a person in controlling access to their personal information. The National Disability Bill focuses on human rights and safeguards against abuse of people who are in vulnerable situations.

REFLECTION POINT

Dynamic evolution of laws and regulations

1 Select either the *Privacy Act* or the National Disability Bill, as outlined earlier. Read about the detailed provisions, including any schedules.

2 Describe in your own words what aspect of service delivery the scheme is addressing, and how the provisions work together to achieve the objective or purpose.

Case law

A separate and independent court system is in place to interpret the legislation and regulation peacefully and fairly. This system is called the **judiciary**, and it is involved in resolving disputes.

Abhorrent and unacceptable conduct by institutions or people can be dealt with by the state, to protect the state and its people. Criminal case law represents the application of criminal statute law to an alleged crime, which is conduct that is so reprehensible that it is deemed by society to be punishable by a criminal law penalty. The judge—or in some cases, judge and jury—decide if the facts as tested in court amount to a certain 'crime'. The judge then decides on an appropriate punishment, in accordance with expected punishments listed in the relevant statute. A criminal case will reflect the public's disapproval of the action carried out, and delivers punishment or penalty to the wrongdoer on behalf of the community.

judiciary
Court system set up to adjudicate and resolve disputes between the state and a person, or between two persons.

Potentially criminal conduct is prosecuted by the state, as the alleged conduct is 'crime against the state'. The person being prosecuted is then usually named as the defendant, and the proceedings are usually conducted in public. This is also why the names of criminal cases that you will see noted in law case citations are the 'state' or the 'crown'—in shorthand, *R* for *Regina*, v 'Person's name'. This is pronounced 'The Queen (or King) and Person's name'.

common law
Fair rules and principles set down in civil courts for the people to follow.

Common law or civil law is the body of determinations and reasoning from courts deciding private matters. The decisions stem from disputes between parties, and the decision captures the essence of what was in dispute and the judicial decision on why certain action or behaviour was acceptable or unacceptable in that context.

One person can bring an action—called 'a claim'—against another person who they say is responsible for harm that has occurred. A company or institution can also be a person, if it is a legal entity. When two persons are contesting an issue, they are named as the two parties to the matter.

In common law, the two parties to the dispute engage in an adversarial process, as each party puts forward their evidence and it is tested before the court. The common law case names reflect the names of the parties, and you will have seen that the case citations include these names. So, when you look up different cases, you will see '*Brown v Smith*', or '*Smith v Health Care Institution*', or even two corporate entities such as '*Company 1 v Company 2*'. The 'v' is spoken as 'and', so a case name is pronounced 'Brown and Smith'. Then the full reference to where the full decision or a report and summary of the case is available follows in a citation, which is like a journal article reference. Reading the headnote in a law report is like reading an article abstract. To understand a case you need to do more than just read the summary paragraph—you need to read a case fully to understand the reasoning behind the decision.

The information that the parties want the court to consider is potential evidence. Evidence should be relevant and admissible, and each party can object and prompt an assessment of admissibility and relevance, testing whether it should be part of the court's consideration in reaching a decision, within the rules of process to be followed in the court in which it is heard. Barristers are the legal advocates who are the experts in presenting and testing evidence before the court. Judges and magistrates conduct the proceedings, and make procedural rulings on evidence during the court hearing.

The contemporary community context always informs the interpretation of the law by the courts. The learned opinion of His Honour Justice Gleeson, the former Chief Justice of the High Court in *Singh v The Commonwealth* (2004) was that: 'Changing times, and new problems, may require the Court to explore the potential inherent in the meaning of the words, applying established techniques of legal interpretation.' (*Singh v The Commonwealth* (2004), at paragraph 18.)

The decisions that are made are available so that justice is open and transparent, and to deter persons in the community from causing similar harm or undue burden to others. Lawyers are experts in finding out what the current law is, and then advising institutions and people of their rights and responsibilities according to that law.

The decisions are made on the evidence, and to the required standard of proof, and both the decision and reasons are usually publicly available. The body of decisions and reasons from the courts is known as case law. If a court is deciding whether a wrong has been committed, and how to address it, it will apply legislation to see if the elements of conduct described in the statutes are proven. It will also be guided by decisions in other court cases involving similar principles, and it will prefer those decisions from a court higher in the court hierarchy in the same jurisdiction. This is to follow precedent (Bogaric, 2013, pp. 1141–50, citing *Broome v Cassell & Co Ltd* [1972], and *Fleming v White* [1981]). So, reading what courts have decided in the past will inform professionals about how their conduct would be viewed if they acted similarly. But remember that if legislation changes, the basic principles that are being applied to the reasoning can change. Also, case law is dynamic and develops over time as circumstances in society change. So, it is more helpful to read the most up-to-date cases from the highest court available. Reasons also refer to precedent that has remained unchanged, so you will find out by reading the whole published judgment and reasons which principles and precedents are still current.

INTEGRATED LEARNING AND PRACTICE

Does the law have a higher expectation of health care professionals?

Yes, the law does have a higher expectation of health care professionals. This is in keeping with the importance of maintaining high standards of ethics in all conduct that affects a client's interests.

The law provides essential guidance on the responsibilities that stem from the trust placed in a health care worker. For instance, the special relationship that a health care worker has established with a patient or client is relevant in both criminal and civil matters.

Ethics responsibilities define the special relationship of trust, and the law formally recognises trust as important because of the role it plays within society.

The trust placed in the relationship can give rise to certain **fiduciary duties**. Fiduciary powers are those given to one person to exercise for the benefit of another. A medical (or health) adviser and a patient have long been recognised as being in a relationship that gives rise to fiduciary duties, given the relationship of influence by the adviser (Finn, 2016, p. 92, citing *Mitchell v Homfray* (1881)). Once someone is designated a fiduciary, the reversal of the onus of proof can apply in some allegations of wrongdoing (Finn, 2016, p. 309). Fiduciary duties are the focus of legal comments, such as confidentiality of information (Breen, Cordner & Thomson, 2016, p. 166, citing *Breen v Williams* (1994)).

In common law matters, judges apply their discretion in considering issues such as:

- undue influence
- conduct that has been unconscionable (or unscrupulous)
- fiduciary duties towards individuals in a dependent position, given a relationship of influence that rises above the obligations.

fiduciary duties
Duties of good faith so that trust, confidence or influence over another person and their trust and confidence in the fiduciary relationship is not abused.

Judges then apply discretionary remedies. A sense that higher principles and expected standards of conduct should apply is available by appealing to equitable principles (Finn, 2016, pp. 2, 4). This means that well established principles of fairness in society are considered by judges, so the person in most power in a relationship is expected to behave honourably. Judges take these standards very seriously, and try to correct the disadvantage a person has been placed in if that trust or confidence is abused. Such settled principles in case law do not need to be set out in legislation, because they are so fundamental and accepted as reasonable standards in law.

Fiduciary duties could additionally be relevant in administrative forums, when departures from acceptable professional standards are considered by employing or contracting institutions and the health profession boards, or health councils and complaints ombudsman, or a complaints commission.

Trust is placed in a health care worker to act in the patient's interests, and not to use the relationship as an opportunity to benefit personally—particularly if it would be to the detriment of the patient. For instance, it would be a serious breach of duty for a health carer to profit from vulnerable and dependent clients—such as older persons in care—over whom a relationship of influence as a medical or health adviser had been established.

For example, a nurse received criminal convictions in a Local Court hearing, and in separate administrative tribunal proceedings she lost her registration and was prohibited from working in any health service for the time period that she remained deregistered. She was found to have accessed confidential information from hospital records, and then visited patients or their relatives at home to request substantial 'loans'. She also had not disclosed her criminal conviction on renewal of her registration. As part of the earlier court orders, she was also required to repay the loans, and an order was issued to take a portion of her wages so the debts were repaid over time (*HCCC v Belkadi* (No, 2) [2012]). Notice that the criminal, civil and administrative hearing systems were all involved in order to mark society's disapproval of the conduct and to protect the public from such activity in the future.

The language in considerations of equity is similar to the expectations expressed in ethics. Equity and ethics have a strong shared heritage. Both reasoning traditions owe much to the philosophers and jurisprudential scholars who debated how to understand obligations and balance individual rights in a collective society setting.

Individuals working in health care are legally responsible when they offer their services. When individuals decide to work in health care, they need to inform themselves of what they can legally do and what they should not do in the course of their work role. As you have already read in Chapter 2, the governance requirements and institutional safety and quality standard processes and protocols in institutions are informed by legal principles. They are a good time saver for the workforce to rely on as a practical legal briefing of requirements. A large organisation will have inductions and briefings for its staff on significant policy updates. Professional associations will likely make discussion papers and resources available. Active learning is always required, as the law and acceptable standards can change. This requires keeping up to date as protocols and procedures change, and attending professional development regularly so that you are aware of significant developments that are likely to affect the way you work. Professionals must ensure their registration and training is up to date. Individuals are only able to offer their services within the scope of their authority—or their conduct may be judged improper in the eyes of the law.

You can extrapolate from case law to work out the accepted standard for a similar situation tested in a court by comparing the circumstances, context and facts of the case and any new situation that arises. So, if you had a hypothetical situation, you could look up case law with similar facts and issues to see which decisions could help you to decide what you should or should not do.

Jurisdictions working together under Constitutional law

A society's government and structure is set out in its constitution—which lists principles that guide the development of more specific laws, rules and standards. In democracies, the constitution usually separates powers explicitly, such as between:

- the parliament—the elected representatives of the people
- the executive—the administrative arm of the government
- the judicature—the court system that adjudicates on disputes within society.

All three bodies play a role in a peaceful and stable society. Legislation, which is developed within parliament, has high status as the guiding set of rules that should be adhered to by citizens, and also as rules to be considered and applied by judges when they make their determinations. Constitutional law and the rule of law work together to create the practical legal framework for the society (see Burton Crawford & Goldworth, 2017).

As you read in Chapter 1 and Chapter 2, aspects of health are governed by federal law, because the powers derive from the Constitution, or the powers have been vested to federal level by the states. The provision of federally funded health services is supported by the Constitution (see section 51(xxiiiA)) in *Commonwealth of Australia Constitution Act 1900* (Cth) (the Constitution). The process of federal assistance in legislating or coordinating to achieve the *Health Practitioner Regulation National Law 2009* scheme, and thus uniformity in the common interest of all states and territories, was informed by the Constitution—which sets out the powers each level of government was able to exercise.

The highest court in Australia is the High Court of Australia. It considers matters of Constitutional law, and may consider appeals involving matters under federal laws from the lower Federal Courts, or matters involving Commonwealth officials, as well as appeals from decisions of the courts of the other states or territories. The court has independent judicial power, and is able to consider if the laws are inconsistent with the Constitution (Creyke & McMillan, 2012, p. 269).

Prohibited conduct that is a crime

Criminal law is shorthand for a jurisdiction's body of rules on prohibited conduct—and what penalties should be applied if it is proven that prohibited conduct has occurred. As a safeguard against misuse of that power, a person is presumed innocent. Neither police, nor prosecutors—on behalf of the state—can alone decide whether someone is guilty. The judiciary decides, in a process that is independent of government. This is to demonstrate the independence of government, executive and judiciary.

These principles of independence are set out in criminal law cases from time to time, such as in *The State of New South Wales v Gregory Wayne Kable* [2013], in which the High Court considered the legal principles of a previous detention order having been made, and special legislation that had been passed, to keep a person in detention when it was thought he may otherwise commit a violent crime. The principles of independence are expressed in the case and the lower level court hearings (such as *Kable v Director of Public Prosecutions* (1995), at page 378). The government makes the laws, the executive brings alleged perpetrators before the courts, and the courts then decide if a crime has occurred, and what the punishment under the **criminal law** should be.

criminal law
Jurisdiction's body of rules on prohibited conduct and omissions and penalties for proven prohibited conduct.

Given the decision on whether someone has been guilty of acting in a prohibited way is so serious—and the potential penalties imposed by society are so significant—the standard of proof of 'beyond reasonable doubt' is applied. This is to be 'certain' (Bogaric, 2013, p. 192, citing *Keeley v Brooking* (1979)). This is a higher standard of proof than in civil matters, in which a balance of probabilities applies. In some situations, a person may lose their freedom and liberty as a consequence of breaching the standards set out in criminal law, so the standard of proof is set at a level that the community considers is proportional to the possible consequences of the finding.

Historically, the 'beyond reasonable doubt' standard evolved when capital punishment and imprisonment were both available as penalties. It will be interesting to see in the future whether a distinct standard of proof for criminal matters is maintained for all 'criminal' matters, particularly when the penalty for lower-level criminal conduct is more like a civil penalty such as a fine, or a prohibition from being in certain locations. This could extend to not working in certain occupations or working within a limited scope of practice—such as only working with adults. Alternatively, the criminal finding could give protection at an administrative level—such as when an institution gives a prospective candidate or volunteer a Working with Children Check.

In jury trials, the panel of jurors decide if the alleged facts are proven. Some matters are heard by a magistrate or judge alone, and others by judges sitting together, who manage the court proceedings and then also decide what penalty, if any, is to be applied. At this stage, the crime a person has committed, its seriousness and the circumstances in which it was committed are considered, and the penalty provisions set out in the legislation are applied. In carrying out this task, a judge weighs up the jurisprudence principles of punishment, deterrence and rehabilitation, being acutely aware of the need to address and forestall further crime, and also being aware how central a person's liberty and freedom is within society.

A society's safety and security may be restored by removing a person from normal interactions within the community, or by applying strict community 'good behaviour bond' expectations which, if breached, will then result in further loss of freedoms within a community.

The considerations of 'harm' done, and potential limits to 'autonomy' are always considered in criminal justice debates. In Chapter 1 you read how Jeremy Bentham grappled with what would be a fair and just structure of societies' rules; today's judges grapple with how to fairly reflect a societies' expectations for fair behaviour between its citizens and also how to redress those wrongs when they occur.

When criminal charges are heard, the mental and physical elements of the alleged criminal conduct are considered by the court. The focus of the physical elements of a crime is on conduct, such as physical or factual evidence of action or inaction. Intention, recklessness, knowledge, or negligence are *mens rea* (or mental elements), and these can be proven by evidence or inferring from the physical element aspect of the conduct that has been proven. In some instances the mental element is sufficient for a crime to be committed—for instance, planning to commit murder, or acts of terrorism. The mental element isn't needed if the law deems an action or consequence to be a 'strict liability', either given the wording of the legislation or the subject matter of the offence.

The physical element of the crime of assault is to touch someone without permission to do so, or an action that causes an apprehension of immediate physical contact that amounts to physical violence. If a person is injured, then a separate crime of assault occasioning actual bodily harm may be committed. This means it is vital to gain permission before touching a person in a certain way.

In a health care context, gaining 'consent' to performing examinations or procedures should be—and is—part of routine practice. All health professionals and carers need to be mindful of the unacceptability of assuming that people can be touched unless they agree to the process that is being conducted in that touching. A recklessness in failing to seek proper consent can be sufficient to prove the mental element of assault on the part of the carer. For example, a gynaecologist was convicted of aggravated indecent assault after a court found he had operated on women and performed more extensive surgery on them than they had consented to (*Reeves v R*; *R v Reeves* [2013]).

Civil actions in tort can also be brought, given unwanted touching without consent, as in the treatment of a person with 'deep sleep therapy' at Chelmsford Private Hospital. The onus of proof that there was consent falls to the professional (*Hart v Herron and Anor* [1996]). The therapy prompted a Royal Commission, so that such practices could be avoided in the future (New South Wales Government, 1990). This fundamental importance of documented consent highlights the importance of adequate records, as you read in Chapter 1, and also of clearly informed decision-making processes. You will learn more about consent in Chapter 8.

Assault was defined early in Chapter 1 as an inclusive term to mean contact without agreement, or the fear of that contact. Battery is a term that is sometimes used for the physical contact aspect of assault.

There are exceptions for instances of emergency, to preserve life, when no informed consent can be obtained. The common law doctrine of necessity also applies for actions in tort (Madden & McIlwraith, 2013, p. 337, citing *Rogers v Whitaker* [1992]). (There is a summary of tort law later in this chapter.) Torts and crime are interrelated, as some breaches in tort are also crimes (Balkin & Davis, 2013, p. 6).

Usually in practice, if consent is given, the action lies in negligence (tort) not in assault and battery (Vout, 2016, p. 730, citing *Sidaway v Governors of Bethlehem Royal Hospital* [1985]). However, consent to use of force is not generally extended to be consent to any bodily harm (Bogaric, 2013, pp. 150–1). Health care is comparable to sporting contexts, in which there is routinely an agreement to be touched in certain ways that will 'injure' a person, but if the physical contact or force is outside the acceptable rules or standards of conduct, then the consent is not valid, and the contact can be interpreted as assault. Consent may be negated—for instance, for elective surgery—if the consented surgery is not performed by an appropriate specialist, or information on pain and scarring was not given (Vout, 2016, p. 730, citing *D v S* [1981]). This area of the law is torts, a private action.

An unfortunate part of health care is that patients can threaten the very people who are trying to help them. Patients can become aggressive towards other patients or staff, particularly in emergency departments and mental health units. Quite frequently, these people are cognitively incapacitated at that time, due to drugs or alcohol or their medical condition—they are unpredictable and not thinking or behaving rationally. When someone has diminished responsibility, they may be unable to form an intention to commit a crime, so the action may be viewed in a different light, at least in terms of individual responsibility for those actions. For instance, murder can be downgraded to a manslaughter charge in some jurisdictions if a defence of abnormality of mind is proven. This defence is available in Queensland, the Northern Territory, New South Wales and the Australian Capital Territory (Bogaric, 2013, p. 539).

Strategies to contain the threat of violence from patients are now routine. Professionals are trained in how to divert a threat by calming a person down. Security staff are available if needed if the threat escalates. You may agree to work in emergency, but you do not agree to be assaulted. The organisation has a duty to reasonably protect its staff and other patients from such incidents, and you and other staff will be trained to restrain a person if necessary so that they do not harm staff or other patients, with reasonable force consistent with self-defence principles—which would be objectively viewed as a reasonable response to the threat posed. A person trained to handle an aggressive situation is then judged by those skills—for instance, when gauging what is reasonable force for someone trained to handle such a situation. The use of excessive force is not supported for anyone relying on self-defence as a defence to otherwise criminal conduct, as set out in crimes Acts or criminal codes—for instance, see *Crimes Act 1900* (NSW), at sections 418–422. The circumstances of security being available to contain the threat would be important in judging whether a health carer needed to contain the threat themselves, or could rely on other more highly trained members of staff to perform that duty. Remember the principles of false imprisonment from Chapter 1—and take care to only use reasonable restriction.

You know from Chapter 1 that a crime does not become a crime under specific municipal law until there is legislation, and that this law then defines the punishment for the crime once it is proven.

It is now a criminal offence to represent that you are qualified in a registered health profession if you are not. This is set out in the *Health Practitioner Regulation National Law*. For instance, see sections 113–120 in *Health Practitioner Regulation National Law (Victoria) Act 2009* (Vic).

In a recent prosecution brought by AHPRA in the Local Court, a man was criminally convicted and fined $30,000—as well as having costs awarded against him—after he used a doctor's medical qualifications to falsely register and practise in Australia. He had worked in Australia, including in hospital roles, and a private company he later worked for queried why his UK registration details matched those of a different person. The AHPRA news report about the successful prosecution noted that the Council of Australian Governments (COAG) Health Council is considering increasing the possible penalties to include imprisonment (Medical Board of Australia, 2017). So, increased penalty provisions are likely. COAG made the following recommendation:

> Health Ministers discussed the adequacy of penalties under the National Law, in light of recent cases of individuals holding themselves out as health practitioners when they are not registered under the National Law.
>
> Health Ministers agreed that new multi-year custodial sentences and increased fines and additional prohibition powers are needed for offences committed by people who hold themselves out to be a registered health practitioner, including those who use reserved professional titles or carry out restricted practices when not registered. This important reform will be fast tracked to strengthen public protection under the National Law. Health Ministers urged all employers of registered health practitioners to ensure that identity verification procedures and other probity checks, are robust.
>
> *(COAG, 2017)*

There have been successful prosecutions of people who have maintained that they were registered after their registration had lapsed. If you look up the results of recent cases on the AHPRA website <http://ahpra.gov.au> under 'Court and Tribunal Decisions', you will see varied examples across a wide range of professions, such as:

- a person describing herself as a midwife when no longer registered
- a student falsely claiming to be a registered nurse
- an unqualified person describing himself as an optometrist.

It is important that you describe your skills and registration status accurately at all times.

Thinking more broadly to the world community, individual criminal responsibility has been increasingly emphasised in international law, and crimes against peace, war crimes and crimes against humanity—such as torture—can be prosecuted in international criminal justice courts. The International Criminal Court complements each member state's criminal jurisdiction, and may hear a case if a state fails to investigate or prosecute an alleged grave crime. Individuals acting either on their own behalf or in the name of a state may be pursued

INTEGRATED LEARNING AND PRACTICE

Development of regulations in response to criminal conduct

An extreme example of criminal conduct by a health professional is that of British GP Dr Shipman who was convicted in 2000 of murdering 15 patients and of forging a patient's will, even though he had denied all charges. He had earlier been obtaining and using illicit pethidine, which his former colleagues discovered in 1975, and he was dismissed from that group practice.

The GP subsequently had a long-term pattern of working alone from his new practice and making unannounced home visits. A local undertaker noticed that many of the GP's patients were dressed in their day clothes—which he found unusual, as people who feel ill normally lay in bed in pyjamas. The deceased patients were sometimes found sitting, fully dressed, in their lounge rooms. Then a different local GP expressed concern about the rate of death certificates she was being asked to countersign, prompting an initial police investigation, which was completed without specific conclusion. The possibly fraudulent inclusion of the GP's name as a beneficiary in a will prompted the eventual successful criminal investigation, and subsequent commission of inquiry (Smith, 2003). Audits of patient files and deaths of other patients led to calls for further charges (Ramsay, 2001, pp. 123–5).

The cover page of the Shipman Inquiry Report notes Mr Justice Forbes' remarks at the sentencing hearing on 31 January 2000: 'None of your victims realised that yours was not a healing touch. None of them knew that in truth you had brought her death, death which was disguised as the caring attention of a good doctor' (Smith, 2003).

The learning from the Shipman Inquiry was used to develop practical safeguards in death certification. Commentary from the UK focused on concern that the activities were not detected sooner, and restoring the public trust in the quality, appropriateness, and **accountability** of professional medical services, and why the existing safeguards such as death certification had failed to detect his criminal activity sooner (Horton, 2001; Baker, 2004). Opportunities for detection are highest when individual actions and judgments are accountable to others. This was emphasised by the Shipman Inquiry chairman, Dame Janet Smith, in her lengthy findings into the practice and death certification process. In the Inquiry, Dame Smith estimated that over 200 patients had been killed, and the inquiry recommended steps to improve accountability of individual professionals and the death certification process (Smith, 2003).

accountability
Process of being open to scrutiny for assessment of conduct of responsibilities.

and held responsible under public international law, following the principle that their international duties to fellow humankind transcend the national obligations of obedience imposed by their own state. This principle was established by the Nuremberg Tribunal, a joint international (Allied) post–World War II tribunal that considered atrocities committed during the Nazi regime in Germany and surrounding countries, with the stated approach that 'crimes against international law are committed by men, not by abstract entities'. The serious abuses of human rights that were seen in World War II in 'medical research' conducted on detained people were prosecuted in the Nuremberg Trials (Crawford, 2012, pp. 671–3). The lessons from this time have informed the development of research ethics safeguards, as you will read in the Chapter 7 'The limits of care'.

Integration of ethics in laws and regulation on medical or surgical termination

The issues of sexual activity, planning children, and pregnancy face most adults, testing ethical convictions in each decision that is made.

INTEGRATED LEARNING AND PRACTICE

Why is where someone lives so important to the type of services they can expect?

Laws define criminal conduct, which can have the effect of prohibiting certain services being offered in the particular jurisdiction in which the laws apply. Consistent with these laws, preventing or aborting pregnancies for medical, emotional or social reasons is heavily regulated.

Unless laws are debated and changed by the people and their elected representatives, certain prohibitions remain. The debates are often grounded in fundamental belief systems, and ethics reasoning and philosophical traditions feature in the discussions. The issues are not resolved easily. Similar debates have been taking place since early days of law and society, and can be expected to be continuing in the future.

Abortion and contraception laws in each country reflect cultural stances and beliefs on the ethics of reproductive choices and the development of personhood. In some cultures, such as in China, abortion has officially been viewed as one of the range of contraceptive methods available. This is partly based on the belief that a human being or person comes into being at birth, not before. The Chinese debate over abortion has traditionally been about the acceptability of late-term abortion rather than the acceptability of abortion itself (Qui, 1996).

The legal stance of each country and each state on difficult issues such as abortion may change from time to time. Also, key players on each side of the debate may alter their views. The *Roe v Wade* court case in the USA made history in the 1970s, when the case for the right to legal abortion was argued for and was won. The ruling essentially limited the power of the state to intervene or interfere to prevent abortion before the foetus was viable, on the grounds of liberty of personal privacy for the mother. In an article published in 1996, the woman whose right to an abortion was at issue in that case discusses her changed views on abortion (*Roe v Wade* (1973); *New York Times*, 1995). She reportedly said she became vehemently 'pro-life' (anti-abortion), in contrast to her former 'pro-choice' stance, and since the case she had campaigned outside abortion clinics to stop abortion. One of the things that reportedly made a difference was that she had become a fundamentalist Christian. This is an example of one of the features of ethical reflection. Over time, and given our understanding, convictions and experiences, we can change our minds.

REFLECTION: PERSONAL CHOICES AND INDIVIDUAL DIFFERENCES

The following scenario can be used to ponder the ethics choices raised by pregnancy. A couple has been trying to have a child for some time. The woman who is trying to conceive is in her early forties. At last, they conceive a child. Routine tests early in the pregnancy reveal a very high chance of both Down's syndrome and various disabilities in the child. The couple pursue further tests, which confirm that the child is likely to have severe disabilities. They now feel torn between their strong desire to have and raise this child, and the fear that they may inflict a life of pain and burden on the child by allowing it to progress to term and be born.

1   What would you think about first in this scenario?
2   Should Down's syndrome be thought of as a 'disability'? What are the other 'diminished capacities'? (Note: Some medically defined disabilities may not be considered disabilities in other contexts, and vice versa. The cultural context of such decisions can make a significant difference.)

In Northern Ireland, assisting in abortion has been traditionally criminalised, in contrast to more permissive laws in England, Scotland and Wales. In recent times, debate began in Ireland on relaxing abortion laws to allow access for more than exceptional cases—such as if the life of the mother is at risk. At the time, no change to the *Abortion Act 1967* (UK) had been made to allow further exceptions, despite a 2015 High Court ruling that not allowing such exceptions would be incompatible with human rights obligations. The Taoiseach (or Prime Minister) Leo Varadkar committed to a referendum in 2018, which promised to clarify whether the people supported a repeal of the ban on abortion (Mulraney, 2017). The debate was evident in the contemporary legal cases as well as media commentary and reports, so it was not surprising that parliament—as a voice of the people—was urged to grapple with the issue.

The earlier background to this debate is contained in a 2015 High Court judgment, in which Judge Horner opined at paragraph 4:

> Any issue involving abortion is always highly contentious. It inevitably raises philosophical, moral, social, religious, political and other matters that are extremely divisive. One of the foundations upon which the common law is built is the principle of the sanctity of life. As Lord Hoffmann said in *Airedale NHS Trust v Bland* [1993] AC 789 at paragraph [30] this "entails its inviolability by an intruder". One of the other foundations of the common law is the principle of personal autonomy, the right of self-determination. Those in favour of abortion in the exceptional circumstances put forward before the Court rely on personal

autonomy. Those against abortion call in aid the sanctity of life. One of the tasks of this Court is to place these principles in their proper context. As Lord Steyn said in the judgment he delivered in *R (Pretty) v Director of Public Prosecutions* [2002] 1 AC 800 at [54] which related to assisted suicide:

> It is of great importance to note that these are ancient questions in which millions in the past have taken diametrically opposite views and still do.

The same sentiments apply with equal force to the issue of abortion (*The Northern Ireland Human Rights Commission's Application* [2015]).

Northern Ireland's existing laws had only permitted abortion in circumstances where the mother's life was at risk, including from suicide, and travel to another jurisdiction was permitted. The legislative ban that had been set by authorities, which were considered better able to judge the 'requirements of morals of their country', was applied in a 2011 case, even though the importance of autonomy and the sphere of private life decisions was acknowledged. The failure to allow for exceptions to the abortion laws for exceptional cases is what was found to be incompatible with human rights conventions in the 2015 case. The case was not considered by the judge to be on a general right to abortion. The judge considered when interference in a private domain is justified. As at paragraph 145:

> An interference having been established under Article 8(1), that is the interference with the personal autonomy of women who are pregnant with SMFs, FFAs or as a result of sexual crime, then the interference has to be justified by the Government. According to Strasbourg jurisprudence (eg see *S and Marper v UK* [2009] 48 EHRR 50), such justification rests on three separate strands. The interference must be:
> a) In accordance with the law.
> b) For a legitimate aim.
> c) Necessary in a democratic society.

Judge Horner found it was not a legitimate aim to keep a prohibition in place, and it was disproportionate to pursue such state interference, 'if a foetus had a fatal abnormality', or if a viable foetus had been 'conceived as a result of a sexual crime'. In those circumstances, the judge found no pressing need for social interference—meaning the restrictive laws—was found (*The Northern Ireland Human Rights Commission's Application* [2015], at paragraphs 6, 38, 129–40, 145–150, noting and also citing *AB and C v Ireland* [2011]). You can read the judgment at <www.courtsni.gov.uk>. Press coverage followed, with reported considerations by the Attorney-General of lodging an appeal against the decision. The Director of the Northern Ireland branch of the Royal College of Midwives was quoted as saying that the decision was welcomed, as it gave legal protection to health professionals, including midwives, who feared prosecution if they offered appropriate care, support and advice to women who were carrying a foetus with a fatal abnormality (McDonald, 2015).

Two prominent ethicists, whose work is frequently referred to by commentators in the abortion debate, and who use the paradigms of classical philosophy, are John Finnis and Judith Jarvis Thomson. Thomson asserts a woman's right to choose, arguing that the potential to develop into a human is not equal to a human, just as an acorn is not equal to an oak tree. Further, she claims that a woman should have the right to choose to allow or not to allow an imposition on her body. She makes an analogy between this choice and the choice that a Samaritan makes in helping another. Thomson uses the analogy—which is now quite famous—of a violinist to highlight how one body may be justly or unjustly imposed on another:

> You wake up in the morning and find yourself back to back in bed with an unconscious violinist, a famous unconscious violinist. He has been found to have a fatal kidney ailment, and the Society of Music Lovers has canvassed all the available medical records and found that you alone have the right blood type to help. They have therefore kidnapped you, and last night the violinist's circulatory system was plugged into yours, so that your kidneys could be used to extract poisons from his blood as well as your own. The director of the hospital now tells you, 'Look, we're sorry the Society of Music Lovers did this to you—we would never have permitted it if we had known. But still, they did it, and the violinist now is plugged into you. To unplug you would be to kill him. But never mind, it's only for nine months. By then he will have recovered from his ailment, and can safely be unplugged from you.'
>
> (Thomson, 1971, p. 48)

Thomson's point is that the woman faces a difficult decision: whether or not to allow another human being the use of her body. She argues that the woman has a moral right to choose what to do on her own terms and in her own way.

Finnis discounts this argument on a number of grounds, not the least being that the concept of rights is a popular concept that is widely used and misapplied (Finnis, 1974). In Hohfeldian terms, a liberty or choice does not equal a claim right, which implies an obligation on another to act. (This is highlighted in Chapter 10, given the distinction between liberties, interests, claims and rights.) Finnis questions Thomson's reliance on a woman's right (to anything), positing that a right does not exist until it has been proven to be a claim right. The notion of when personhood begins seems to be central to the debate between Thomson and Finnis; the earlier the point at which personhood is said to come into existence, the harder it is to discount that being's 'right' or 'claim' to life.

Throughout the parry between Finnis and Thomson, the different ethical frameworks of utilitarianism and deontology are apparent. According to **utilitarianism**, serving the greater good may justify inflicting harm on others, depending on the circumstances and on the consequences for the mother, the potential child and society. Under deontology, intending harm is of the utmost ethical gravity, regardless of whether a good outcome may be achieved. Bad actions cannot justify good outcomes.

The current abortion law in Australia is that abortion is regulated, and participation in early termination is allowed if refusing would expose the pregnant woman to serious risks, such as to life, or to physical or mental health. The number of weeks of gestation before an abortion is presumed illegal is different in different jurisdictions, so the legislation for each jurisdiction should be referred to, as well as the regulations supporting the legislation that set out the required process and documentation of the justification for the procedure (Breen, Cordner & Thomson, 2016, pp. 480–2).

utilitarianism
An ethics theory in which the outcome of actual or proposed action is the focus, and the acceptable course of action is that in which the greatest good for the greatest number is achieved.

In Queensland, the original law from 1899 remained in force until 2018, prohibiting abortion as a crime excepting procedures to prevent a serious danger to a woman's physical or mental health. The Queensland Law Reform Commission's report (2018) considered replacement of the *Criminal Code* provision with a health regulation, prompting preliminary discussion of a Bill in parliament, and ultimately a narrow conscience vote in favour of the proposition to remove abortion from the *Criminal Code*. A move from criminal to the administrative regulatory provisions would be philosophically significant. As you have learnt, the criminal law focuses on prohibiting certain behaviour that is regarded by society as reprehensible, and punishment can be given to protect the community and also mark society's disapproval so that others are deterred from similar conduct. An administrative approach is not generally punitive, and can provide a practical and pragmatic way of limiting unacceptable conduct, providing safeguards for individuals and society in limiting unacceptable conduct and encouraging and facilitating careful considerations about the conduct.

Health care workers will make their own ethics decisions about whether or not to be involved. If there is a service that an individual health care worker feels unable to provide, they should at least refer the client to someone who can explore the decision.

Government agency decisions and supporting discussion documents can provide an interesting public record of community sentiment and shifting ethics debates on basic bioethics issues. Their rulings provide the benchmark for subsequent administrative implementation of treatment processes.

For example, consider the morning-after pill, an emergency contraceptive that is routinely available over the counter in some countries. When a New York judge supported its over the counter availability in a 2009 judgment, the focus was on the administrative justification for excluding 17-year-olds from access, given that the Food and Drug Administration (FDA) had already decided that such women could access the treatment safely, with appropriate consent (*Annie Tummino et al v Frank M. Torti* (2009)). So, the legal focus of the decision was effectively on safety and autonomy. The ethics debate of personhood and acceptability was assumed to have taken place elsewhere, when the FDA granted general approval for the contraception. A comprehensive critical review of the controversy surrounding the earlier approval process had been undertaken (Brooks, 1993).

The same issue with the morning-after pill was debated extensively in Australian parliaments in 2006 before being passed to the Therapeutic Goods Administration (TGA) to decide on. You can see those debates for both Federal Senate and House of Representatives sittings in February 2006 in the official record, *Hansard*. The reading of the Bill and the speeches given in parliament are interesting. The issues raised include:

- philosophical reflections on personhood and the intervention of humans in conception
- religious expressions of doctrine and rules of conduct
- practical concerns about the risks that are posed and benefits to be gained.

In Australia, publicly available information on websites is that emergency contraception pills can now be sought from a local pharmacist. They are more effective taken the day after unprotected sex, but some can be taken up to three or five days after sex, and are designed to reduce the risk of pregnancy (healthdirect.gov.au & thewomens.org.au). Regarding the morning-after pill, the Pharmaceutical Society of Australia provides information on:

• the pill and its potential side effects
• the requirements for pharmacists before providing the pill, including professional standards considerations
• the steps in assessing the patient's needs and providing counselling supported by written information
• referral information for sexual assault services.

The pharmacist must note the relevant state or territory legislation as well—for instance, on the age of a minor who can be supplied with the emergency contraception (Pharmaceutical Society of Australia, 2015).

Emergency contraception is available in many countries. In the USA, there is awareness that availability could always be reconsidered in the Senate. Abortion laws are regularly redebated at the level of state legislature in the USA, and each debate generates further professional comment and discussion (Tanne, 2006). So, the parliamentary debates in each country can provide an ongoing interesting insight into community sentiment and ethics debates on basic bioethics issues, as well as noting current practices.

Private agreements and obligations under contract law

When parties agree how to act towards each other in a way that is legally enforceable, the agreement is termed a *contract*. If there is a breach of a contract, an innocent party can bring a civil action in **contract law**, to be compensated for the consequences of a contract not being performed to completion. The aim is for the party to be placed in the same position as if the contract had been properly performed. This principle underlies the development of the law of contracts (*Robinson v Harman* (1848) and *Butler v Egg Pulp Marketing Board* (1966), as cited in Davis, 2012, p. 684). The party claiming they deserve to be compensated would also have a responsibility to take reasonable steps to prevent a loss occurring if they could, and unexpected losses that could not be reasonably predicted would not be able to be recovered.

contract law
Principles of legally enforceable agreements and procedure for testing breaches in a civil court.

Understanding basic principles of contract law is useful in many agreements that we enter into in our lives, and in all forms of business practice. The principles clearly identify what each party promises to do: and that they agree to be legally obliged to carry out their promises. The elements of a contract are: 'intention to create contractual relations; agreement, which consists of acceptance of an offer; and consideration' (Davis, 2012, p. 7).

A contractual capacity to enter into the type of contract being considered is needed for an intention to create legal relations—that is, to create an agreement that is legally enforceable. Whether parties intend to be immediately bound by the terms of the contract is a central issue, particularly for informal contracts. The purpose of the contract must be legal for it to be legally enforceable. Express or implied terms can be identified in a contract, and the scope of the agreement must be sufficiently certain and complete—at least in its essential terms—for it to be relied on. An offer and acceptance amounting to genuine consent to the terms of the contract is in place, and either a formal contract is in place, signed and attested, or for simple contracts—which can be oral or in writing—valuable consideration must be expressed. Consideration demonstrates the reciprocal exchange—what each party will do as part of the enforceable agreement, such as pay money or perform services.

Contract law principles are largely found in case law, so reading cases to understand the basic propositions is very important in developing an understanding of how those principles are likely to be applied in new situations. Considerable case law explains each of the above elements (Davis, 2012).

When you sign an employment contract, you are formally agreeing to take on certain roles in a health service. As consideration, you offer your availability, skill and labour. Your potential employer offers conditions of employment, including a certain salary and conditions. Your representations about the level of your skill and training are relied on for the offer of employment to be valid, and it would be voidable if you were found to have misrepresented yourself on your CV. Take great care with your CV. It is essential that it is accurate, complete—and in no way misleading. Take similar care with the way you describe your experience when applying for a new job. Each representation that you make has legal significance as part of the negotiation process that culminates in an employment contract. The notice period that you or your employer should give is usually outlined in your contract, either in the main agreement, or in the conditions of that employment.

REFLECTION POINT

An accurate and complete CV

1   Draft your CV or résumé and, after pairing up, question a colleague about aspects of their documented skills and experience.

2   Consider if any changes should be made to your CV to describe your knowledge, skill and experience.

INTEGRATED LEARNING AND PRACTICE

Why must my CV be accurate?

1   Revisit the chapters up to this point. Note all the reasons why you should represent your training and skill accurately and honestly.

2   Support your answer with at least five standards drawn from law, ethics and regulation.

Remember that the representations you make to your employer will be relied on to offer services to the public. Patients receive a health care service, and your work is part of the process to deliver the service. Goods and services can be dealt with contractually. A client enters into an agreement to pay for services received from the health service. Health care providers can be sued in contract if they do not deliver the services they have agreed to provide, and the patient as a result can demonstrate some type of loss. Health services also rely on equipment providers so that services offered are of an acceptable standard. Protection is available under the Australian Consumer Law, and contract law principles, in the *Competition and Consumer Act 2010* (Cth), Schedule 2: *Australian Consumer Law* (ACL).

Misleading and deceptive conduct is prohibited in this uniform legislation (*Australian Consumer Law*, section 18; Corones, 2011). Representations that will be relied on in a contract should not be misleading or deceptive in any way.

To be of fit quality to be sold for the purpose it is offered—that is, merchantable quality— is essential for products such as pacemakers as patients rely on them, and the manufacturer accepts a significant responsibility for its quality given the role of the pacemaker in regulating a person's heart rhythm. In one class action case, the risk of premature battery depletion was sufficient to be a legally significant risk, even if the battery had not failed. In order to test each pacemaker it had to be removed from the patient (*Medtel Pty Ltd v Courtney* [2003]).

You should remember the ethical importance of honesty, veracity, integrity and professionalism in all of your professional representations, both for your representation of yourself and your skills, and for the services you offer or carry out.

Respectful conduct and reasonable care for others under torts law

A tort is a type of wrong that is specific in a legal sense. It is a wrong that has occurred against a person or the interests of a person. This can be a wrong:

- to their interests in their own physical security
- to their reputation
- to their property.

tort law
Common law principles of wrongs committed against a person or the person's interests and the process of proving those wrongs in a civil court.

The person who is wronged can seek redress or compensation from the person who was responsible for the wrong occurring by bringing an action in **torts**, guided by the principles of the common law of torts, as found largely in case law (Vout, 2016, p. 5).

An inviolate interest in one's own body is supported in law and has a long history in common law. Blackstone, quoted from 1830: 'The law cannot draw the line between degrees of violence, and therefore totally prohibits the first and lowest stage of it; every man's person being sacred, and no other having a right to meddle with it, in the slightest manner'. (*Blackstone Commentaries* [1830], cited in Balkin & Davis, 2013, p. 36).

The injury in trespass is a breach of a right, and it is not necessary that a person suffers actual damage in terms of their physical person or property as a result for it to amount to an 'injury' that can be the subject of a legal claim against the wrongdoer.

Every human being of adult years and sound mind has a right to determine what shall be done with their own body, and a surgeon who performs an operation without his patient's consent commits an assault. An operation performed without consent is an assault. This

REFLECTION POINT

Respect for a person's inviolability

1 From the suggested cases, take note of still relevant historical cases that are cited in the published reasons for decision on the importance of the legal principle of inviolability. (Alternatively, you could take notes from a different case you have found.)

2 Why is such an old legal statement still applied in such a different modern context?

was established in the US case, *Schloendorff v Society of New York Hospital* (1914), as cited by Madden & McIlwraith, 2013, p. 20; also citing an Australian case approving this principle, *Secretary, Department of Health and Community Services v JWB (Marion's Case)* (1992) at paragraph 234.)

Traditionally, trespass to the person is a tort of battery if it is done by touching someone without consent intentionally, negligently or recklessly (*Christopherson v Bare* (1848), as cited in Balkin & Davis, 2013, p. 35), and to cause a person fear of being touched is the tort of assault. They are now collectively referred to as assault, which is a form of trespass to the person. A person who is assaulted can seek common law redress from an identified assailant if the touching was intentional, direct, and there was no lawful justification for the physical interference with that person.

You read about assault and battery as a criminal law concept. It is a tort as well as a crime. It is a private interest that is so important that the state protects all citizens in their right to be free of fear from assault and battery.

Consent can be implied, such as holding out an arm ready to receive an injection, or to allow a blood sample to be taken for testing (Balkin & Davis, 2013, pp. 134, 137).

There are some things that can't be consented to, arguably on public policy grounds (*Pallante v Stadiums Pty Ltd* [1976] at 340, as cited by Balkin & Davis, 2013, p. 141). Surgery or examination can be consented to, and it is the consent that makes acceptable what would ordinarily be unlawful trespass. However, a surgeon who performs the wrong operation, which wasn't consented to, is liable for trespass (*Chatterton v Gerson* [1981] at 443, as cited by Balkin & Davis, 2013, p. 134).

Ordinary contact in everyday life is to be expected, and is not sufficient to be a tort, as there is some implied accepted interference (*Cole v Turner* (1704) and *Collins v Wilcock* [1984] at 1177 per Goff LJ, as cited by Balkin & Davis, 2013, p. 37). Brushing against someone in a crowded corridor, or in a crowded lift, is part of what we agree to. Offering a person assistance to walk or stand up, or physically catching a person who is in danger of falling is uncontroversial. Common sense is used to decide if the type of touching involved intrusion to that person's physical security beyond what is normally acceptable.

The onus is on the person who makes the physical contact to prove that there was consent, so it is essential that you take the time to gain and document an informed decision before proceeding. Keeping extensive documentation is essential for many procedures, and you will read one health service's advice on this in Chapter 8 'Lifelong practice in decision making'. A health professional's recollection that consent was given is not sufficient. It must be transparent and objectively assessed that this process of seeking and obtaining consent has occurred. The medical record is a start on proving that you have obtained consent, and the notes may be essential if you do need to formally defend any aspect of the care that you have provided. The explanation that is documented to have been given must in fact have been given for the consent to be valid (*Chatterton v Gerson* [1981] at 443, as cited by Balkin & Davis, 2013, p. 137). The importance of record keeping and your professional responsibilities in contributing to accurate records was discussed in Chapter 1, and regulations in relation to documentation of consent are further discussed in Chapter 8.

Negligence is an area of tort law that routinely causes professionals in practice to actively reflect on whether they are practising in an acceptable way. Professionals are obliged to offer their skill to an appropriate level, if they profess a skill and offer it to patients or clients or more broadly to the public, so accepting a duty of care. Duties can be enshrined in statutes, which means that a statutory or strict duty could be applied in deciding if a breach of duty occurred. Negligence claims must be brought within three years of the harm being caused, unless an extension is granted. There is a length period since a harm was caused—for instance, for children—who can bring a claim up to three years after they turn 18 years old (see Statutes of Limitation in each jurisdiction).

Common law duties encompass the vast majority of duties that apply in professional contexts. Health carers who do not uphold their duty of care can be sued if a person to whom the duty is owed suffers harm as a result because of breach of duty. All practitioners and health care workers need to exercise the skill and judgment they have been called upon to use in being asked to provide a health service. Whether their actions are reasonable in the circumstance will be judged against legal requirements, as well as the opinion of their peers of good repute, taking into account the health carer's training and level of experience, on what is regarded as 'competent professional practice'. (For example, see section 50 *Civil Liability Act 2002* (NSW)). An employer is vicariously liable for their employees' negligence, provided the employees were acting within their authority and within the scope of their role. But outside that role, the institution or employer is not vicariously liable—for example, for criminal conduct, or the nervous shock arising from it (Madden & McIlwraith, 2013, p. 94, citing *New South Wales v Lepore* [2003]).

Providing information and giving advice as part of an informed decision-making process by the patient can be the subject of negligence claims. The acceptable standard for disclosure of information is a matter for evidence, and then the information that was provided is also assessed factually. (You will read more on the standards of information disclosure in Chapter 8.) The current law is that patients should receive information on material risks in undertaking certain courses of treatment.

Whether the information disclosed should be objectively that regarded by peers as accepted practice (called 'the Bolam standard') or more subjectively what is relevant and 'material' risk to each patient has been tested in many negligence cases over the last 20 years. England applied the Bolam standard, given a majority judgment in *Sidaway v Governors of Bethlehem Royal Hospital*. The minority judgment argued that in some circumstances, the

Bolam standard of disclosure should not apply, as information about substantial risks could be necessary for a patient's informed decision. More recent UK cases have upheld a higher standard of disclosure (*Sidaway v Governors of Bethlehem Royal Hospital* [1985], cited in Samanta & Samanta, 2014, pp. 49–51). In contrast, they point out that in the USA, the more patient-centred approach has applied for some time, as established in a 1972 case (*Cantebury v Spence* (1972)).

The Australian High Court case *Rogers v Whitaker* [1992] HCA 58, on disclosure of material risks, has been affirmed in a more recent High Court case, *Rosenberg v Percival* [2001], so the principle to uphold was then as follows: if a reasonable person in the position of the patient would attach significance to a risk, or if a treating professional is aware, or should be reasonably aware, that the patient would regard it as significant, it is material. The High Court commented that the test is partly objective and partly subjective (Madden & McIlwraith, 2013, p. 26).

Some limits to civil liability are defined in legislation. (For example, see the *Civil Liability Act 2002* (NSW).) If a plaintiff has contributed to their own injury in any way, such as accepting a significant risk, then compensation under the Civil Liability Act will be limited or proportional.

In matters of technical conduct of procedures, the emphasis is more on the professional view of acceptable standards. If there is absence of other reasonable explanation, this would amount to a **prima facie** case of negligence. Negligence applied in the case of a swab left in a patient who had undergone an operation; as the operation was in the exclusive control of the health care staff and health care organisation, the presence of the swab was sufficient to show breach of duty and causation of injury sufficient to show the surgeon's negligence without calling further evidence, if the surgeon was in control of all relevant stages of the treatment (*Mahon v Osborne* [1939], as cited by Balkin & Davis, 2013, p. 304).

prima facie Conclusion supported by first observation or apparent evidence.

A defence of what reasonable peer professionals would have made known and discussed can now be relied on by professionals in a civil claim, given the provisions in the Civil Liability Acts or equivalent Acts as follows (as cited in Kerridge, Lowe & Stewart, 2013, p. 210):

- *Civil Liability Act 2002* (NSW), section 5O
- *Civil Liability Act 2003* (Qld), section 22
- *Civil Liability Act 1936* (SA), section 41
- *Civil Liability Act 2002* (Tas), section 22
- *Civil Liability Act 2002* (WA), section 5PB
- *Wrongs Act 1958* (Vic), section 59.

The history of the area of negligence starts with a classic case, *Donoghue v Stevenson* [1932], and the contaminated contents of ginger beer bottle. A duty of the manufacturer was described to any eventual users of the product—the consumer, and not just the party the manufacturer sold the product to. The duty is therefore viewed as extending beyond contractual agreement. Reasonable care should be taken for the welfare of those who would foreseeably be affected by the action of the manufacturer offering the product as safe. This duty is not to injure your 'neighbour'. 'Neighbour' in this sense means the person you don't have a particular contractual agreement with but who you live alongside in your community, and who you should therefore have in mind as being affected by your actions, in a fair assessment of the totality of your relationship. This broader view of duty to neighbour allows application to new situations and new duties that haven't been considered before (Stewart & Stuhmcke, 2017, pp. 160–1, citing *Donoghue v Stevenson* [1932]). The potential liability of manufacturers of medical devices to eventual users of those products is a potential area of application of negligence—for example, hip replacement parts, implanted pacemakers, hoists used for patient care, and many more pieces of equipment (including those not invented yet).

Negligence is relied on in product liability cases, including for risks posed by manufacturers, as the courts have maintained the general duty of a manufacturer to the end user. In one case, a person successfully sued as a new drug was found to have contributed to his heart attack (*Peterson v Merck Sharpe & Dohme (Australia) Pty Ltd* [2010]). The drug was subsequently withdrawn from the market.

There is a further shared scheme across Australian jurisdictions—the *Australian Consumer Law*—which makes clear the rights of consumers not to be injured by unsafe products, and that products should be fit for the purpose they have been offered (*Competition and Consumer Act 2010* (Cth), Schedule 2: *Australian Consumer Law*).

Maintaining a safe environment is a duty that an organisation has for both clients and employees, and this can be the focus of negligence claims if someone is injured as a result of a failure to do so. Someone being injured due to slipping on a floor is a classic example of injury in a public area—such as in shopping centres. Hospitals face a huge challenge to clean but also keep areas safe for workers in potential accidents, and visitors onsite, as well as for patients in their care. If a floor is wet due to a spill or because it has just been cleaned, you will likely notice a sign warning of the danger being placed there, as the warning minimises the danger for everyone—and also shares the responsibility for taking caution on the wet floor. The practice of warning people of a danger stems from the principles identified in tort law—to warn of material risks.

When a hospital cleaner was injured changing a continuous towel dispenser because the split pins holding the roll were missing, the hospital (the employer) was partly responsible in negligence (25 per cent) because of a failure to warn employees about the risks, and also a failure to ensure the pins were in place. The supplier was held 75 per cent responsible for the injuries caused to the employee due to negligence (*Richards v Hunter Area Health Service* (1998) Australian Occupational Health & Safety 53–372, cited in *Product Liability Australia, Liability in Tort*, at section 3.30, p. 5036).

The fairness of decisions affecting individuals under administrative law

Administrative regulations are derived from legislation. They are the scaffold for the government, or executive, to keep a society safe and orderly, by regulating conduct within a community.

In applying regulations, decisions need to be made by administrative authorities in a timely and efficient way, and also in a measured way that is comprehensive, fair and procedurally appropriate. **Administrative law** is concerned with the scope of administrative decisions that can be made, and the way those decisions are reached.

As a community endorsed system of governance, the implementation of administrative law depends on three principles. They are:

1 *administrative justice*—safeguarding of individuals' rights and interests affected by the decision

2 *executive accountability*—with potential for explanation and justification of decisions made

3 *good administration*—through rational, fair, consistent and transparent decision-making processes (Creyke & McMillan, 2005, p. 14).

There is a presumption that administrative decisions can be reviewed, to the extent that the correct test, or application of legislative or regulatory provision, has been applied in the administrative decision that has been made (as in *Minister for Immigration and Ethnic Affairs v Wu Shan Liang* (1996)). The general principle is that if an error is found, a court can remit the decision back to the administrative forum, to revisit the proper application of the relevant principles.

Further guidance is found in constitutional principles. A government should not take coercive action in the absence of clear existing legal authority to do so—such as express and unambiguous language. Governments also need to be sure that in interpreting legislation and regulation to define their legal authority, they are not abrogating—or doing away with— fundamental rights, freedom and immunity (Creyke & McMillan, 2005, p. 234).

Examples of administrative decisions that affect a health care worker are:

- decisions made on a person's initial registration as a registered health professional
- decisions to place conditions on someone's registration
- decisions to cancel a person's registration.

You read about this aspect of administration and regulation in Chapter 2 'Standards for professional training and practice'. Principles of natural justice apply to administrative decisions, and a person should be given the right:

- to respond to any complaints
- to be given notice of any hearing or deliberation
- to comment and be heard on matters that materially adversely affect them—such as conditions placed on how or where they practice their profession.

Decision makers should declare any potential conflicts of interests in being part of the decision process, and they should remain free of actual bias or influence that is inappropriate. This applies to all administrative decisions that affect the rights, interests and expectations of the individual citizen, rather than policy matters applying to members of the public in general (*Kioa v West* (1985), at paragraph 31, Mason J, as cited in Boland [2017]).

Decision makers should consider relevant issues, as set out in the scope of their decision remit, and should not be influenced by irrelevant issues. The reasons for the decision should be clearly documented. That is why these administrative decisions are accompanied by a document

administrative law
Principles and procedures of fair administration and administrative decision making for matters particularly affecting an individual's interests.

entitled the decision and reasons. The protective nature of these decisions is paramount—the interests of the community and safety of the public guide the decision making.

Similar principles of natural justice apply in issues of local or institutional regulation. If an employee is to be sanctioned for their inappropriate conduct in a work setting, they should be afforded the right to respond to a complaint, and be afforded a fair and reasonable decision process as it affects their employment and other rights, interests and expectations, such as future employment prospects and possibly their reputation in work settings.

We understand that a basic level of administration and regulation is essential, to safeguard the public. As you read in Chapter 2, restriction of persons being able to work in health care is accepted as a public necessity, because of the immense risk posed by people working in the field who are not adequately prepared, or have become unsafe.

The discussion of public law in Chapter 6 shows how legal principles are reflected in practice in the complex issues faced by society and health practitioners and health care workers.

REFLECTION POINT

Soaps, drama and law

As a review of legal concepts that you have just learnt about, watch 10 minutes of a contemporary film or modern serial set in a hospital or medical setting. As fast as you can, list potential legal issues for the characters, separated into the areas of law that you have now encountered. This is a fun speed test of noticing everything within a new prism of potential legal implications. Try out your speed-spotting with a friend or colleague—and then trade off your dot points in 30 seconds to see who found the most issues (or the best quality issues).

Research skills: Cases

Kay Tucker, Law Library Manager, Monash University

Finding a case is usually straightforward if you have a specific citation (where the case is published) or other details such as the party names, Court or Tribunal and the year of the decision. To identify cases on particular topics and issues, the easiest way—as with legislation (see p. 7)—is to use books, journal articles or legal commentary services as your starting point. These point you to the precedents (which are cases that have established a principle of law) and provide good examples of cases that consider a particular legal issue or set of facts. Read these precedents to understand the points of law and use them as authority when writing your advice or assignment.

To help you access Australian cases and find out more about them, there are two main subscription databases:

+ CaseBase (LexisNexis)
+ FirstPoint (Westlaw).

Both databases provide specific search boxes for you to enter one or more parameters—such as Case name, Catchwords and Summary, Jurisdiction—as well as a more general Terms box, which searches through the entire case record.

Searching in the Catchwords section is more efficient than a general terms search, and ensures that you will retrieve cases directly on point for specific legal areas and principles. A good way to get to know the legal terminology used by the Courts is to look at the Catchwords of a case you've been given or directed to, then use those terms to search for more cases that consider the same legal principle.

For example (using CaseBase), searching the phrase *medical negligence* in the Catchwords/Summary box results in around 400 hits, as opposed to twice that number when searched in the Terms box. You may then wish to focus on a particular subset of these results to find cases that involve—for example, the occurrence of brain injury or brain damage—so add the term *brain*. You may further be interested in the damages sought and obtained, so limit the results to those with the term *damages*, bringing you to around 30 cases. There are various additional limiters available, including Date range and Court. Selecting the High Court of Australia brings you to the case *Tabet v Gett* (2010) 240 CLR 537.

In the case law databases, you can usually link to a version of the case to read in full. First, you should take note of the information provided by the database about the case. Along with the citation and practical court details, you will see the litigation history (if the case has come on appeal from a lower court or if there was a later appeal), and other cases considered by the judges in coming to their decision and subsequent or later cases that have in some way considered the case. Looking at these will help you to determine whether the case is still 'good law'—that is, has it been used in a positive way by being Followed or Applied by later cases. Note also whether the case has been Reversed or Overruled. This information will help you to determine whether the case might be useful for your purposes.

Another useful feature of the databases is the provision of references to case notes and journal articles that discuss, explain or comment on the case. Read some of these to help you understand the case and its wider implications. They often reference similar cases and other useful sources.

There are likely to be instances where a Catchwords/Summary search doesn't work well. You may have more luck with a search of the full case, particularly where the search concerns the facts of a case or the term is more obscure. You can search the full cases in the subscription databases Lexis Advance and Westlaw AU if you have access, as well as on free websites.

The best free sites are AustLII <www.austlii.edu.au> and BarNet Jade <https://jade.io/t/home>. Both websites provide cases from a wide range of courts and tribunals. AustLII includes many Tribunals, Commissions and Boards, as well as Commonwealth, State and Territory courts. For example, you might need to find written findings of the Coroners' Court of Victoria, Medical Practitioners Board of Victoria, Nursing and Midwifery Tribunal of New South Wales, or the Pharmacy Tribunal of New South Wales. A number of these resources have been grouped together to form the Australian Health

Practitioner Law Library <http://www.austlii.edu.au/au/special/healthprac/>. The coverage on AustLII is often not comprehensive, so check the specific court or tribunal page for the date of the most recent document added and the years of coverage.

To search AustLII, use the default standard search of full text documents or go to Advanced Search for more options. Enter your terms—for example, the phrase 'mental capacity', or a more complex string such as 'medical negligence NEAR child*' (* is a wildcard that instructs the search to include variations of the word, i.e. *child* or *children*). An Advanced Search of this set of terms in All Case Law Databases results in around 70 hits. The default order of results, Relevance, displays the High Court precedent *Cattanach v Melchior* [2003] HCA 38 at the top. View results 'By Database' to see the results from particular courts. Note that AustLII provides the judgment in the version sent by the Court (called an Unreported Judgment). For High Court judgments, the CLR (Commonwealth Law Reports) citation—in our example, 215 CLR 1—is added for reference purposes. If you decide to use the case, try to check the citation in CaseBase or FirstPoint and read it in the CLR—available on the Westlaw database—if you can, as these are the authorised reports for the High Court. Each of the superior courts has its own 'authorised' law report series.

More tips:

- When a judgment is handed down, it is assigned a Medium Neutral Citation from the Court. For example, [2003] HCA 38 is the 38th judgment from the High Court of Australia in 2003. This citation stays with the case and is a useful finding tool—particularly for very recent cases.

- Cases are often published in a number of different places, including freely available websites, and print and electronic 'law reports'. Make sure that you check in CaseBase or FirstPoint to see whether there is a reported or 'authorised' version of the case. This is the version you need to cite.

- There is an accepted style to citing Australian cases, prescribed in the Australian Guide to Legal Citation. You need to include the party names, the year, law report abbreviation and starting page number, as well as any pinpoint citations to particular pages or paragraphs that you use. Use the Monash University Legal Abbreviations website to find the meaning of a case abbreviation: <https://guides.lib.monash.edu/legal-abbreviations>.

References

Melbourne University Law Review. (2018). *Australian Guide to Legal Citation* (4th edn). Melbourne: *Melbourne University Law Review/Melbourne Journal of International Law*. Retrieved from <https://law.unimelb.edu.au/mulr/aglc>

REFLECTION: SEARCH FOR YOUR OWN CASE

1   Search for your own case, using one of the methods described in 'Research skills: Cases'.

2   When you have read a case—and the judge's decision and reasons for that decision—write notes about what was unacceptable conduct when judged in the legal forum.

3   Share your example with a group, if possible, and see if you can find a pattern in terms of:

   a   basic setting of minimum standards and safeguards

   b   protection of the public

   c   compensation apportioned for unfortunate mistakes

   d   punishment for grave and intentionally disruptive or destructive behaviour.

4   Reflect on how such standards have come to be accepted as community expectations and standards.

REFLECTION POINT

Learning from case law

As a review of concepts covered in this chapter, try the following reflection exercise.

Look at the law databases that are available to you to find a case about a dispute in a health care context. Make a note from the Headnote of the case about which area of the law is being considered.

Always remember that a professional is open to a 'higher' moral aim than that required by law. It is also possible for individuals to behave differently and never really have their behaviours tested by the legal limit, because they rise well above that level. Personal ethics and professional ethics are evident in the objectives chosen by those individuals, and the way they strive to meet optimal standards.

REFLECTION: NOTICING LEGAL PRINCIPLES IN PRACTICAL DOCUMENTS

This exercise reviews how the law contributes to the setting of standards in health care.

1   Either now or later on, consider the provision of health services in an institutional setting.

   Source a policy or procedure requirement in a governance document. Critically analyse the policy or procedure and summarise how it reflects standards that have been derived from law.

+ continued

> 2   Alternatively, find a patient consent form, and find which aspects of an informed decision-making process are documented on it. Gather any information sheets you can find related to a specific procedure. Choose five aspects of the documentation you have, and summarise the legal significance of those steps.

Summary

You have now built on your understanding of the role of law in providing peaceful and orderly structure for the community. You can now appreciate the different contributions made by areas of the law, such as criminal law, tort law and contract law. Some of the principles and standards derived from these areas of law apply to everyone in society, and some elevated standards are particularly important for health care professionals because of the special role that they are given in society.

You have learnt about acceptable standards in reproductive health, and understand how the place you live provides practical limits to the standards that are then set and the choices that can be made for personal and professional health care matters. You will remember that the earlier chapters included the legislative examples of the laws, for instance those that provide for Medicare. You will remember the legislation you looked up when you searched for 'health' in your own parliament's website, including the uniform registration schemes for registered health practitioners and students.

STUDY QUESTIONS

Prepare paragraph length answers, with references, for the following questions.

1   How are my obligations towards my patients defined by law?
2   Why must I ask permission before touching a patient?
3   Why do we spend time talking through the treatment options and side effects, and why does it take longer with some patients than others?
4   Why is it important for a CV to be comprehensive and accurate?
5   Think back to your earlier reading. Summarise and explain the legal, regulatory and ethics requirements for record keeping, and outline how health records may be relied upon in subsequent legal and administrative proceedings.

SAMPLE ESSAY QUESTIONS

1   Describe the role of criminal law, tort law and contract law in our society.
  - Source and describe one finding from criminal law, and one finding from either torts or contract law (or that includes both). After reading each case, write a Headnote in your own words for the cases you have found.
  - Critique the cases, and comment on whether they satisfy the role of law that you have outlined.

2 'Law and ethics work together to balance the freedoms of individuals and the structuring of a peaceful and orderly society.' Discuss.

REFERENCES

[ ] Abortion hero turns pro-life. (1995, 12 August). *Sydney Morning Herald* [reprinted from *New York Times*], p. 17.

[ ] *Product liability Australia: Liability in tort*, Butterworths LexisNexis, [looseleaf service], as at 16 May 2018.

Australian Health Practitioner Regulation Agency. *Court and tribunal decisions*. Retrieved from http://ahpra.gov.au

Australian Parliament. (2006). *Hansard*. House of Representatives, 16 February 2006; Senate, 29 March 2006. Retrieved from www.aph.gov.au/hansard

Baker, R. (2004). Patient-centred care after Shipman. *Journal of the Royal Society of Medicine*, 97(4), 161–5.

Balkin, R.P., & Davis, J.L.R. (2013). *Law of torts* (5th edn). Australia: LexisNexis Butterworths.

Bogaric, M. (2013). *Ross on Crime* (6th edn). Sydney: Thomson Reuters.

Boland J. (2017, 22 November). *Quality decision making under the Health Practitioner National Law: A judge's perspective.* Paper presented at the Medical Council of NSW Seminar, Quality decision making, risk assessment, and the impaired practitioner, Sydney University.

Breen, K.J., Cordner, S.M., & Thomson, C.J.H. (2016). *Good medical practice: Professionalism, ethics and law* (4th edn). Kingston: Australian Medical Council Ltd.

Brooks, M.J. (1993). Commentary: RU-486: Politics of abortion and science. *Journal of Pharmacy & Law*, 2, 261–92.

Burton Crawford, L., & Goldworth, J. (2017). *The rule of law and the Australian Constitution*. Sydney: Federation Press.

Coalition of Australian Governments (COAG). (2017). *Health Council Communique 24 March 2017*. Retrieved from http://mentalhealthcarersnsw.org

Corones, S., & Clarke, P.H. (2011). *Australian consumer law* (4th edn). Pyrmont: Thomson Reuters.

Crawford, J. (2012). *Brownlie's principles of public international law* (8th edn). Oxford: Oxford University Press.

Creyke, R., & McMillan, J. *Control of Government Action*. (2005). Australia: Lexis Nexis Butterworths.

Creyke, R., & McMillan, J. (2012). *Control of government action: Text, cases & commentary* (3rd edn). Australia: LexisNexis Butterworths.

Davis, J.L.R. (Ed.). (2012). *Contract: General principles: The laws of Australia* (2nd edn). Pyrmont: Thomson Reuters.

Finn, P. (2016). *Fiduciary obligations*. Sydney: Federation Press.

Finnis, J. (1974). The rights and wrongs of abortion. In M. Cohen et al. (Eds), *The rights and wrongs of abortion* (pp. 85–113). Princeton: Princeton University Press.

Horton, R. (2001). The real lessons from Harold Frederick Shipman. *Lancet*, 357, 82–3.

Kerridge, I., Lowe, M., & Stewart, C. (2013). *Ethics and law for the health professions* (4th edn). Sydney: Federation Press.

Madden, B., & McIlwraith, J. (2013). *Australian Medical Liability* (2nd edn). Australia: LexisNexis Butterworths.

McDonald, H. (2015, 1 December). Northern Ireland law on abortion ruled 'incompatible with human rights'. *The Guardian*. Retrieved from http://theguardian.com

Medical Board of Australia. (2017, 3 April). *AHPRA successfully prosecutes NSW fake doctor and welcomes proposed new powers*. Retrieved from http://medicalboard.gov.au

Mulraney, F. (2017, 26 September). *Ireland will hold an abortion referendum in 2018*. Irish Central. Retrieved from http://irishcentral.com/news

New South Wales Government, The Honourable Mr Acting Justice J.P. Slattery, Royal Commissioner. (1990). *Report of the Royal Commission into Deep Sleep Therapy*. Sydney, New South Wales Government.

Office of the Australian Information Commissioner (OAIC). (2018). *Notifiable data breaches scheme*. Canberra: Australian Government. Retrieved from www.oaic.gov.au

Pharmaceutical Society of Australia. (2015). *Guidance for provision of a Pharmacist Only medicine Levonorgestrel: Approved indication: emergency contraception*. Retrieved from http://psa.org.au

Queensland Law Reform Commission. (2018). *Review of termination of pregnancy laws: Report*. Report No. 76, June 2018. Brisbane: Queensland Government.

Qui, R-Z. (1996). Bioethics in an Asian Context. *World Health*, 5, 13.

Ramsay, S. (2001). Audit further exposes UK's worst serial killer. *Lancet*, 357, 123–5.

Samanta, J., & Samanta, A. (2014). *Medical law concentrate*. Oxford: Oxford University Press.

Smith, J. (2003). *The Shipman Inquiry. Third report: Death certification and investigation of deaths by coroners*. Cm5854. Whitehall, London: Secretary of State for the Home Department and the Secretary of State for Health.

Stewart, P., & Stuhmcke, A. (2017). *Australian principles of tort law* (4th edn). Sydney, Federation Press.

Tanne, J. (2006). South Dakota abortion ban encourages other states. *British Medical Journal*, vol. 332(7542), 626.

Thomson, J.J. (1971). A defense of abortion. *Philosophy and Public Affairs*, 1(1), 47–56.

Vout, P. (2016). *Torts: The Laws of Australia* (3rd edn). Pyrmont: Thomson Reuters.

LEGISLATION

Civil Liability Act 2002 (NSW)

Civil Liability Act 2003 (Qld)

Civil Liability Act 1936 (SA)

Civil Liability Act 2002 (Tas)

Civil Liability Act 2002 (WA)

Commonwealth of Australia Constitution Act 1900 (Cth) (the Constitution) compilation prepared 4 September 2013

Competition and Consumer Act 2010 (Cth), Schedule 2: *Australian Consumer Law* (ACL), Retrieved from
http://consumerlaw.gov.au

Crimes Act 1900 (NSW)

Health Practitioner Regulation National Law Act 2009 (Cth)

Health Practitioner Regulation National Law (Victoria) Act 2009 (Vic)

*National Disability Insurance Scheme Amendment (Quality and Safeguards Commission and Other Measures) Bill
2017* (Cth)

Privacy Act 1988 (Cth)

Privacy Amendment (Notifiable Data Breaches) Act 2017 (Cth)

Wrongs Act 1958 (Vic)

CASES

AB and C v Ireland [2011] 53 EHRR 13.

Airedale NHS Trust v Bland [1993] AC 789.

Annie Tummino et al v Frank M. Torti (Acting Commissioner of the Food and Drug Administration), US District
Court for the Eastern District of New York, Brooklyn New York, Edward R. Korman, United States District
Judge, Judgment dated 23 March 2009; Memorandum &Order No 05-CV-366 (ERK) (VVP).

Breen v Williams (1994) 35 NSWLR 35.

Broome v Cassell & Co Ltd [1972] AC 1027.

Butler v Egg Pulp Marketing Board (1966) 11 CLR 185.

Cantebury v Spence (1972) 464 52d 772 (DC).

Chatterton v Gerson [1981] QB 432.

Christopherson v Bare (1848) 11 QB 47.

Cole v Turner (1704) 6 Mod Rep 49.

Collins v Wilcock [1984] 1 WLR 1172.

D v S (1981) 93 LSJS 405.

Donoghue v Stevenson [1932] AC 562.

Fleming v White [1981] 2 NSWLR 719.

Hart v Herron and Anor [1996] NSWSC 176 .

International Military Tribunal (Nuremberg) 41 AJIL 172 (1947)

Kable v Director of Public Prosecutions (1995) 36 NSWLR 374 .

Keeley v Brooking (1979) 143 CLR 162.

Kioa v West (1985) 159 CLR 555.

Mahon v Osborne [1939] 2 KB 14.

Medtel Pty Ltd v Courtney [2003] FCAFC 151; 130 FCR 182; 198 ALR 630.

Minister for Immigration and Ethnic Affairs v Wu Shan Liang (1996) 185 CLR 259.

Mitchell v Homfray (1881) 8 Q.B.D. 587.

New South Wales v Lepore [2003] HCA 4.

Pallante v Stadiums Pty Ltd [1976] VR 331.

Peterson v Merck Sharpe & Dohme (Australia) Pty Ltd [2010] FCA 180.

R (Pretty) v Director of Public Prosecutions [2002] 1 AC 800.

Reeves v R; R v Reeves [2013] NSWCCA 34.

Richards v Hunter Area Health Service (1998) Australian Occupational Health & Safety 53–372.

Robinson v Harman (1848) 1 Ex 850.

Roe v Wade (1973) 410 US 113

Rogers v Whitaker [1992] HCA 58.

Rosenberg v Percival [2001] HCA 18.

S and Marper v UK [2009] 48 EHRR 50.

Schloendorff v Society of New York Hospital (1914) 211NY 125.

Secretary, Department of Health and Community Services v JWB (Marion's Case) (1992) 175 CLR 218.

Sidaway v Governors of Bethlehem Royal Hospital [1985] AC 871.

Singh v The Commonwealth (2004) 222 CLR 322.

The Northern Ireland Human Rights Commission's Application [2015] NIQB 196.

The State of New South Wales v Gregory Wayne Kable [2013] HCA 26.

CHAPTER 4

An ongoing dialogue relying on ethics traditions

LEARNING OBJECTIVES

- To understand the choices available to you in ethics reasoning frameworks.
- To learn to recognise ethics reasoning in health standards.
- To develop skill in ethics reasoning as part of your reflective practice.
- To integrate ethics reasoning further in your reflection exercises.

KEY TERMS

absolutism	normative ethics
casuistry	principle
consequentialism	proportionism
conviction	relativism
descriptive ethics	religion
doctrine	respect for persons
doctrine of double effect	slippery-slope argument
duty of care	

CASE EXAMPLE

Utopia: Something for everyone

The new state that you encountered in Chapter 1 now has a name. Utopia hopes to offer something for everyone.

To control or allow freedom still has the planners perplexed. They brief you again as a consultant to add some ethics reasoning to the debate.

As you think about choices in ethics reasoning frameworks, summarise how you could support control or total freedom, using ethics reasoning tools.

Thinking about principles and choices in reasoning

You started learning about ethics in earlier chapters, covering key terms such as the following. You can find definitions for them in the glossary.

autonomy	good	obligation
belief	human rights	principlism
beneficence	ideals	professional
bioethics	impropriety	professional code of ethics
character	insight	propriety
code of conduct	integrity	reflection
communitarianism	justice	responsibility
deon	libertarianism	rules
deontology	medical ethics	utilitarianism
duties	morals	values
fit and proper person	non-maleficence	virtue
goals	norms	

You will be discovering new ethics terms in other chapters, so you could add to this list as you go.

As you learn more about ethics reasoning in this chapter, remember that you can choose from many different ethics reasoning frameworks for your own reflection on health care issues. Learning about the different main forms of ethics reasoning can help you with your reflection on your responsibilities as a health care professional. Considerable philosophical discussion and ethics reasoning has been devoted to identifying, understanding and upholding obligations in a health care context.

The following examples of forms of reasoning, classic debates and contemporary philosophical discussions have been chosen to highlight the forms of ethics reasoning available to you.

Expressing professional goals and duties is quite complex. Some are broad notions; others are more specific. There has been a move in recent times to simplify the ethical goals and duties for health care into broad **principles**. Principlist frameworks for decision making are a modern phenomenon. They provide tools for summarising the obligations and aspirations of health care workers.

Beneficence, non-maleficence, autonomy and justice are the most widely used **principles**, as defined by American ethicists Beauchamp and Childress. Beneficence is the obligation to do good, to care for people, and non-maleficence is the paired obligation to do no harm to them. Autonomy is the principle of self-rule, of clients making decisions about their own lives. Justice is the fair distribution of resources, particularly when the pool of resources is limited (Beauchamp & Childress, 1994, p. 38). You might remember using the principles of Beauchamp and Childress in Chapter 1 as a tool to summarise issues in professional codes.

principle
A fundamental proposition, from which goals or duties can be derived, or under which goals and duties can be described.

A British ethicist, Gillon, proposes similar principles of respect for autonomy, beneficence, non-maleficence and justice, but provides a slightly different definition of 'respect for autonomy', which he defines as 'the moral obligation to respect the autonomy of others in so far as such respect is compatible with equal respect for the autonomy of all potentially affected' (Gillon, 1994, p. xxii). In essence, Gillon's definition builds a social context into autonomy.

Slightly different principles have also been used to think about ethics duties and conduct in health research practice. These research principles have been termed the Belmont principles because they were originally coined by the US National Commission for the Protection of Human Subjects of Biomedical and Behavioural Research, in the Commission's Belmont Report. In the Commission's terms, the Belmont principles are:

- beneficence—a dual obligation to do no harm and promote the wellbeing of individuals, and also to maximise the potential benefit to society
- **respect for persons**—an obligation to uphold the autonomy of individuals
- justice—an obligation to share the benefits or burdens of research fairly in society (US Department of Health, Education, and Welfare, 1978, pp. 4–10).

respect for persons
The principle of respect for persons, generally used for research participants.

The Belmont principles are used as a tool in Chapter 7 to highlight ethics issues in research.

There is broad agreement in the principles suggested by Beauchamp and Childress, Gillon and in the Belmont Report, as summarised in Table 4.1.

TABLE 4.1 SUMMARY OF ETHICS PRINCIPLES

Beauchamp & Childress	Gillon	Belmont
beneficence	beneficence	beneficence
non-maleficence	non-maleficence	(beneficence includes do no harm)
autonomy	respect for autonomy	respect for persons
justice	justice	justice

The principles suggested by Beauchamp and Childress, Gillon and in the *Belmont Report* have gained support because they provide a form of shorthand for thinking about ethics issues. The principles are used as tools to collect and summarise issues expressed by professionals, clients and the community as being of concern. The principles are used as tools for ethical analysis and comparison. They do not, in themselves, give ultimate guidance on 'right' or 'wrong' behaviour.

Beauchamp and Childress defined their principles of beneficence, non-maleficence, autonomy and justice despite their own personal theoretical differences. Beauchamp's stance can be broadly described as utilitarian, whereas Childress's stance is, generally speaking, deontological. Remember that the principles complement rather than supplant ethics theories and forms of reasoning (Beauchamp & Childress, 1994, p. 45). A utilitarian concentrates on the outcome of behaviour for the greatest number, and aims for the happiness (or utility) of the greatest number in society. Utilitarianism is a theory that is compatible with **consequentialism**, an ethics theory that focuses on consequences, and nominates utility as the outcome that should be assessed. A deontologist, on the other hand, looks at the fundamental rule (or deon) that should be applied, in all situations, to ensure an ethical process. In **absolutism**, a rule-driven process is the focus of analysis. Deontology is an ethics theory that is compatible with absolutism, describing the process of identifying rules and the derivation of those rules for use in guiding ethically acceptable processes.

Deontology and utilitarianism are very commonly taught frameworks, as they are useful to illustrate that ethics reasoning can lead to different conclusions, so that two people can choose a quite different yet reasoned course of action, and both can be ethical. Utilitarianism rights and virtue theory—and maybe other Kantian ethics—are explained by Beauchamp and Childress, who also comment on convergence and useful compatible reasoning that can be applied by people who subscribe to the different theories (Beauchamp & Childress, 2013).

Some support for the principles of beneficence, non-maleficence, autonomy and justice can therefore be found in different ethics theories and frameworks.

For a libertarian, it is assumed that in allowing autonomy, each person acts to pursue their own wellbeing and happiness. Under John Stuart Mill's theory, liberty should be limited to a certain extent to allow for justice and the fair distribution of burden and benefit. Individual liberty is limited when exercising liberty may unreasonably infringe on others; liberty would be denied in circumstances in which other individuals were severely harmed or their similar liberties were threatened (Mill, 1975, pp. 94, 96). In contrast, the central issue in Immanuel Kant's theory is the individual pursuit of morality and the identification of the categorical imperative. The categorical imperative is to: 'Act only on that maxim which you can at the same time will to be a universal law' (Honderich, 1995, pp. 435–9, at p. 437).

Freedom underpins Kant's theory, as it is needed for individuals to develop and act on their moral laws. A duty to uphold freedom entails respect for oneself, and respect for others. Although Kant rejects a perfect duty to benefit others and not to harm them, he maintains that a duty to benefit oneself and to refrain from harming oneself is part of the fundamental duty of respect. As respect for others is also fundamental, duties to benefit others and refrain from harming others stem from allowing them freedom to safeguard their own wellbeing. Justice implies that we fairly respect everyone's need to develop their own moral selves. It also implies the ultimate good of 'moral perfection'. The way of achieving moral perfection, according to Kant's theory, is to treat individuals with respect, and to extend that respect to

consequentialism
An ethics theory in which the consequences of actions are the focus, both on the actor and others affected by the action.

absolutism
An ethics theory in which a rule or rules are identified as fundamentally important, and of unvarying significance.

all people equally, under a framework of justice as fairness. In other words, moral perfection stems from treating individuals with respect, and not as a means to an end (Sullivan, 1989, pp. 46, 104, 105, 203, 207, 208, 234.).

INTEGRATED LEARNING AND PRACTICE

Am I allowed to think for myself in my own way?

Yes, you are allowed to think for yourself! The most important part of ethics is that it is a toolkit of reasoning styles, and if you are ready to actively reflect, that is the best first step.

No law or regulation tells you how to think through an ethical issue, but they do remind you that there are some limits to what you decide to do and how you then act— and may even offer you some protection if your reasoning leads you to act bravely to try and help someone in need.

As simple shorthand points, the principles of beneficence, non-maleficence, autonomy and justice have the potential to be very useful. Many students and health professionals use them precisely because they are easily grasped and applied. While you cannot expect them to provide answers for all of the ethical dilemmas that you might face, they will always provide a starting place for reflection on professional ethics in health care. Each principle has its merits, and how much you emphasise each principle depends on your preferred form of ethics reasoning.

In many practical situations, ethics reflection using your chosen ethics framework will help you to decide if it is necessary or preferable to give priority to one or more of the principles. Considerable thought and discussion will be needed in situations in which the principles conflict, as different theories would prioritise the principles quite differently. For instance, while the libertarian's central value of individual freedom emphasises autonomy, a communitarian's concern with achieving good for all (in a fair manner) emphasises justice. A deontologist who is ready to guard against a harm that is unacceptable given an identified rule or deon—even when the patient has indicated a willingness to be harmed, or there is a good that must be promoted—emphasises beneficence and non-maleficence.

You have a choice about whether or not to take on care responsibilities—for example, whether or not to disclose your health care skills in everyday situations in which they may be called upon, and whether or not to disclose the extent of your capabilities in the course of caring for a client. On a group holiday, would you disclose that you are clinically trained? Would you be prepared to adopt your professional role if it could be helpful in the course of the trip—for example, if someone had a stomach upset, broke an arm or suffered a serious allergic reaction? Think about what you would be prepared and able to do in such situations. Of course, answering this depends on your training and skills, what resources you have around you, how serious the situation is, and who else is available to care. (Legal protection when taking on treatment responsibility in emergency situations was discussed in Chapter 3.)

Pondering the duty to do good

The definition of beneficence has some force because it creates a responsibility. Once you settle on the scope of what you define as beneficent, you may be obliged to assist in that way. On a broad level, once you train as a health care professional, you may be obliged to use your training where your skills are needed. That responsibility can be interpreted as an obligation to assist and rescue whenever anyone is in need.

Consequentialism or utilitarianism theories are teleological—the 'right' thing to do is that which maximises the good. The outcome of an action is what is ethically important. The greatest good for the greatest number is pursued. The good can be a specific utility or felicity (or happiness). Utilitarian theory aims for the smallest possible amount of harm and the greatest possible amount of benefit. For utilitarians, beneficence involves maximising benefit and minimising harm.

In some frameworks, a health care worker's own interests do not necessarily receive priority if the greatest good for the greatest number is the prime consideration. Australian philosopher Peter Singer believes that beneficence means that you must always act to prevent what is bad, unless something of comparable moral importance must be given up by performing the action—such as leaving yourself worse off than your potential clients. In Singer's framework, other people's interests are equal to our own (Singer, 1979, pp. 13–19).

This is not quite a positive duty—which is an obligation to actively seek out ways of doing good—but it is a duty to intervene to prevent harm occurring. For example, if harm is about to be experienced by someone because of lack of food, shelter or medical care, then preventing the consequent harm may require positive action—such as giving them some of your food, which would imply some degree of self-sacrifice. Another example of this prioritisation of duty to others is the way in which religious orders, missionaries and volunteers offer to place themselves in living conditions similar to their clients, and suffer great physical ordeals so that they can improve the lives of others. It often takes particular skill and special commitment to work in dangerous or exacting conditions. For instance, the rescue training for the ambulance paramedic service is described on one ambulance service website <http://ambulance.vic.gov.au> as intense, and physically and mentally demanding. Ambulance officers need the capacity to 'remain calm, think clearly and act quickly in stressful situations' (Ambulance Victoria, 2016).

It is up to you to decide whether you think the level of service promoted by Singer is an obligation or a sacrifice. If you see it as a sacrifice, then you would view those who make this sacrifice as Samaritans. More importantly, not to do it would not reflect badly on you at all.

The limits of a **duty to care** are more palatable to the professional if Singer's position is seen as a sacrifice, and this seems to be the professional consensus. Few health care workers would envisage their responsibilities to extend to 24-hour vigilance, or treatment for all people in all parts of the country or world. Being a counsellor doesn't necessarily mean that you are obliged to work in crisis situations that you find too stressful. You can fulfil your obligations to beneficence by finding your own niche, and satisfying yourself that the work in crisis situations is being done by someone else. However, there is value in following ethics

duty of care
An obligation to take reasonable care in dealings with a person, once there is an undertaking to provide care or advice, or contribute to such specific benefit for a specific person.

reasoning through to its natural extreme conclusion. Even if you do not agree with the ultimate position, it can help you to reflect on what you are able to accept, and the reasons why you feel comfortable with that position. In shorthand, the duty can be expressed in both ethics and law as duty of care, at least once that role or duty is accepted.

Beauchamp and Childress explored the obligation to be beneficent, and they suggested that it could only be determinate, and amount to a duty to rescue the other person, if their action (with their skills of course) was highly likely to be successful, and also essential, either alone or with others to prevent significant loss or damage to the other person. Further, the benefit to the other person should outweigh burdens to the carer or rescuer (Beauchamp & Childress, 2001, p. 171). Risk to self and burden is an important consideration, before obligation to rescue is accepted.

This position is echoed in codes of conduct or standard operating policies in modern workplaces, which emphasise safety to self and others in the course of your work. For instance, Paramedics Australasia outline understanding 'the need to establish and maintain a safe practice environment', including health and safety legislation and policies (for workers), and to identify and manage risks to safety, as a competency and therefore as part of the scope of practice of paramedics' roles and responsibilities and practice (Paramedics Australasia, 2011, Competency 3.a.2, pp. 5, 11),

You can nevertheless expect that your commitment to beneficence will be tested in your routine job, in unusual times of crisis.

REFLECTION: STAY OR GO IN A RISKY SITUATION

The following facts have been changed slightly from a real example from early 2003, when the severe acute respiratory syndrome (SARS) epidemic was reaching its peak.

At the time, it was unclear whether the epidemic of the flu-like illness was peaking, but it was clearly racing through populations in Hong Kong and regions of China, people had died in Singapore and Canada, and there were isolated cases in the USA and Europe. The sudden acute illness was affecting frontline health workers significantly, and schools were being closed and sections of the community quarantined. Daily updates on the number of people who had contracted suspected symptoms—as well as the number of people who had died from suspected or confirmed SARS—were issued by the World Health Organization (WHO) and local health authorities.

A local practice receptionist and health nurse, living and working in Hong Kong, with two young children, became worried that her work was becoming increasingly busy and demanding. She had seen her hours increase dramatically as people flocked to the local doctor to have any symptoms checked, and to ask about the symptoms of SARS. One of the practice doctors, an expatriate Australian, decided to take his family home, thus leaving fewer doctors and an increased workload for the practice. Those remaining were under stress, and were increasingly worried about their families if they should contract an illness from one of the patients. As the receptionist, she was the first to see

+ continued

any patients. She felt she had to make a decision for her family's sake on whether or not to keep working. What should she do?

How could you advise her to go about making her decision? If she is solely a receptionist, does she have the same higher duties as a health professional? How far do those duties extend if she is practising as a nurse? And what do you say about the doctor who returned home? Advise them. Try applying two frameworks to see if the resulting advisable actions are different.

Note the different extent of professional responsibilities and duties, and the varying weight placed on context, broader family duties and responsibilities by different ethics reasoning frameworks.

Under utilitarianism, a limited good is shared by maximising distribution on utility grounds. Deciding what you can do as a health care worker depends on what can be achieved by what your team or institution can offer to patients. The crucial test is whether it can bring about good—whether it really is beneficent. This decision as to whether or not it is good involves taking into account the other options available to the client. What you have to offer may not be appropriate. Jennett (1989) has provided a test—which is essentially a set of guidelines— for deciding when a specific treatment is inappropriate. He proposes that if the treatment satisfies any of the following five criteria, then it should not be used:

1 It is unnecessary because the patient is not seriously enough affected to need it, or the desired objective can be achieved by simpler means.
2 It would be unsuccessful because the patient has a condition too advanced to respond to or benefit from treatment.
3 It would be unsafe because the risks outweigh the probable benefits.
4 It would be unkind because the quality of life following the treatment is not likely to be good enough or long enough to justify such treatment.
5 It would be unwise because it would divert resources from activities that would benefit others to a greater extent.

This test has been used in individual treatment decisions, as well as in resource debates, because it takes into account the good that may be achieved for one person, as well as the good that may be achieved through the same or other means for others. You will read more about health care resource distribution debates in Chapter 5 and Chapter 10. It is possible to reject such utilitarian assumptions when making ethical decisions, as ethicists did when responding to a classic hypothetical scenario on predictive cancer testing (which is discussed later).

Professionals resolve ethics issues within their own practice with team and peer assistance, but sometimes they seek ethics committee assistance, particularly when there is a complex issue involving a large team, or conflicting views between carers and family.

In the USA, committee involvement in ethics decisions is more common, as ethics consultants are employed in large hospitals. The consultants sometimes have beepers and are on call for urgent consideration of ethics issues. Outside the USA, ethics committees concentrate more on policy formation in order to guide clinicians in complex cases in the future. These are not necessarily dramatic issues. They could be as 'simple' as when to allow care of a child to proceed without accompanying parents or guardians, or when to suggest a child be offered the opportunity to speak on their own with their carer. Or how to ensure specific groups of clients make the best use of the available services, given cultural or physical limitations. In some jurisdictions, clinical ethics committees provide case consultations.

Under deontology or absolutist frameworks, certain absolute rules guide conduct. Some acts must be done—because that is necessary to uphold a particular rule or rules—and some conduct is wrong and therefore must not be done—for example, because a particular rule or rules would be breached. The rules are commonly thought to be handed down from God, such as the sanctity of life.

Religious philosophies and ethics

Early Western writings on ethics were more obviously intertwined with religious philosophy and theology than is the case today. These writings struggled with the power of God, and the nature of man as related to the world and to God. Western philosophers transformed and challenged the church, particularly throughout the Reformation, and doctrines about man's manipulation of life emerged (Honderich, 1995, p. 761).

The religious philosophies of non-Western cultures are currently receiving attention in the context of health care ethics. Robert Veatch has written extensively on this matter (Veatch, 1989). Given the multicultural nature of many modern Western societies, it is increasingly common to find summaries in textbooks of the implications that different non-Western philosophies have for health care.

Some non-Western philosophies and **religions** give specific guidance on how medical practitioners should treat their patients. For instance, under Chinese medical ethics, which have Confucian, Buddhist and Taoist affiliations, modesty and hard work are valued. Under the teachings of Islam, a health professional should treat the person's body and mind, should encourage what is good, and should restrain people from doing what is bad. Virtue and equal treatment of rich and poor is emphasised, and certain rules are laid down, such as not procuring abortion (Devereux, 1997, pp. 14–23).

religion
System of faith and belief according to recognised sacred teachings.

If you are religious, your religion can—and probably does—affect your work as a health care worker. It is one of the things that forms your values and how you try to relate to others. It would be artificial to have two moral or ethical standards—one religious standard for purely religious life, and one professional standard for work. In Chapter 2, you may have noted that religion is one of the influences that helps define you as an individual. There are times when your religion will prompt you to examine your place in current health practices, either as providers or as consumers of services—for instance, abortion, euthanasia and blood transfusions. (Abortion was discussed in Chapter 3; euthanasia and blood transfusion are discussed later in this chapter).

Commenting on euthanasia from a Singaporean perspective, researchers noted that the vast majority of the Singaporean population was religious. Therefore, Singaporeans would be expected to react adversely on religious grounds to euthanasia, or any other issue (Singh & Gan, 1996, p. 40). Singh and Gan summarise the key Singaporean religious views, and identify the crucial rules or laws in those religious perspectives.

- Christians and Buddhists tend to value both life and non-interference with life affirmatively—Christians, because they believe life has divine origin; Buddhists, because they believe life has spiritual destiny.
- Muslims tend to view suffering as a mitigation of suffering in the hereafter, in accordance with Islamic law.
- Jews tend to hold the sanctity of life to be infinite, in accordance with Jewish laws.

Most legal systems uphold the right of individuals to hold religious beliefs, but not to impose them on others.

Traditionally opposing frameworks

Contemporary philosopher Robert Nozick has argued against libertarian rights prevailing. He is viewed as a deontologist, favouring a variety of theories that support actions that have been reflected on as right in themselves, independent of the end result or consequential state of affairs (Honderich, 1995, pp. 187, 629). His book *The Nature of Rationality* concentrates on the rationality of decision making and belief, with rationality seen as a special feature of being human, which is then used to formulate principles that can guide action (Nozick, 1993).

Deontological rules translate into duties to act or refrain from acting. Acting and not acting can have moral importance. There is also a philosophical debate about whether actively causing harm, or allowing harm to occur, such as through not intervening, is equally morally reprehensible.

'Smith and Jones' is a shorthand way of referring to a well known scenario illustrating a particular type of philosophical conundrum: the moral import of acting or not acting—of killing or letting die. In one version of this scenario, a cousin (Smith) actively drowns his younger cousin (Jones); in the other, Jones watches and does nothing while Smith drowns. Inheritance is a key part of the scenario: in both versions, one person stands to gain from the other's misfortune. Rachels argued that the bare difference between killing and not killing is not, in itself, morally relevant (Rachels, 1975).

REFLECTION: REFLECTING ON FICTION

A murder scene from a novel by P.D. James (1989, pp. 92–3) may help you decide if there is a moral distinction between acting and not acting, when harm seems to be the outcome of not acting.

In the scene, two children are playing in the garden while their father clears away part of the shrubbery. The father is using a sharp-bladed hook, called a billhook, to cut and pull away the overgrowth. Suddenly, the children hear him yell in pain and call for help. They both look from a distance and see him bleeding heavily, with a large gash on his thigh.

The older child, a boy, drags his sister after him, but instead of pulling her towards their father, he pulls her out of sight and into the orchard. She asks him to let her go so they can get help, but he holds her still against a tree. They wait there for a few minutes, until the brother releases her, and says that they can go now. When they reach their father he has died. The boy simply says that she has nothing to fear from now on.

- List why you think each each child in this scenario is morally responsible (or not responsible) for the harm, and why.

REFLECTION POINT

Options for 'action' or considered inaction

There are times when you, as a health care worker, have a choice about whether or not to act. As an exercise, role-play a health care situation in which there is a choice of acting or not acting, and demonstrate why you think each person in your role-play is (or is not) morally responsible.

There are a number of philosophical **doctrines** we can use to help decide if harm is morally our responsibility. One is the **doctrine of double effect**, a classic deontological tool, which poses a distinction between what one foresees and what one intends. Harm may be morally forgivable if it is foreseen, but not if it is also intended (Honderich, 1995, pp. 204–5). The responsibility for something bad occurring—even though a good was aimed for—is a key issue for health care workers.

The doctrine of double effect can also assist workers in their reflection. For example, a psychologist who encourages a client to face their phobias, intending, in the long term, to lessen their fears, may in fact cause the client to experience short-term anxiety. The psychologist can be forgiven if they had not intended to cause that anxiety, even if it was foreseen as part of the healing process. However, if the psychologist intended to cause anxiety for its own sake, they may be regarded as unethical because of the intention to cause harm.

The doctrine of double effect may also be relied in more extreme classic scenarios. For example, a pregnant woman with a cancerous uterus may be told that, in the absence of intervention, there is a high likelihood that both she and her unborn child will die. The woman may decide to have a hysterectomy, and it would be an unintended—but foreseen—consequence that the unborn child would be aborted. Under the doctrine of double effect,

doctrine
Tenet or lesson held out or taught as a true guiding rule.

doctrine of double effect
Ethics doctrine in which the intention of likely positive effects is considered to morally excuse certain foreseen negative effects.

it would be unethical if the bad effect (the abortion) were the means to the good effect (the curing of the cancer). It could not, however, be said of this situation that the abortion would be the means to the curing of the cancer. Rather, it would be the hysterectomy—in conjunction with further therapy—that promises to achieve that good effect. The doctrine of double effect attempts to achieve a balance between the good pursued and the harm that may accompany an attempt to do good. The action taken—in this case, the hysterectomy—must be good in itself, just as treating the woman for her cancer is good.

Some modern philosophers, such as Philippa Foot, reasoned that the crucial point is whether something is deliberately allowed, and this concept of deliberately allowing something encompasses both intended and foreseen consequences (Foot, 1985). Such philosophers would encourage us to acknowledge that harm from actions is often unavoidable, before weighing up the rights of the parties to decide whether we are entitled to bring about some benefit for one person when another may be harmed. Professor Foot has been described as a naturalistic ethicist, who has worked on virtue theory, and has explored the limits of utilitarianism (Honderich, 1995, pp. 283–4).

In Chapter 9 'Timeless quandaries at the beginning and end of life', you will read more about the timeless philosophical issues surrounding personhood and life, in contemporary law, ethics and regulation positions on reproduction and beginning of life. Later in this chapter, you will examine current discussion of laws and guidelines for dying with dignity and the end of life. Deontological positions continue to be prominent in these discussions.

A break with tradition to embrace pragmatism

There are further, more pragmatic ethics reasoning frameworks available to you.

Laws or other guidelines or standards often express a community's principled approach. **Descriptive ethics** can simply note the position taken in such rules, as it is a named interpretation of a social behaviour that has been judged to be right (to be encouraged) or wrong (to be discouraged).

A starting point in **normative ethics** is to 'state and defend the basic principles of morality' (Kagan, 1992, p. 223).

Relativism

Relativism is an example of an approach to the search for minimum acceptable standards that is often conducted when two groups differ on the appropriate course of action in treatment. Relativism is not compatible with deontology—in which rules are universally applied—but it can be used in combination with other moral theories, such as utilitarianism or communitarianism. Relativism takes note of the rules or values that are appropriate for the context in which decisions are made.

descriptive ethics
An ethics tradition demonstrating or noting the stance adopted, and not necessarily the reason for the stance.

normative ethics
An ethics tradition in which moral positions that are held are demonstrated and reasons for the adoption of those positions are also explored.

relativism
An ethics theory in which divergent perspectives are canvassed, with a view to establishing courses of action that are acceptable to those perspectives in their given context.

Under relativism, the question of what to do is defined with reference to the relevant acceptable boundaries for a particular context or culture, rather than by referring to strict rules. These boundaries are relative—that is, they are fluid and can change.

Harman is a philosopher who has defended relativism, a theory that suggests that there are no hard and fast rules in ethics. Rather, ethics can change depending on the perspectives of key participants in a dilemma and the stance of the group to which they belong. Not all people agree with relativism.

However, it is useful to think about relativism, because it stresses how an agreement can be reached between people with different perspectives on what might be best, or right. Harman claims that a judgment of proper conduct by one party towards another depends on the agreement between the two parties (Harman, 1975, p. 3). In a professional–client relationship, both parties should agree that what is being undertaken is proper. In the context of a health care team, the team should also agree that it is proper—but remember that they might agree for different reasons. Reaching this agreement does not necessarily mean minimal standards. In any contractual situation, an upper level, beyond a bare minimum, can be negotiated.

Proportionism

Proportionism acknowledges rules and values—but does not regard them as universal. It is quite a pragmatic theory, which, without using binding principles as a guide, takes into account the human nature of the person, the situation, and the intention behind the person's actions. Proportionism aims for a broad idea of good.

Doing the best one can is a common pragmatic approach to ethics. The proportionist would require that best is pursued in full knowledge of the ethics choices and practical alternatives. Proportionism is essentially a compromise between the extremes of absolutism and relativism.

As an individual's treatment progresses, circumstances and achievable outcomes change. A pragmatic approach such as proportionism looks for an acceptable resolution of difficult ethical dilemmas, rather than the 'right' thing to do. This relies on your own confidence in certain decisions. If a variety of ethics theories and reasoning would support a certain decision, your confidence would increase. If there is divergent opinion on what is best to do, your confidence would decrease but you could still choose a 'best' answer from among the alternatives, based on the weight of the reasons. Canvassing divergent options and divergent views from stakeholders, or interested parties, is the hallmark of pragmatism and proportionism, because a resolution is chosen, while still recognising that not all people will view it as 'right' or 'best'.

A user-friendly process for decision making in paediatric critical care nursing has been described by Daniel Wueste. Wueste's process takes into account the developing nature of medical indications and social circumstances of each case, and that the views of stakeholders on what is best to do can change over time, given what is at stake. At each decision point— such as whether to operate to correct serious birth defects; whether to offer transplantation;

proportionism
An ethics theory in which rules and values can be used as guides, but their application takes into account the practical alternatives in a given situation, with allowance for human nature.

and what to do when parents become less than compliant with management, perhaps due to social difficulties—resolution is aimed for not only with the greatest convergence, but also with confidence in an overriding argument if there is divergence (Wueste, 2005).

Proportionism acknowledges that individuals and communities will have different perspectives on the most acceptable course of action, and a pragmatic way forward is sought.

Communitarianism

Communitarianism places the community at the centre of a value system and its corresponding ethical analysis. While the individual members are acknowledged, it is the good of the community, its goals, and the threats it faces that are the key considerations. Communal and public goods are emphasised, and community views must be sought to unravel difficult issues.

Casuistry

casuistry
An ethics theory in which previous decision are analysed in terms of values, and factual and cultural contexts, and used to guide future decisions.

Casuistry is also a pragmatic addition to ethics. It emphasises the importance of understanding value-laden decisions in their appropriate factual context and culture. Starting with individual cases of conscience—and considering a proposed action—the question is whether that action would be in conflict with a law. It owes its early history to pastoral care assistance by priests; it then fell out of favour, but re-emerged in modern medical ethics discussions (Honderich, 1995, pp. 124–5). Legal case law reasoning traditions, such as discussed in Chapter 3, seem to be remarkably close to casuistry. Legal case law reasoning starts with the facts and context, and relates them to precedent. Precedent is law derived from previous decisions in cases involving the same or similar circumstances, or the application of statute law. To apply precedent in a legal context is to use a type of case-based legal decision making that applies certain legal principles derived from an accumulated history of case law to the particular facts of the dispute. In a similar way, thinking through each new ethics case prompts you to reflect on whether the same precedent applies, given the slightly varied facts and circumstances.

Applying different reasoning in practical situations

This section contains a few starting analyses to demonstrate the direction that ethics analysis can take, depending on which theoretical frameworks you use in your reflection. There is a reminder along the way to remember to check if any particular laws or regulations could help to focus your pondering, or highlight limits to the practical decisions you could make. You can use each of these reflections and examples as an exercise to expand on the analysis you started at the beginning of the chapter, and add your own ideas to complete your reflection. Ideally, you could return to your notes to keep adding ideas as you read further chapters.

REFLECTION: MULTIPLE ISSUES

Patients rarely have just one medical or health concern. Their social context is also complex. How you define 'health' will lay the foundation for your reaction to this case with Ms Tan. But first, consider whether your definition of health is as broad as that of the WHO, which includes the physical, mental and social wellbeing of a person. The definition of health, and the good to aim for as a health care worker, was discussed in Chapter 2, and is a central focus of Chapter 10 'Regulation and availability of health and community services'.

When you first met Ms Tan, she was 14 years old. She has a slight mobility disability from a congenital spinal problem, and a mild intellectual disability. With the aid of an interpreter—English is her second language—you arrived at a course of treatment and management for her recently diagnosed asthma in close consultation with her other health care workers and her parents. Now, three years later, Ms Tan returns. She has left school, is working part-time, and has more ambitious life priorities, in keeping with a young adult. She asks for your help in continued treatment, but also in gaining more independence from her family. She feels that they closet her because of her medical problems.

Deontological theory would emphasise the duties owed to Ms Tan as an individual, especially the duty to further good for her and limit harm coming to her, particularly intentional harm. There may be some rules that would preclude doing what she asks—and you would need to name them and support them with your argument before applying them strictly.

If you adhere to the ethics theories that place the most weight on patient autonomy, such as libertarianism, upholding Ms Tan's choices will be important to you, even if you do not agree with the choices she makes. You will be concerned with establishing that Ms Tan has capacity—or, as termed in earlier writings, is competent—to make certain relevant decisions and life choices. The issue of capacity is covered in Chapter 8 'Lifelong practice in decision making'.

Ms Tan's cultural and family contexts are especially relevant if you rely on proportionism and communitarianism frameworks. Both theories balance goals, such as life and health goals, with individual variation and choice in relation to these goals, according to cultural and societal limits.The question of whether allowing the choices Ms Tan wants to make will result in good for her, her family and society is a key factor in utilitarianism. This is because the good that is aimed for also has a societal context— that is, it has ramifications beyond Ms Tan as an individual.

So, while all theories rely on an obligation to care on the part of the health worker, they give startlingly different reasons for the existence of that obligation.

In this instance, contemporary legislation, regulation and policy is a practical guide. Australia has also made a commitment in principle to the international community to work towards full and equal civic participation for persons living with disability, as a signatory to the International Convention on the Rights of Persons with Disabilities (CRPD) (United Nations, 2006). This Convention is an expression of commitments made in previous human rights conventions, collected in one United Nations statement of

+ continued

rights for people with disability, to comprehensively reaffirm a commitment to promote and protect the rights and dignity of people with disability in society.

The Convention obliges member states to guard against discrimination, including in civil and economic life, and health services. The rights and integrity focus and respect for individual economic, social, cultural rights and the right to development is fundamental in many ethics reasoning frameworks, with the common ground between them expressed in the principlist expression of autonomy or respect for person. Australia signed the CRPD on 30 March 2007.

It is hoped that enhancing accessibility and choice of services and community activities for people with disability will become a routine part of all mainstream services and sectors, and this is set out by the Australian Government Department of Social Services in the National Disability Strategy 2010–2020.

The CRPD is welcomed by advocacy groups, but many consider more work is needed so that people are better protected from discrimination, abuse and violence, and unreasonable exclusion on the basis of their disability (Attard & Price-Kelly, 2010).

1   Can you think of a recent Commonwealth program that aims to support people with disability to participate more fully in the community?

2   Brainstorm the changes you have noticed in your community or health setting because of the program you mention in your answer to Question 1.

3   Suggest a reasoned action you could use to respond to Ms Tan's request.

Consider how a practitioner's experience will affect the reasonable expectations placed on them, even when a ward is busy.

PRACTICE EXAMPLE

Reasonable care

Jennifer Haines

Jennifer has been a Registered Nurse for 40 years and spent most of those years practising in critical care areas, ICU, CCU, Neurosurgery ICU and Emergency Department.

An experienced nurse of 30 years, Nurse A started her shift at 2200 hours. She was given a handover that indicated that one of her patients was deteriorating. The last observations done at 2000 hours show the patient had a temperature of 37.6°C and a small downward movement in blood pressure. Other than take the patient's temperature at 0200 hours, when it was 37.9°C, Nurse A did no further observations of the patient that night.

Nurse A wrote a note in the patient's progress notes at 0200 hours that all was stable with the patient. However, she didn't read the patient's notes. If she had read the notes, she would have found out that three doctors had documented that they were to be contacted immediately if the patient became febrile.

Nurse A did her first full set of observations on this patient at 0600 hours. By that time the patient was very hot, their pulse was racing, and they were profoundly hypotensive, tachypnoeic and desaturating on pulse oximetry. Nurse A called the doctor, who took an hour to arrive. The doctor diagnosed peritonitis and transferred the patient to ICU. The patient died later that morning in ICU.

1   Did Nurse A exercise reasonable care, skill and judgment for a nurse of 30 years experience? Why or why not?

2   What other actions should Nurse A have taken?

3   What professional standards apply to this situation?

4   What does this case teach you about your own future practice?

One situation nurses may face is when the patient's family demands medical treatment that the medical team considers medically inappropriate. Such a situation can raise a reconsideration of appropriate care and decision making for that care.

Seeking to offer the best appropriate care

PRACTICE EXAMPLE

Fiona Foxall

Fiona has been a Registered Nurse for almost 35 years and worked predominantly as an intensive care nurse in the UK and Australia.

Mr Cho is an 82-year-old man with a long history of emphysema and right-sided heart failure, considered to be as a result of cigarette smoking. He gave up smoking six years ago. He was diagnosed three years ago with vascular dementia and his resultant confusion is worsened by his poor command of English. Suki, Mr Cho's granddaughter, is his primary carer and she speaks English fluently.

Mr Cho has been admitted to a haematology ward in a very unwell state following a diagnosis of acute lymphocytic leukaemia, and it has been determined that he is suffering from pneumonia. The haematologist caring for Mr Cho has explained to Suki all the treatment options he considers reasonable for an individual of Mr Cho's age and general medical condition.

Suki is distraught and unable to fully comprehend all that is happening. She tearfully asks for all treatment options to be administered to her grandfather. She states that she believes there are other treatments available and wants her grandfather to survive at any cost—she also says that she believes that this is what her grandfather would want.

+ continued

The limits of treatment believed to be appropriate in Mr Cho's circumstances are repeatedly explained to Suki, as well as the potential difficulties that he would face should he receive aggressive treatment. However, Suki persists in demanding that all available treatments be administered to her grandfather.

1 Can Suki demand that treatments considered medically inappropriate by the doctor be given to her grandfather?

2 What are the legal issues raised by this situation?

3 What are the ethical issues raised by this situation?

4 In view of these legal and ethical issues, what would be the best course of action to resolve this situation?

The next Practice example provides concrete examples of beneficence and non-maleficence, balancing out doing possible harm with doing good.

PRACTICE EXAMPLE

The relationship between beneficence and non-maleficence

Jennifer Haines

You are treating a patient for a pressure area sore that is large and painful. They must be moved every two hours, which causes them discomfort even though they are given pain relief—which is arguably causing them harm. Pressure area care is necessary to promote healing—which is doing good.

• Is the conflict of these principles justified? To what extent?

You can apply a similar reasoning process to many practical procedures in nursing and other health care practices.

REFLECTION POINT

Translating conventions into policy and law

The process of signature and ratification is explained in a brief paper entitled *The Convention on the Rights of Persons with Disability*. This paper is available on the Australian Human Rights Commission website: http://humanrights.gov.au

1 Note your reaction to the process of translating conventions into policy and law. How does the process of translating conventions into policy and law protect each community's independence and sovereignty?

2 Is this protection important in your opinion?

A policy maker is aware that there can be many different ways of translating principles into practice, and sensitivity is needed so that the policies can be as effective as possible in diverse community contexts. The next Reflection prompts you to think about the community's capacity to support expensive treatment options.

REFLECTION: COORDINATING CHOICES

Imagine you are involved in a care program that is coordinated, in conjunction with many different health care providers in your local area. The money available for care is controlled by a central coordinator—in this case, a nurse—and the money is hypothetically capped for each chronic health problem.

Your client, Mr Helm, is in his mid-forties and has many complex medical problems resulting from a car accident five years ago. This accident left him with internal injuries. A new drug has just finished being tested, and has been registered. There is a possibility that the drug could significantly help your client, but it is not known if the results, as published in your professional journal, apply to him. The drug is also very expensive. Mr Helm does not know about the new drug. He comes to see you as part of ongoing rehabilitation, and expresses dissatisfaction with the current treatment plan. He wistfully says that he wishes there was something else he could try.

Coordinated care places emphasis on working as a team. In relation to any particular client, the objectives of care, arrived at by the team, are crucial. Discussing what each member of the team is aiming for is important, as you have read in earlier chapters. (Working models of managed or coordinated care are discussed in Chapter 10.)

Libertarian theories, in particular, would allow as much choice as possible to be made by the individual patient. The professional may be obliged to promote such a choice if they adhere to libertarian or other autonomy-based theories. Apart from issues of ability to make treatment and life decisions, there is an issue of information disclosure here. The professional holds information that may be relevant to the patient's choice. The importance of the patient knowing the relevant information before treatment decisions are made is discussed in Chapter 8. Paternalism—which contrasts sharply with libertarianism—may be at work if the practitioner or health care worker is withholding so much information that it effectively nullifies patient choice.

Deontology would ask whether the possible treatment really is better for this client. Research is essentially a balance of risks and benefits, as discussed in Chapter 7 'The limits of care'. This is the case in drug development and research, as outlined in the section on drugs in Chapter 7. Is a new untried treatment better than the myriad of treatments—and side effects—currently available to Mr Helm? This value judgment clearly needs to be made with professional clinical expertise and with the relevant medical facts available.

In the case example about Mr Helm, the facts are scant. If the risks include significant harm, the ethical obligation to care may translate into an obligation to protect rather than chance further injury. The chance of further injury can be hard to predict in situations where complex conditions are treated with multiple powerful

+ continued

drugs. You may like to consider whether you are sufficiently knowledgeable or skilled to deal with that drug, or with the combination of it and other medications that Mr Helm is currently taking (and will, no doubt, continue to take). The limits of skill are a central issue in caring, and this was the subject of the reflective exercise 'Learning and limits' in Chapter 2.

The obligation to provide the best available treatment is double-edged. You may have an idea of what is best, but is it 'available'? Certain utilitarian theories that hold that a good should be available to the greatest number of people gives society the ethical authority to limit the availability of resources. Under these theories, limiting the access that certain individuals have to certain resources is justifiable if those individuals consume 'too much' of the health care budget.

In addition to considering whether a community can afford to offer or deliver certain care, it may be prudent to consider whether there is community support for types of treatment or intervention being available at all.

REFLECTION: GAUGING A COMMUNITY'S COMFORT LEVEL

Innovations in medicine and health care pose challenges. Transplantation medicine has advanced, and surgery that is possible challenges us to consider whether it is acceptable.

The trial of facial transplantation for people who had experienced devastating facial disfigurement was considered early in the twenty-first century. In England, the Royal College of Surgeons (RCS) considered and reported on their position. The RCS discouraged full face transplants due to an anticipated inability to assess the physical or psychological safety of the process. In view of the difficulty in assessing the risks, they concluded that there would be a less than satisfactory consent process (Royal College of Surgeons, 2003).

As you will read in Chapter 8, informed decision making depends on the availability of good quality information on the risks and the likely benefits. The view of surgeons differs from country to country. The first partial face transplant was performed in France in 2005, for a woman with severe disfigurement from dog bites. It was reported that the surgical team waited for ethical reasons, but were ready and technically confident. The donor had agreed to be an organ donor, and the additional permission was sought from the donor's family for the face transplant. That permission was granted (Spurgeon, 2005).

There are implicit cultural tolerances of body parts beyond organs being 'retrieved' and used for others. Think about what you—and those working with you—would accept. If you are facilitating the group discussion, expect to hear different views, and encourage people to express those different views. Perhaps put up a body chart—if this is culturally acceptable for your group—and take a show of hands on what body parts should or could be transplanted. The aim is to gather as many views as possible within a short space of time—say, 10 minutes in total.

Later, on your own, try to describe differences in what each of you would accept in terms of different types of organ, tissue and body part transplantation. Identify cultural, religious, and personal limits to what each person would accept. There are some cultural taboos and religious prohibitions that guide everyday life for many people. Try to list as many of these as you can for yourself, then next to each one list medical interventions that you have heard of that would not be acceptable for you. Then consider if you would be prepared to offer them to someone else, even if they were not preferable or acceptable for you.

Questions of personhood may affect your reasoning on what part of a body, if any, could be used in transplantation or if alternative means of regeneration of tissue should be pursued. Issues of personhood are explored in Chapter 9. Considering the availability of organs for transplant, you may like to reflect on whether it is a gift from an autonomous person and their relatives, or if it is a community resource. This is explored further in Chapter 10. A utilitarian and a consequentialist would regard it as a resource, to be used for the end result that promises the greatest benefit for the greatest number. You could find out a little more about communitarian ethics, and consider whether you would be comfortable to apply what a community regarded as the best way forward in this instance. A communitarian would regard it as a resource, as under that framework, the community value is the most important arbiter of acceptability. On the other hand, a virtue ethicist would afford the professional involved far more importance in actively defining what rules or laws could be useful as safeguards, before perhaps negotiating a way forward.

In some ethics theories, reaching agreement on what is 'right' or 'ethical' may not be crucial. Some theories, such as proportionism, emphasise acknowledging difficult situations, diverse views, and guiding values and rules, and then simply doing the best you can in the sense of finding a path that is practical in a given context, and allowing for the fallibility of human nature. It is a pragmatic approach, and is ideally chosen with a knowledge of the ethical choices—including rules and values—and balancing those with what is practically achievable. Refer back to Chapter 2 for the use of community consensus in libertarianism and deontology.

Individuals' beliefs and convictions can affect the availability and delivery of many health care processes. Anticipating this diversity of opinion and conviction—and understanding that some people will not feel able to take part in certain processes—is part of effective health care delivery planning.

REFLECTION

Religious conviction and actions

Consider the following situation, which is adapted from a media report.

A taxi driver was allegedly called to pick up a package from a blood service and deliver it to a hospital. The package contained blood. The blood was urgently needed for an operation—but it never arrived. The blood was allegedly found abandoned near the driver's taxi depot, with the packets pierced and unusable.

What do you think?

If the driver did in fact dump the blood, and tamper with it, did he have a right to act on what seems to have been his religious convictions that use of blood was fundamentally wrong?

Conversely, did those who gave it to him have an obligation to ensure that he was agreeable to delivering the blood before they entrusted it to him?

Would any of your own convictions or religious beliefs prompt you to decline to take part in some health services? If so, explain what the objection would be, based on your conviction or belief.

conviction
Firmly held belief.

Any practices that challenge religious convictions can raise dilemmas for individuals holding those particular **convictions**. Any part of practice that challenges religious convictions is also ethically suspect for individuals who adhere to those faiths. For instance, Jehovah's Witnesses believe that it is wrong to place foreign blood matter into a person's body. Thus, for strict Jehovah's Witnesses, taking any part in a process that aims to place blood or blood-derived products into people poses a dilemma. Subsequently, problematic medical practices include not only blood transfusion, but any collection or use of blood products.

The hypothetical in 'Religious conviction and actions' stimulates discussion of what the bounds of acceptable behaviour are, who determines these bounds, and which should prevail: community expectations or moral and religious conviction? Bear in mind that the taxi driver is not a health professional. He has not sworn to abide by a code of ethics. He has not agreed with the charter of the hospital. Yet he, like many other non–health professionals, is involved in the delivery of health care services. He, like the millions of hospital support-staff (and ancillary staff) around the world, is one of the people who make the system—and the current set of health services—succeed or fail. You might like to consider whether any of the responsibilities and ethical aspects of practice discussed in Chapter 2 are relevant to the tax driver as a non-professional, and how rules and codes could apply. Kantian ethics would suggest that a categorical imperative should be universal in order to be a robust rule that should be pursued. If you feel unhappy with the consequences of the taxi-driver's action, and that this outweighs his personal convictions or desires, then you may be leaning towards the utilitarian reasoning frameworks. Jurisprudence scholars and philosophers might also point to the criminal law as an expression of penalty for conduct that a community finds unacceptable. As noted in Chapter 2, the community is able to define a limit and create a rule that has philosophical significance in many ethics reasoning frameworks.

You could look up recent standard operating procedures—it is likely you will find that it is no longer acceptable for a health service to use taxis for such deliveries.

People can express their professional autonomy by non-performance of certain procedures. Perhaps the taxi driver's action was an example of this: an expression of his choice not to be party to something he regarded as unacceptable. Is that any different from the way that some health care institutions do not provide abortions? Would the taxi driver be morally part of something that was sinful if he had delivered the blood for others to then use? Think about the difference between not being party to something, yet allowing it to continue to happen, and actively stopping such procedures from happening under someone else's purview. The difference between allowing a harm and actively causing it has relevance in many deontological and virtue ethics discussions.

Integrated contemporary ethics debates

Ethics tools and reasoning frameworks are evident in contemporary ethics debates, as well as in debates on law reform. This section contains an example of contemporary use of classic philosophical and ethics reasoning frameworks in thinking about end of life issues. You will find yourself thinking quite closely about the way ethics contributes to the setting of standards and the navigation of such complex professional practice issues.

Suicide

Suicide is the killing of oneself. Arguments about whether or not suicide is a legitimate action tend to centre on whether a person should interfere with their own life. Arguments against the legitimacy of suicide often rely on the 'God-given' sanctity of life; those supporting its legitimacy often rest on the principle that one's own life is a natural extension of autonomy (Honderich, 1995, p. 859). Proponents of each of these positions seem to agree that suicide attempts by people without capacity, who by definition are not acting autonomously, should be thwarted. Depressive symptoms, for instance, can often be seen in people who attempt suicide. Health care workers whose clients manifest suicidal tendencies often intervene to treat or refer the client for their depression, to ensure their safety and help them to return to competent decision making.

REFLECTION: FINAL PLANS

Ponder the following dilemma, which was written as part of a study about ethics in a general practice setting. The vignettes in the study were constructed in response to the ethics concerns of general practitioners and consumers, and were determined from a survey (Berglund et al., 1997).

+ continued

A 52-year-old woman has breast cancer with bony secondaries—meaning that the cancer has spread to the bones. She is not currently in pain and could, with treatment, have a good quality of life for two or more years. She tells her GP that she will not take the medication and that, after getting her affairs in order, she is going to kill herself. The GP discusses this with her, and suggests that she seek counselling, but the woman refuses.

Some six months later, the woman is found dead in bed, having overdosed on medication prescribed for a recent hip fracture.

1   Even if suicide is not illegal, aiding suicide still could be in many jurisdictions. Did the doctor aid the suicide?

2   Is the choice the woman's alone?

Euthanasia

Euthanasia literally means an 'easy death', or a 'good death'. It has been hotly debated, particularly in Australia with the debate over the Northern Territory law giving people a right to a physician-assisted death (*Rights of the Terminally Ill Act 1995* [NT]). Supporting patient autonomy—in part through comprehensive patient understanding of the extent and significance of their illness—was debated, as a safeguard that the decision to die is voluntary, and whether it was sufficient as the primary reason to allow voluntary assisted dying.

Participants in the original Northern Territory debate used key ethical terms in very different ways, as is demonstrated by a piece of research informed by a social constructivist perspective. By examining written comments and interviews about the issue in Australia, Oosterhof and colleagues found that while key players in the euthanasia debate relied on moral arguments—especially the concept of autonomy—they applied these arguments and concepts quite differently (Oosterhof, Scholten-Linde, Houtepen & Berglund, 1996). This analysis highlights the usefulness of reflection on the debate, as well as the importance of actually debating such a complex and emotive issue.

The passing of this Act was followed by the lengthy development of protective guidelines before a handful of people used the Act to gain medical assistance to die. The death of the first person to make use of the provisions under the Northern Territory Act was reported in the media. Although the first media report on his situation stated that he wished to remain anonymous, his name was revealed and his explanatory letter referred to in many subsequent media reports. The first media report was in 1996 (Alcorn, 1996). The general practitioner who cared for the person assumed significant notoriety, as he was willing to explain and promote the rationale of allowing an individual choice of this sort (Slaytor & Lesjak, 1997).

Subsequently, a private member's Bill, known as the Andrews Bill, designed to overturn this legislation, was introduced into the Commonwealth Parliament. Eventually the *Euthanasia Laws Act 1997* (Cth) overturned the Northern Territory law in the

Commonwealth Parliament, removing the right of the territory to legislate on euthanasia, so the Act was without effect.

The Commonwealth Act meant that euthanasia then returned to being judged as equivalent to murder or manslaughter. The initial Northern Territory Act and the process involved in its inception and its eventual defeat involved people at all levels of the community in active debate about euthanasia. Productive ethical reflection and debate does not only involve canvassing viewpoints—we also need to spend time defining the terms and clarifying what we are discussing. Poor definition of terms was one criticism that was made of the Andrews Bill. In particular, as noted by Cica, this Bill's failure to adequately define what is 'the form of intentional killing called euthanasia' may have skewed the debate (Cica, 1997). Although some attempt was made in 2018 for the Commonwealth to give up its restriction on the legislative authority of the territories (Judd, 2018), the Parliament did not proceed further with that Bill, so the situation remained unchanged. In theory, the Northern Territory law remains in place, and there may be further calls for a Bill to be put forward in Commonwealth Parliament to remove the effect of voiding the legislation.

Bills on dying with dignity are debated from time to time in other jurisdictions, such as in South Australia in 2016 and Victoria in 2017. Parliamentary debate provides an interesting insight into current discussion at community and government representative level on voluntary euthanasia, when a draft piece of legislation, called a Bill, is presented for discussion to parliament (*Voluntary Assisted Dying Bill 2017* (Vic)). Victoria's legislation passed both houses in 2017, after a series of debates and amendments were made to the proposed Bill (*Voluntary Assisted Dying Act 2017* (Vic)). You can look up the Victorian Parliament website to see that it was debated in the Council in the sittings 31 October 2017 and 2–3 November 2017; and in the Assembly in the sitting 17–19 October 2017. A State's law has a different status to a Territory's, as a State is self-governing over many matters.

After the law had been passed in Victoria, accompanying voluntary assisted dying regulations were developed to take effect on the date the law is in effect, 19 June 2019. The purpose of the regulations is to facilitate the objectives of the legislation that has been passed, setting out practical administrative requirements for the safe and effective delivery of the health service that has been permitted by law. The safeguards and administrative processes were developed within the Department of Health and Human Services, and with the benefit of expert input and wide consultation.

Recommended safeguards were set out in an advisory panel report. The recommended Victorian safeguards include regulations to ensure the following:

- voluntary access and eligibility criteria
- that the person themselves initiates a request, which is witnessed by independent witnesses
- that the person takes time to consider going ahead
- assessment processes
- that the person is informed of the diagnosis, prognosis and treatment options
- self-administration of medication

- delegated management for returning the unused medicine
- practitioner choice and protection within the legislation
- reporting obligations
- criminal sanctions related to falsifying records or inducing a person to act
- oversight by an independent statutory body (Victorian Government, 2017, pp. 180–2).

The regulations were then developed, to include practical safeguards such as:

- the person making two separate requests for a permit to access assistance to end their life
- a waiting time between first and final requests
- documentary evidence on the person's disease and diagnosis available to the Department Secretary who would grant the permit
- the person having decision-making capacity
- a plan for the disposal of the unused medicine with a designated responsible contact person.

Practical requirements, such as labelling the lethal medicine and safe storage box 'This substance will cause death', were set out (Dow, 2018; Victorian Government, 2018). One of the community safeguards is that the person has resided in the jurisdiction for a period of time. From a practical perspective, this means that the jurisdiction requirements, and reassurances, in documented form that will be sufficient, will be available to administrative decision makers in deciding to issue a permit.

This jurisdictional requirement is not always implemented in other countries. For instance, a Swiss hospital reportedly decided many years ago to allow patients from other jurisdictions with the intention of committing suicide to use their beds, with the explicit help of assisted suicide groups. A patient with an incurable disease, and of sound mind, could be admitted if a persistent wish to die had been expressed, and they were able to carry out the final act themselves. The hospital was reported to state their overriding principle of respecting the patient's wishes as determining their decision (Chapman, 2006).

As for any health decision that is made by a patient involving an ethical or moral element—even if legislation permitting voluntary assisted dying was passed in a jurisdiction, and regulations supported a practitioner involvement—a practitioner may decide not to contribute to the process. In addition, hospitals and health services can choose whether or not to support their practitioners and resources being involved in the delivery of particular services. As is the case relating to abortion, if the practitioner does not wish to assist in the process, they would be obliged to refer the patient to someone who would be prepared to discuss or investigate the issue. This discretion is part of the notion of professional caring. It is up to each professional to decide what type of care they are prepared and willing to offer—in other words, to define beneficence in their own terms. (See the discussion of beneficence in this and earlier chapters.) There may be a fundamental objection, or a more practical concern with the adequacy or nature of administrative and protective safeguards that were in place.

Other states, such as Queensland, are likely to bring on debates on the issue. When a Member brings a Bill to parliament, the debate on the floor of parliament is initiated, and time is set aside for that discussion.

REFLECTION: PRINCIPLES IN REGULATIONS

The process under Victorian legislation and regulation is represented in the flowchart in Figure 4.1 (Victorian Government, 2018).

FIGURE 4.1 PROCESS UNDER THE VICTORIAN ASSISTED DYING REGULATIONS

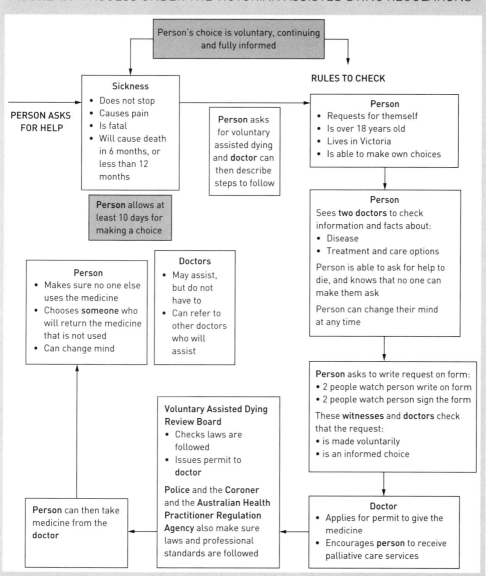

The Victorian voluntary assisted dying framework became publicly available in late 2018 (Victoria State Government, 2018). The steps represented in the flowchart are mainly drawn from the Easy English document about the voluntary assisted dying laws.

+ continued

There is a sense in the *Voluntary Assisted Dying Act 2017* (Vic) of the importance of establishing with sufficient certainty evidence:

- that the patient's illness is terminal
- that it is the patient, and not some other party, who is seeking the 'treatment'
- that there has been considered reflection—on the part of the patient—in reaching the final decision of their life.

As an exercise in identifying the nature of the key ethical issues in the process, tag the boxes in the flowchart with the principles of beneficence, non-maleficence, autonomy, or justice. The competent and autonomous nature of the decision is a crucial link in each step.

Euthanasia can mean many things; most notably, it can be 'active' or 'passive', 'voluntary' or 'involuntary'. Active, voluntary euthanasia, which is what the debate is currently about, is 'the deliberate hastening of death, on request by a person, to ease distress' (Baume, 1996).

In an early article on euthanasia, Anthony Flew argues that the will of even one individual who wants euthanasia can create a legal right to euthanasia. This argument relies on the importance of upholding a person's liberty, and on the suffering that would occur if their life were to continue (Flew, 1970).

Caution is often advised to safeguard against the possibility that euthanasia might occur in connection with less-than-extreme illnesses, or against the occurrence of active, involuntary euthanasia, in which people's lives may be ended against their will (Murphy, 1996). These concerns have been expressed in relation to euthanasia in the Netherlands, where euthanasia was illegal for some time, but prosecutions were not required by law.

Medically assisted euthanasia is now legal in Belgium and the Netherlands, and is regulated. Patients state their wish repeatedly, to their doctor, with whom they must have an ongoing relationship. Their doctor then seeks a second opinion and investigates alternative treatments that may provide potential improvement in the patient's condition, and notifies the review committee of the patient's request. Each case is subject to a review process before final plans are proceeded with (Smets et al., 2009). The **slippery-slope argument**—an argument that relies on the notion that allowing something in one situation opens the way for the same action to be used unacceptably in different situations—is often used in debates about euthanasia.

slippery-slope argument
An argument that small 'slips' in standards will lead to larger 'downward slides' and a degradation of standards, so that any small slips should be vigorously guarded against.

A cross-sectional survey of physicians asking about the use of euthanasia, physician-assisted suicide and other end of life practices in the Netherlands—and statistical analysis of all deaths and causes of death in the Netherlands in 1990, 1996, 2001, 2005 and 2010—has been reported in a leading American medical journal. In 2010, almost 20 years after the euthanasia legislation was enacted, euthanasia was the cause of 2.8 per cent of deaths, without significant increase if rates back to 1995 are considered, and continuous deep sedation up until death was more frequently used in 2010 (12.3 per cent of deaths in 2010, compared with 8.2 per cent of deaths in 2005). Other means of death were very rarely used and less often than before, including ending of life without a patient's consent (0.2 per cent in 2010), or a patient's decision to stop eating and drinking (0.4 per cent in 2010); of the latter, half had made an unsuccessful euthanasia application. The authors commented that the law had increased the transparency of end of life practices (Onwuteaka-Phillipsen, 2012).

There is also concern that a more fundamental discussion over adequate resources for services would be neglected. Part of the debate over the Northern Territory legislation was about whether fewer patients would be asking to die if more could be done to offer dying patients effective care and comfort in palliative care. This was echoed in the debate in the Victorian Parliament. In addition, there were calls for a closer examination of the social causes of suffering so that they could be addressed. Inappropriately relying on assisted dying as a solution to such problems, such as inadequate caring for the aged and elder abuse, would in itself be a slippery slope, as argued by leading bioethicists (Somerville, 2016).

The form of euthanasia that was supported in the now inactive Northern Territory Act can be called suicide or physician-assisted suicide. The procedure involved the patient initiating the process by pressing computer responses to confirm that they wished the fatal medication to be administered. Of course, the doctor had aided the process by setting up the equipment and preparing the fatal compound.

The first documented physician-assisted suicide took place in the USA in the 1990s. A former physician was with an Alzheimer's patient who had travelled across the USA to seek his help to die. The article that first reported this suicide is a useful starting point for discussion. The photo in the article shows the suicide 'device': three intravenous (IV) bottles connected up to a drip. The process is set up by the physician, then the drip is started by the patient pushing a button. The process begins with a harmless saline solution. This solution is then increasingly infused with two drugs to induce unconsciousness, and finally, heart-cessation and death. This article reports that the former physician, 'a long-time advocate of euthanasia, said he took the action partly to force the medical establishment to consider his ideas. He said he knew he might face arrest' (*New York Times*, 1990).

REFLECTION: ASSISTING WITH FINAL PLANS

Whether patients are entitled to ask for help with their final plans, or similar help, and whether doctors or other health care workers should provide it, are crucial questions. Examining ethics-related codes can help you to identify the controversial points in the euthanasia debate. Take one consumer code of rights and responsibilities, such as that set out for the Australian public health system in the *Australian Charter of Healthcare Rights*, available through the Australian Commission on Safety and Quality in Health Care website: <https://www.safetyandquality.gov.au>. You could also use the Australian Medical Association (AMA) Code of Ethics for this exercise, as a physician is involved under legislative provisions in all jurisdictions.

+ continued

> Try to identify points of possible support or opposition to the action that the former physician in the USA reportedly undertook. This exercise highlights the emphasis on patient autonomy, in both consumer and professional codes. It also underlines the importance in the context of euthanasia of assessing how ill someone is, and whether treatment options are available or have been tried.
>
> Regarding the dying patient, the AMA code of ethics states: 'Remember the obligation to preserve life, but where death is deemed to be imminent and where curative or life-prolonging treatment appears to be futile, try to ensure that death occurs with dignity and comfort' (AMA, 2006). There is a fine balance between allowing and promoting patient choices—and a patient's life-wishes—and bringing harm to patients.
>
> You will likely discover that there are some principles that can be interpreted as being in favour of professional assistance in euthanasia, and others that can be interpreted as being strongly opposed.

Some circumstances—such as where the client is too young to express a choice, or is otherwise incapable of doing so—can generate debate that runs for decades. This happened in a case in the early 1980s, where a newborn infant with Down's syndrome received only nursing care and painkillers, under medical instructions. The doctor was acquitted of attempted murder, and a debate began over issues of personhood, disability, treatment decisions and, more broadly, euthanasia. The case is the basis of Raanon Gillon's classic book *Philosophical Medical Ethics* (Gillon, 1986).

It is perhaps not surprising that debate over euthanasia polarises people's viewpoints according to their preferred ethics frameworks. Neil Brown has suggested that the debate is characterised by a split between utilitarians—who may consider actions that, although concerning or even harmful, will result in a desired end—and deontologists, who will always act to preserve rules such as the integrity and sanctity of life (Brown, 1996).

Summary

You should now feel more confident in recognising ethics reasoning that is drawn from certain ethics frameworks. You have learnt that ethics reasoning can be found in places other than ethics texts. It is alive and well in policy and laws—and is certainly active in the discussion and debates that are part of lawmaking and law reform. You have learnt from contemporary ethics debates on suicide and voluntary euthanasia that a jurisdiction's laws and regulatory frameworks represent community ethics positions, and that the legal limits are continually shaped by ethics issues and positions that are adopted by stakeholders in the debates. The debate is at the same time contemporary and timeless, as similar themes emerge in both ancient and modern discussions. Ethics frameworks can help—and the choice is yours to apply your own chosen framework in your reflection and reasoning.

STUDY QUESTIONS

1 Briefly describe the reasoning process used in three of the following ethics frameworks: deontology, utilitarianism, normative ethics, proportionism, relativism, casuistry.

2 Select one framework and comment on the 'Final plans' Reflection dilemma to suggest what, if anything, the GP should have done.

3 Choose an integrated issue from an earlier chapter. Select your preferred ethics reasoning process and apply it to suggest your preferred way forward.

SAMPLE ESSAY QUESTIONS

1 Research contemporary initiatives in elder care, and safeguards in relation to elder abuse.

2 Describe the current standards, and comment on the contribution of law, ethics and regulation in the formation and implementation of these standards.

REFERENCES

[ ]. Death with Dignity. *CCH Australian Health and Medical Law Reporter* (sections 22–268). CCH Australia: Sydney.

Alcorn, G. (1996, 26 September). Mercy death world first: Cancer sufferer first to die under Northern Territory euthanasia law. *Sydney Morning Herald*, p. 1.

Ambulance Victoria. (2016). *Become a paramedic*. Doncaster, Melbourne: Ambulance Victoria. Retrieved from https://www.ambulance.vic.gov.au/paramedics/become-a-paramedic/

Attard, M., & Price-Kelly, S. (2010). *Accommodating violence: The experience of domestic violence of people with disability living in licensed boarding houses*. People with Disability Australia. Retrieved from www.pwda.org.au

Australian Commission on Safety and Quality in Health Care [ACSQHC]. (2018). *Australian Charter of Healthcare Right*. Sydney: ACSQHC. Retrieved from http://safetyandquality.gov.au

Australian Government Department of Social Services. (2017). *National Disability Strategy 2010–2020*. Sydney: Department of Social Services. Retrieved from www.dss.gov.au

Australian Medical Association [AMA]. (2006, rev. edn). *AMA Code of Ethics*. Canberra: Australian Medical Association. Retrieved from http://amaq.com.au

Baume, P. (1996). Voluntary euthanasia and law reform. *Australian Quarterly, 68*(3), 17–23.

Beauchamp, T.L., & Childress, J.F. (1994). *Principles of biomedical ethics* (4th edn). London: Oxford University Press.

Beauchamp, T.L., & Childress, J.F. (2001). *Principles of biomedical ethics* (5th edn). New York: Oxford University Press.

Beauchamp, T.L., & Childress, J.F. (2013). *Principles of biomedical ethics* (7th edn). London: Oxford University Press.

Berglund, C.A., Pond, C.D., Harris, M.F., McNeill, P.M., Gietzelt, D., Comino, E., Traynor, V., Meldrum, E., & Boland, C. (1997). The formation of professional and consumer solutions: Ethics in the general practice setting. *Health Care Analysis, 5*(2), 164–7.

Brown, N. (1996). The 'harm' in euthanasia. *Australian Quarterly, 68*(3), 26–35.

Chapman, C. (2006). Swiss hospital lets terminally ill patients commit suicide in its beds. *British Medical Journal, 332*, 7.

Cica, N.T. (1997). *The euthanasia debate in Australia: Legal and political issues.* Topics for Attention Issues paper No. 2. Canberra: Australian Institute of Health Law & Ethics.

Devereux, J. (1997). *Medical Law: Text, Cases and Materials.* Sydney: Cavendish.

Dow, A. (2018, 26 September). 'This substance will cause death': New euthanasia rules announced. *The Age.* Retrieved from www.theage.com.au

Flew, A. (1970). The principle of euthanasia. In A.B. Downing (Ed.), *Euthanasia and the right to death* (pp. 30–48). Los Angeles: Nash Publishing.

Foot, P. (1985). Killing and Letting Die. In J.L. Garfield & P. Henessey (Eds), *Abortion: Moral and legal perspectives* (pp. 177–85). Amherst, Massachusetts: University of Massachusetts Press.

Gillon, R. (1986). *Philosophical medical ethics.* Chichester, UK: John Wiley & Sons.

Gillon, R. (Ed.). (1994). *Principles of health care ethics.* Chichester: John Wiley & Sons.

Harman, G. (1975). Moral relativism defended. *Philosophical Review, 84*, 3.

Honderich, T. (Ed.). (1995). *The Oxford companion to philosophy.* New York: Oxford University Press.

James, P.D. (1989). *Devices and desires.* London: Penguin.

Jennett, B. (1989). Quality of care and cost containment in the U.S. and the U.K. *Theoretical Medicine, 10*(3), 207–15.

Judd, B. (2018, 15 August). ACT, NT push for control of euthanasia laws as private Bill to restore rights reaches Parliament. *ABC News.* Australian Broadcasting Corporation. Retrieved from http://abc.net.au

Kagan, S. (1992). The structure of normative ethics. *Philosophical Perspectives, Ethics, 6*, 223–42.

Mill, J.S. (1975). On liberty. In *Three Essays* (pp. 92–114). London: Oxford University Press.

Murphy, T.F. (1996). Physician-assisted suicide and the slippery slope. *Department of Medical Education Bulletin, 3*(2), 1.

New York Times. (1990, 7 June). Doctor helped woman commit suicide. *Sydney Morning Herald*, 12 [reprinted from the *New York Times*].

Nozick, R. (1993). *The nature of rationality.* Princeton: Princeton University Press.

Onwuteaka-Phillipsen, B.D., Brinkman-Stoppelenburg, A., Penning, C., de Jong-Krul, G.L.F., van Deiden, J.J.M., & van der Heide, A. (2012). Trends in end-of-life practices before and after the enactment of the euthanasia law in the Netherlands from 1990 to 2010: a repeated cross-sectional survey. *The Lancet, 380*(9845), 908–15.

Oosterhof, J.E.J., Scholten-Linde, J.L.H., Houtepen, R., & Berglund, C.A. (1996). *The interpretation of morality: Cross-purposes in the Australian euthanasia debate.* (Unpublished Masters paper). Sydney: University of New South Wales.

Paramedics Australasia. (2011). *Australasian competency standards for paramedics.* Ballarat: Paramedics Australasia. Retrieved from http://paramedics.org

Rachels, J.A. (1975). Active and passive euthanasia. *New England Journal of Medicine, 5*, 39–45.

Royal College of Surgeons of England. (2003). *Facial transplantation: Working party report.* London: Royal College of Surgeons.

Singer, P. (1979). *Practical ethics*. Cambridge: Cambridge University Press.

Singh, K., & Gan, G.L. (1996). An Asian perspective on euthanasia. *Australian Quarterly, 68*(3), 36–45.

Small, M. (2007, 24 October). *The Convention on the Rights of Persons with Disability*. Australian Human Rights Commission. Sydney: AHRC. Retrieved from http://humanrights.gov.au

Smets, T., Bilsen, J., Cohen, J., Rurup, M.L., Dekeyser, E., & Deliens, L. (2009). The medical practice of euthanasia in Belgium and The Netherlands: Legal notification, control and evaluation procedures. *Health policy, 90*(2–3), 181–7.

Slaytor, E., & Lesjak, M. (1997). Euthanasia seminar. Public Health Association of NSW. *News, 11*(2), 7.

Somerville, M. (2016, 12 December). Margaret Somerville: Post-truth, euthanasia and elder abuse: The storm. *The Catholic Weekly*. Retrieved from www.catholicweekly.com.au

Spurgeon, B. (2005). Surgeons pleased with patient's progress after face transplant. *British Medical Journal, 331*(7529), 1359.

Sullivan, R.J. (1989). *Immanuel Kant's moral theory*. Cambridge: Cambridge University Press.

United Nations General Assembly. (2006). *Convention on the Rights of Persons with Disabilities and its Optional Protocol*. Annexed to resolution 61/106, Adopted by consensus on 13 December 2006, Ratified 2008. Geneva: United Nations.

United States Department of Health, Education, and Welfare. (1978). *Ethical principles and guidelines for the protection of human subjects of research*. [The Belmont Report]. Publication No. OS 78–0012. Washington DC: US Department of Health, Education, and Welfare.

Veatch, R.M. (1989). *Cross-cultural perspectives in medical ethics*. Boston: Jones and Bartlett.

Victorian Government. (2018). *Understanding voluntary assisted dying: Community and consumer information;* & *Voluntary Assisted Dying Laws: Easy English*. Melbourne: The Department of Health and Human Services. Retrieved from www2.health.vic.gov.au

Victorian Government. (2017). *Ministerial advisory panel on voluntary assisted dying: Final report*.Melbourne: Victorian Government. Retrieved from www.health.vic.gov.au/about/health-strategies

Wueste, D. (2005). A philosophical yet user-friendly framework for ethical decision making in critical care nursing. *Dimensions of Critical Care Nursing, 24*(2), 70–9.

LEGISLATION

Rights of the Terminally Ill Act 1995 (NT)

Euthanasia Laws Act 1997 (Cth)

Voluntary Assisted Dying Bill 2017 (Vic). Retrieved from http://hansard.parliament.vic.gov.au

Voluntary Assisted Dying Act 2017 (Vic)

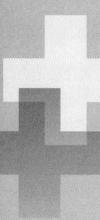

CHAPTER 5

Respect for a patient's journey

LEARNING OBJECTIVES

- To appreciate the significance of demonstrating respect for a patient in their health care journey.
- To practise defining the objectives of care.
- To be able to define and explain standards of information disclosure.

KEY TERMS

dignity

paternalism

respect

substitute decision maker

trust

veracity

wishes

Becoming unwell and seeking treatment

When you meet a patient or client for the first time, you meet a new person. A first guiding rule is to **respect** people for who they are, as an individual.

respect
Hold in high regard and esteem, and to refrain from interference with a respected person.

REFLECTION POINT

People you meet

Take a moment to think about the last client—or person—you met. What did you notice about them? What did they tell you about themselves? What makes this person different from other people? What makes them who they are?

1　Make a note of what you noticed about the last client—or person—you met.

2　What do you think people notice when they meet you for the first time?

When a person falls ill—or has a need for a health service—they are coming to terms with that illness or need and, at the same time, entering a health service, meeting you, and seeking your help.

INTEGRATED LEARNING AND PRACTICE

Why is the way you greet a patient important?

Ethics standards emphasise respect for a person and maintaining their dignity.

Legal principles support the clearly defined interactions in caring relationships between two persons, as duty of care is then assumed, and a process of communication begins which may lead to formal agreement to further interaction or treatment.

Regulation around respectful interaction is evident in patient and institution charters. Introducing yourself at the start of every shift is part of institutional policy, as part of a handover and as a demonstration of taking responsibility for aspects of care—for instance, if you have been allocated patients on a ward. It also shows that you are respecting the rights of patients to know how their care is being managed.

The principle of 'respect for persons'—otherwise known as the principle of autonomy—is about respecting the **wishes** and **dignity** of each person. Many people, when asked to respond to the question 'How do you respect people?', would write issues such as 'acknowledge them as people', 'listen to them', 'treat them with dignity', 'ask for and listen to their opinion', and 'give them privacy'.

wishes
Desired states, thought or actions that would bring happiness if attained or realised.

In practice, the principle of 'respect for persons' often revolves around individuals' freedom to plan and choose what will happen to them—that is, their right to be autonomous. 'Autonomy', derived from the Greek terms *autos* and *nomos*, means self-rule. In the context of health care this refers to the client having a degree of power over treatment decisions. A frequent misunderstanding among students is that it is about professionals deciding what should be done in any given treatment situation. While there is such a thing

dignity
Quality of worthiness.

as professional autonomy, the terms 'autonomy' and 'respect for persons' generally refer to client autonomy.

To be able to uphold people's autonomy, to uphold respect for persons, you need to know a little about them. But first, you need to put them at ease. Clients entering your health care service are likely to feel sick, anxious or scared—or all three. As a competent professional, you should strive to put people at ease. Once you have done this, you can begin to hear the client's story and understand them as a person. You need to know what has happened, what their symptoms feel like, what the client values, and what they would prefer. First things first: What is the problem? What brings them to a health care context? How urgent is it, and how much time do you have to work through the possible options in care?

PRACTICE EXAMPLE

Culturally competent palliative care

Susan Alexander

Susan has been a Registered Nurse for 12 years, working predominantly in palliative care and academia, and has a strong interest in professional issues.

Melanie is a 68-year-old patient who identifies as an Australian Aboriginal. She has recently been diagnosed with bowel cancer that has metastasised to her liver and lungs, and is currently hospitalised because of malnutrition and worsening dyspnoea. A CT scan has also revealed possible metastases to the brain.

The Western biomedical model of health suggests that patients be informed compassionately—but honestly and directly—about a terminal diagnosis. The ethical principle of autonomy supports this approach. However, people of Aboriginal and Torres Strait Islander descent prefer a non-direct approach when discussing such matters. They may even prefer for somebody else—for example, an Elder or community leader—to be advised, who will then advise the patient. Instead of using terms such as *death* and *dying*, it may be preferable to use terminology such as *bad news*, *sorry business* or *finishing up*. This approach still complies with autonomy because the patient is making decisions about who will be informed and the manner in which information is delivered. It is also complying with beneficence and non-maleficence, as harm can be caused to people if their cultural requirements are overlooked.

Melanie has requested the assistance of an Aboriginal Health Worker (AHW) who will contact her community Elders. The AHW will also contact a traditional healer, because Melanie has strong beliefs in the power of bush medicine. Although Melanie has not had a direct conversation with her oncologist, she realises she is seriously unwell and has requested that the Elders and community leaders begin planning for the return of her spirit to the land of the ancestors.

1　As a health care professional, reflect on your own responses to the idea that a person may require the services of a traditional healer while an inpatient in a modern, technologically advanced health facility.

2　Preferred terminology has been suggested. What other communication strategies would you adopt to optimise communication between yourself and Melanie?

3　What are some of the sources that you can access to develop your own knowledge of culturally competent health care?

Each client should feel that they are being respected. Each member of the team will contribute to that objective, with your input and guidance.

CASE EXAMPLE

Anh has yet another appointment

Anh's life seems to be full of tests and appointments and procedures at the moment. Next for him on his calendar is a pre-admission check and an ECG test, before a routine surgical procedure.

Anh had been thinking about an unusual, slow-growing lump at the top of his thigh for some time, but he was busy with other tests and a few heart issues, and put off doing anything about it. Now that things had settled down, he decided to ask his GP about it. A couple of ultrasound scans later, and with the lump likely to be lipoma, the next decision was whether to have it removed or keep an eye on it over time with more scans.

Given his preference, Anh's GP referred him to a surgeon, who agreed that surgery was an option, if the lump had become uncomfortable. Anh decided to go ahead as a public patient. He completed some pre-admission paperwork, with previous details, medical history and consent to the procedure. A few weeks later, Anh was asked to come to a pre-admission clinic the next week, as the medical director thought, given his cardiac history, he would benefit from this further assessment.

Arriving at the clinic, Anh waited at the desk with two others ahead of him, then he was greeted with a smile and his name was found on the list very quickly. The receptionist explained that he would see an anaesthetist and a nurse, and the visit would take one to two hours in total. He sat and was soon asked by the anaesthetist to come and talk to her in a private room. She introduced herself and patiently asked details about previous adverse reactions to medications and checked recent cardiac summary reports. She spoke with Anh about choices in anaesthetic approach, including that a general anaesthetic might not be needed. They agreed it could depend on the surgery logistics, so it could be discussed further on the day with the anaesthetist and surgeon as well.

+ continued

Anh was asked to return to the waiting area. He noticed that interpreters were waiting also and they and the patients they were accompanying to the clinic were greeted respectfully, so he guessed that was all pre-arranged and routine. On the wall in the waiting room he read a sign 'What can I expect from the Australian health system?' He agreed they got a tick for all areas listed: access, safety, respect, communication, participation, and privacy. He noticed the name on the sign, and that the main points came from a charter—the *Australian Charter of Healthcare Rights*. Within another 15 minutes, the nurse introduced herself and asked Anh to come to her private room. His blood pressure (BP), height, and weight were recorded. Clear information about the day of the procedure was given to him verbally and in writing. An ECG test was done, and the results shown to a doctor before Anh then left, with an 'All OK' message given to him. He thanked the nurse and the receptionist as he left.

Thinking about why the appointment process was so smooth and good, he reflected that the clinic was orderly and calm. Only as many people as could be seen were checked in, and the administration was efficient. Enough time was given, and each health carer was very clear and confident in their role. No one seemed rushed. He had already noticed the Patient Charter, and he also saw a printed message that the hospital was accredited according to the Australian Council on Healthcare Standards (ACHS) standards as he left the front door of the hospital. He left the visit feeling respected, safe and reassured.

Reflect on why Anh's visit was so positive. Think back to the issues on quality and safety and competence that you read in Chapter 2 'Standards for professional training and practice', as well as the principles of acceptable therapeutic interactions in Chapter 3 'How the law shapes health care' and Chapter 4 'An ongoing dialogue relying on ethics traditions'. You will be reading more on the integration of interpreter services, given the fundamental importance of patient information and consent processes, in Chapter 8 'Lifelong practice in decision making'.

CASE EXAMPLE

Monica's new journey has begun

Monica was worried that an occasional shaking in her legs when she stood still could be something serious. Her GP referred her to a private specialist neurologist, who asked for some tests to be done—pathology blood tests, brain CT scan, electrical impulse study—before Monica was due back to discuss the result.

The gap—that is, the amount above the Medicare rebate—for the first specialist appointment was about $200. The gap for the brain scan was similar. Monica waits to book the next test, so that all of the bills won't need to be paid in the same month. She booked in for the electrical impulse study as soon as she could afford to, knowing that it was important to rule out certain serious possibilities.

The waiting room was crowded and appointments seemed to be double-booked or running behind. The receptionist was distracted and curt—probably just overwhelmed.

Monica was surprised when a junior doctor came to collect her. He introduced himself, sought her consent to start the testing, and then commented that so many people with tremors can't stand up properly as their condition worsens, so he wanted to check if Monica could stand up for a few minutes for the testing. The initial readings were conducted. As the doctor started, he added, 'You'd be surprised, some people can fall over if you ask them to stand at all.'

The specialist doctor she has booked in to see joined the assessment for the last 10 minutes. After he introduced himself and double-checked the initial readings, both doctors turned their backs on Monica to concentrate on the machine readings. After a little while they exclaimed to each other, 'That's good!'... and after a short pause, 'Now you can clearly see the XYZ pattern ... there!' After a few moments, Monica realised that a good reading may not be 'good' news for her, even though their technical skills in capturing it were clearly top notch. She felt devastated, and isolated, and was quiet for the rest of the test.

She returns to the neurologist to discuss the findings, aware that the gap was now near $1000.

What would improve Monica's journey so far? The journey is a series of small steps, and all practical suggestions would be welcome. You may remember from Chapter 2 that communication issues are one of the most common complaints made about practitioners, health care workers and health services. Try to offer some suggestions from Monica's perspective.

Look at the Consumers Health Forum research, with a survey finding that out-of-pocket medical bills exceeding $10,000 have become common for some conditions, for surgery, and for other treatment and diagnostic tests (Consumers Health Forum of Australia, 2018). You will see scenarios dotted throughout this chapter that should prompt you to start thinking about different people and different situations in health care. It is quite routine in health care for situations to develop over time, and for different ethical challenges to emerge at different points of the process of care. Make your preliminary notes on this case—and the other cases when you read them—then return to them when you want to add more ideas to your analysis. You could use the cases as revision exercises for issues raised in other chapters.

Remember that when making your decisions in the future, you can rely on a rich tradition of reflection and analysis that can be found in the ethics writings of others. Listen to and learn from the decisions made by those who have worked in health care before you or who work alongside you, and actively reflect on your practice. The wisdom that you will build will serve you well in making robust decisions in your everyday practice.

The start of each journey is a significant moment for a patient. The initial decision to tell others about private information, to allow someone to touch us to see what is wrong, and to tell others something that is personal is at the heart of health care. We all have different thresholds of privacy, as the next Reflection exercise shows.

Getting to know clients is—at the same time as you begin to understand what has happened to them—is crucial. Unless you know a little about the client, it may be difficult to respect and promote their autonomy. You might need to know whether, for instance, when faced with difficult decisions, they would simply prefer to be left alone to think things through, or whether they would like to talk things over straight away. You might need to ask directly to find such things out, and you might need to undertake gentle questioning or negotiating to come to an understanding of what treatment or management plan the person would like or prefer—given a reasonable choice—and how they would like to receive it. Some standards of disclosure of treatment information rely on this mix of questioning and negotiating. You will read more about them later in this chapter.

REFLECTION: MAKE A WISH

We all have different thresholds in relation to being able to think about what we want, being able to express it, and being able to ask for something. We also have different thresholds as to how inclined we are to further other people's wishes. This is at the heart of who we are, and consequently is crucial to how what we want might be achieved. This brief exercise illustrates how very different we are from each other.

In a group setting, ask the following question of the person sitting next to you: 'If you could wish for anything, what would you wish for?' Make it clear that you want them to tell you only one wish! Then change roles, so that both of you get to tell each other your wish.

Some people have trouble thinking of a wish. Should you, if you believe in autonomy, help them to think about what they want? Or is it their right not to think of anything? If they have thought of something, but feel shy, should you help them to tell you? Or should you leave them be? You will be able to read a more detailed discussion on privacy later in this chapter, as well as in Chapter 6.

Once the wish is expressed, group members should think about whether it is in their power to grant the wish they heard fully, or whether they could help the person part way towards their wish.

In other words, do they agree it is a good wish, and do they feel able or obliged to help? Ultimately, do they feel obliged to help the person in their pursuit of that wish? Their answers will indicate something about how much they value autonomy in its own right. To further autonomy as an absolute right is to further the client's wishes regardless of whether it would be the professional's preferred wish.

Even if patients seek health care on their own behalf, be aware that individuals can approach their own role in their health care quite differently. Researchers have long recognised different types of consumers, including:

* the modern consumer—who makes demands and is assertive
* the traditional client—who feels powerless and relies heavily on trust (de Ridder et al., 1997, p. 557).

Some researchers have questioned whether clients want to be involved in decision making at all (Deber et al., 1996).

The Consumers Health Forum of Australia (CHF) is the national peak body for consumers. The CHF advocates for 'safe, quality, timely health care' supported by the best health information and systems the country can afford, advocating that consumers should learn how to take charge, by learning what to know and what questions to ask. You could go online to see short clips and featured stories on the CHF website <www.chf.org.au>.

Bear in mind that although the health care encounter may not have been initiated by the patient themself, they are still *the patient*, not the person or persons who organised the health care encounter on their behalf.

Clients expect to receive help when they are sick, and they expect to receive help so that they do not become sick. Our society is set up to provide this within reasonable limits, and you have chosen to train so that you are able to contribute to the health care endeavour. When you become a health care worker, others expect certain things of you—and you have taken on the responsibility of meeting those reasonable expectations.

In broad terms, we are all part of a reciprocity of interactions, expectations and benefits. This reciprocity was explored by the philosopher Hume. Hume made a distinction between natural virtue and artificial virtue. However, Hume's use of the word *artificial* did not imply that he thought artificial virtues lacked virtue. He used the word *artificial* to indicate actions that furthered the system of reciprocity that underpins society and aims to ensure the wellbeing of every individual (Honderich, 1995, p. 380).

All members of society expect to receive the benefit that living in our society promises. What consumers want is a reliable health system that is there when they need it. As a health professional, you play a role in delivering those benefits to others. To be successful, you will need to communicate clearly to clients what it is reasonable for them to expect, and what responsibility can be shouldered by the health professional. They do need to present to you for care first though—or do they?

What is your reaction to the next Reflection? Try to take the suggested analysis a little further.

REFLECTION: WORRIED ABOUT MUM

Ms B has recently moved from the country to an outer suburb of a large city to take up a student place at a college. She has two small children, and is receiving a government study subsidy and family support benefits. She is enrolled in a diploma course and hopes eventually to be able to support herself and her children, for whom she is the sole carer.

Ms B wants to arrange routine immunisation for her children, and visits a local GP. She takes their record of immunisation with her, which is entered in the back of the children's Child health book. This book, kept by Ms B, contains entries of the child health nurse visits from when they were babies, and the immunisations they had received. The children are examined, and a history of their health and previous illnesses is taken by

+ continued

the GP and noted in their new medical records. Both children appear to be well, and are given the vaccines that are due for them according to the recommended immunisation schedule. The vaccines were only given after checking that they didn't appear to have been given any of them previously—this was done both by asking Ms B and by reading the entries in the immunisation records.

Ms B is advised when to bring the children back for their next booster. A record of immunisation is entered into the Child health book, and also in the GP's own records. The GP bulk-bills for the children's consultation—not asking for money from Ms B for the consultation or vaccines—noting the Medicare and the Health Care cards that Ms B produced at the reception desk earlier.

The GP also asks Ms B whether she already has a GP for her own health needs since she has moved. The GP has noticed that Ms B appears to be thin, tired and withdrawn, that her teeth look chipped and damaged, and that her gums look swollen. She doesn't appear to be well. Ms B replies that she hasn't been to a GP as yet because she hasn't been sick. Then she volunteers that she was in an 'accident' in the country and is waiting for dental care. She says she can't afford to go to a private dentist, and had been on a public waiting list but hadn't yet heard whether an appointment was available. The GP offers the number for a local public dental clinic, and suggests that if Ms B rings, she may be able to have her appointment moved to that clinic.

Ms B returns at the next scheduled time. Both the children have a cold, and can't be immunised that day. The GP examines them, and rules out more serious febrile illnesses, but explains that the process of immunisation can have more serious side effects if a child is unwell, so it is safer to return the next week.

A week later, when Ms B returns with the children, she apologises that she has forgotten to bring their Child health books. The GP suggests that Ms B drop the books in to reception some time, or just to bring them along on a subsequent visit so the details can be updated from the GP's records. Both children have recovered, and receive their next booster. Ms B volunteers that a date for her dentist appointment hasn't been set yet, but that it seems possible to move it. She seems resigned to wait her turn. The GP worries that in the meantime there may be more gum deterioration, but feels that public dental care is really outside her control. She suggests that Ms B come for a check if she feels she has unusual tooth, mouth or jaw pain, or for other health issues.

Ms B continues to return at the relevant times for the children, but does not present as a patient herself. The GP continues to worry about Ms B's overall health—particularly given her heavy study load and sole caring responsibilities.

If you were Ms B's GP, what would you feel you could or should do? You could:

- find out about Ms B's entitlements to care under the current system

- check up on immunisation and treatment availability

- consider the immunisation strategies supported in state health budgets (as you will read in Chapter 10)

- note the immunisation regulations that are in place at a federal level (as discussed in Chapter 3), and whether the mandatory aspect of those are being upheld by Ms B

- investigate entitlements and interests (which are discussed further in Chapter 10)
- find out if Ms B is your patient yet, under the Medicare billing approach you read about in Chapter 1. If she is not your patient, do you still have a duty of care?
- think about your ethical obligations to care (as discussed in Chapter 2 and Chapter 4). If you decide your obligation extends to Ms B, should your approach be paternalistic, libertarian—or rely on a different ethics reasoning framework?

Dental health is a concern to the health departments, and different policy options have been explored.

The National Advisory Council on Dental Health (the 'Council') was established as a time-limited group to provide strategic, independent advice on dental health issues to the federal government, as requested by Minister for Health and Ageing. The Council's priority task was to provide advice on dental policy options and priorities for consideration in the 2012–2013 Budget. Apart from limited public dental services for those eligible, there is a concern that low-income workers who are ineligible for concession cards and lack private health insurance cover visit the dentist infrequently (Australian Healthcare and Hospitals Association, 2011, p. 5).

Encouraging someone to come along to a clinic or to make use of the opportunity for health education is a broader aspect of working in the health sector. Health promotion initiatives in the community are an important part of encouraging people to seek appropriate health care.

Trust and treatment relationships

As a health care worker, you are able to offer certain treatment options within recognised constraints. Some of those options are predetermined for you (as discussed further in Chapter 10 'Regulation and availability of health and community services'). Some options are decided by the type or level of training and skill that you have achieved, as discussed in Chapter 2 'Standards for professional training and practice'. Some options are decided by you, using your considered professional judgment, in consultation with the client. It is a delicate and complex partnership that requires an atmosphere of mutual respect and attention if it is to develop in a healthy way.

You routinely make promises in everyday life. For instance, you promise to do the washing up. You promise to meet your friends at a certain time and place. Do you keep your promises? Think of an occasion when you did not keep a promise that you had made to a friend or family member. How did the other person react and feel as a consequence? How did you feel?

Promises that are made without your intention to keep them place other's **trust** in you at risk. How much is in your power to promise is also crucial. Do you give others the impression that you can do more than you can—and so not keep promises? When someone

trust
Confidence in another person, or persons within an organisation, to act in an expected manner.

asks you for a favour to help them achieve a wish of theirs, should you promise to help regardless of whether you agree with their wish? Or is it less hurtful in the long run to state your disagreement, and your unwillingness to actively help? If you do agree—but doubt how much you can do—a useful technique is to say, 'I will try my best' rather than promise absolutely, making it clear that while you would hope to fulfil their wish, you may not be able to. You will have plenty of practice at this as a health care professional. Wishes are not acted on without professional consideration of objectives and logistics.

You need to find a way to engage in a care relationship if that is what the person wishes, and work together so that the expectations of clients and carers are similar and you understand each other's responsibilities. Professional responsibilities have been expressed, and are continually developing, in professional codes, as discussed in Chapter 2.

Patient responsibilities and expectations are now visible in patient codes, statements of patient rights, accreditation manuals and patient handbooks—for instance, the *Australian Charter of Healthcare Rights* (ACSQHC, 2018):

Those rights include:

• Respect—'I have a right to be shown respect, dignity and consideration.' This means that 'the care provided shows respect to me and my culture, beliefs, values and personal characteristics'.
• Communication—'I have a right to be informed about services, treatment options and costs in a clear and open way.' This means that I receive 'open, timely and appropriate communication about my health care in a way I can understand' (ACSQHC, 2018).

There is increasing emphasis on the active obligation of clients to be a part of the management plan, to take responsibility for attention to their treatment, and to take responsibility for their recovery and future health. The availability of information about professions and institutions may be crucial in forming appropriate client expectations.

Clients and health professionals engage in client–carer relationships with certain expectations of each other. One expectation held by carers, is that clients will **trust** you and will reveal their problem in detail, so that their care can progress. Disclosure on the part of the clients depends on trusting the carers and health care institutions.

In your health care relationships, your patients make decisions all the time about what secrets to tell, what to let you see, and how much they to trust you as health care worker to use that information constructively, and to respect it as private and confidential.

An appreciation of privacy is expected in relation to physical body exposure. A health care professional becomes used to draping patients so as to expose only as much of their body as is necessary, and to letting patients dress and undress in as much privacy as is possible. A respectful process of assessment is evident in the following policy guidelines, to:

• 'examine least intrusive areas first (i.e. hands, arms)'
• [carry out] 'painful and sensitive assessment last (i.e. ears, nose, mouth)' (Royal Children's Hospital Melbourne, 2017).

The relationship between a counsellor and client could be a useful way for you to think about meeting and getting to know your own clients or patients. A good counsellor–client relationship involves establishing trust and ground rules before tackling the difficult issues that have prompted the client to seek counselling. The initial stages of a counselling relationship have been identified as:

- meeting the client—during which time both the counsellor and client are on their 'best behaviour'
- discussion of surface issues—in which the client feels able to discuss everyday issues
- revelation of deeper issues—which occurs in the context of a developed relationship in which the client feels confident and trusts the counsellor (Burnard, 1994, pp. 96–7).

The counsellor's skill is in setting the client at ease through the initial stage, and gradually encouraging self-revelation (Burnard, 1994, pp. 96–7). It is a subtle art, and one that counsellors must master, as trust is required for an ethical relationship to develop. So much depends on understanding both your client and the problem at hand. You may, like counsellors, have the luxury of more than one meeting to achieve this. If you don't, your bedside manner is all the more important.

Defining objectives of realistic care

As discussed in earlier chapters, doing good can be defined differently by different professions, and the health system may only be obliged to deliver that good if someone has a right to it under the model of justice that operates in our society. However, bear in mind that ethics is an ideal and optimal standard of behaviour—so even if there are constraints, it is plausible to aim to maximise what is regarded as good. The principle of beneficence implies an ideal level of care. It goes beyond what is accessible or affordable, or a just claim. The decision to take on the responsibility of caring for someone underpins health care.

The heart of beneficence, of taking on a responsibility to care, is in considering the micro level of what is beneficial for the client, and in working towards the delivery of that benefit through the partnership between the health care worker and the client. The legal regulatory and ethical issues provide context for the type of care that can be negotiated, and the role of each carer in negotiating and delivering that care.

REFLECTION POINT

Ideals of care

Reflect on what sort of care you would like to provide, given an ideal environment for providing that care. Complete the following statement:

In an ideal world, the sort of care I would provide is …

Health professionals routinely take on new patients or clients, or refer them on to others if they feel they either:

- can't provide the care sought to the standard required
- can't provide care as effectively or timely as another professional.

There are many choices to be made in providing care, and many possible directions in treatment and care that could be negotiated.

In a practical context, what is usually negotiated is realistically achievable rather than ideal care.

Consider the situations in the next Reflection. See if you can develop the analysis a little further now, or perhaps make some notes now and return to it later after further reading.

REFLECTION: CARE AND UNDERSTANDING

Example 1

An 87-year-old man, Mr M, is in a nursing home. He is in reasonable health for his age apart from chronic hip pain and forgetfulness of recent events. Mr M was admitted after the death of his wife from cancer. The local GP said that Mr M had been about to have hip surgery but had postponed it to a few weeks after his wife's funeral. The nursing home is preparing Mr M for the trip to hospital for a hip replacement. Each time the process is explained to him, he forgets by the next day. The operation is booked for one week's time.

What should the nursing home staff do, and why?

Example 2

A nurse in the short stay unit of a tertiary hospital ask an elderly man what he has come for today. He says, 'I can't tell you. They don't tell you much anymore.' Further gentle questioning reveals that the man really doesn't know why he is there. He feels he hasn't been told. After asking her supervising nurse what she should do, the senior nurse tries also, with the same response. 'Ah, dementia,' she says, in earshot of the patient, but talking to the other nurse, as she walked back to her other duties. 'You won't find out more from him.'

Suggest how the situation could be managed.

Two models that summarise issues into meaningful clusters are those by Jonsen, Siegler and Winslade (1998), and the guiding rules proposed by Jennett (1989). These are clinically focused, and seem to be compatible with an analysis undertaken primarily by the clinician. If you were to start with Jonsen, Siegler and Winslade's model in your analysis, you would first try to understand the 'medical indications'—or what the medical situation facing the patient is. Then you would look for evidence of client preferences, consider quality of life and, finally, contemplate contextual features like the resources and so on. Note that you would summarise the issues in a different sequence than if you were using Beauchamp and Childress's model. Of course, some of the same issues would appear. The primary starting point is the health or medical issue to be dealt with, so the process is health–carer driven and seems, in that sense, to favour a carer's view of the important features to consider. This is similar to the 'enhanced autonomy' model for decision making, in which the decisions to be made are limited to those judged to be appropriate by the clinician. This seems a sensible emphasis, given that the health professionals are making themselves available to offer benefit to their patients.

Jennett's guiding rules—which you read about in Chapter 4 'An ongoing dialogue relying on ethics traditions'—could also help when deciding if a specific treatment is appropriate. If you were to apply Jennett's guiding rules, you would explicitly consider whether to apply a specific action or treatment option. So, it is important to identify the likely treatment options, and then analyse each one. You would consider whether the proposed treatment is appropriate, or rule it out if it is unnecessary, or likely to be unsuccessful, unsafe, unkind, or unwise. Some of these models emphasise judgments of care and likely benefit, some emphasise likely harm, and some emphasise issues of resources and justice. So, again, the elements that you would discuss if you used Beauchamp and Childress's principles appear in your analysis. Notice again, though, the emphasis of care issues, and a clinician's interpretation of those issues. There is little explicitly on autonomy built in to this rule-of-thumb analysis, except that each treatment is an 'option' or choice potentially to be offered to the patient.

A relativistic approach would gather up more issues to ponder than either of these models, or at least, emphasise the personal, cultural and community context of the issue, and acknowledge diverse perspectives on the definition of the ethically tricky issues and resolution of them. Mr M's own perspective, including his view of the facts and his preferences, is important—but not more important than the views of the health carers or the community that is providing the health care options under contemplation. He may also just need a little more time to settle and regain his equilibrium after his sudden and tragic loss. He is likely to be grieving for some time.

There are guidelines available to consider 'fitness to sign', and these are noted in Chapter 8 'Lifelong practice in decision making'. A legally robust decision is needed, particularly before elective surgery proceeds. Considering the legal aspects of decision making will highlight further issues. As you will read in Chapter 8, a possible shared or substitute decision-making process may be possible, but there are likely to be limitations to what can be agreed to, bearing in mind the necessity of the surgery for the best interests of the patient in their current circumstances. What lies ahead in rehabilitation should also be considered, as commitment to recovery and exercise and possible further treatment is foreseeable. Who will make those decisions?

Rapid identification of agreement with objectives of care

In many situations, health care workers think and act fast to identify the objectives of care and begin therapeutic intervention. There are practical regulations that support this in certain defined necessary and urgent circumstances—for instance, quick checks of whether a person is able to consent, and mechanisms for substitute decision making if they are not.

When people are rushed into hospital and some particular treatment needs to be given urgently, a mini-mental test is sometimes used to see if that person is able to consent to the treatment. If they are found to be not competent at that time, a relative's permission may be sought or an appointed guardian may be contacted.

Paul Appelbaum and Thomas Grisso are eminent commentators on consent to medical treatment. They completed a study of patients' abilities to consent to medical treatment in two hospitals in Massachusetts and Pittsburgh, USA. As you will read throughout this book, the current term for this ability is 'capacity for informed decision making'. Appelbaum and Grisso's sample included people who were hospitalised with acute, life-threatening conditions. They found that, like other patients, the acutely ill patients were able to give informed consent. Their judgment of ability to consent was made on the basis of the following four abilities:

1   Ability to communicate a choice.
2   Ability to understand relevant information.
3   Ability to appreciate the nature of the situation and its likely consequences.
4   Ability to manipulate information rationally.

Appelbaum and Grisso used specific psychometric instruments—techniques developed to test psychology and cognition—to measure these abilities (Appelbaum & Grisso, 1997). Their point was that even serious illness may not make people totally incompetent to consent. Appelbaum and Grisso's view is that the capacity to consent should be preserved and enhanced, because of its fundamental importance in maintaining the integrity we derive from determining our own lives.

Even if it is established that the client has limited capacity or competency, it may still be possible for them to make certain decisions—and this is valued highly in law and in current regulations. Social workers and residential carers of clients with cognitive or developmental disability advocate maximal autonomy for the client. There is a recognition that this is necessary because of the pursuit of autonomy, but also because exercising one's own life preferences support physical wellbeing and social integration (Newton et al., 1996). This recognition means that in the fields of social work and residential care, an awareness of the importance of autonomy and empowerment has for a long time routinely accompanied training in ethics or philosophy (Henry et al., 1996). The importance of autonomy was also addressed in a scenario in Chapter 4, and has been supported by international conventions.

substitute decision maker
Person who makes a decision on behalf of another, acting as a proxy or surrogate.

Bernat and Peterson have written on the issue of a nominated **substitute decision maker**, also called a 'surrogate decision maker', who may take over decision making for a patient who lacks decision-making capacity after surgical complications. While the patient may have consented to the actual surgery, once different post-operative decisions need to be made, the surrogate's decision comes under ethics scrutiny, particularly if it involves the refusal of further life-sustaining treatment. The authors argued that changed circumstances or complications make the surrogate's decisions more pertinent, and ostensibly different from the general consent to post-operative care that was given in a routine way by the patient prior to surgery. The expectation is that the patient's known views on incapacity and long-term disability would affect their surrogate's subsequent decisions in the circumstances of critical care. If the views are not known, standards of best interests can be expected to apply first (Bernat & Peterson, 2006).

Reflecting on potential dilemmas prepares you for how you might react, and what your options are. Taking on responsibility for caring was discussed extensively in earlier chapters, as it is an important preliminary decision point. Emergency or critical situations make a decision to care quite crucial. Any other help available and the seriousness of the patient's condition make a difference in deciding whether a health care worker should attend and assist.

The levels of duty to care can be debated in legal terms as well as in ethical terms. The commitment to help others (the 'Good Samaritan' principle) is recognised in such situations, and this means that even a professional who helps out without proper equipment and resources will, generally, be protected from being judged on the basis of professional standards that would otherwise apply. There is some latitude allowed to the health care worker because of the immediacy of the situation. As you read in Chapter 3, it is not an assault to touch and treat a person in an urgent life-threatening situation. The urgency of the situation allows for the presumption that care will be desirable, and may be necessary, as a life-preserving measure.

REFLECTION: QUICK DECISIONS

Try resolving this dilemma. The essential elements of this vignette actually took place, although the story has been slightly altered.

A person who is serving a custodial sentence is booked in for a minor operation. On the day of the operation, the inmate is transported from jail to the hospital in a prison van, with two corrective services officers in attendance. The hospital is undergoing extensive renovations, and the parking close to the hospital is very tight. The prison van is parked a block away from the hospital, and the corrective services officers accompany the inmate—who is soon to be a patient—to the hospital on foot. At the corner of the hospital block, just after crossing a road, the inmate attempts to escape. He runs away from the hospital, not back across the road, but down a side street. He is recaptured by one of the corrective services officers after suffering a gunshot injury, and is taken to the hospital.

Referring to legal, regulatory and ethics standards:

1   What should the person be treated for?

2   Do you think the person's consent to the original operation is still valid?

3   Should the person be treated only for the gunshot wound?

4   What should the health care workers do?

You could canvass the interests at stake, in terms of individual autonomy, the receipt of care and service, and the public's interests in efficient care provision. Is the fact that the patient is an inmate relevant in health care ethics? Why or why not?

Quality of life and perspective

Jonsen, Siegler and Winslade's (1998) model of ethical decision making centres on understanding the nature and extent of a medical condition and the realistic negotiation of care. Jonsen, Siegler and Winslade's model has the following main elements:

- medical indications
- preferences of clients
- quality of life
- contextual features.

Quality of life is a key part of the decision making in their practical model. Jonsen, Siegler and Winslade stress that quality of life is not just a summation of medical indications and what the future has in store for someone physically. They argue that the value that a person places on certain aspects of their wellbeing and life is part of their experience of the quality of living (Jonsen, Siegler & Winslade, 1998, p. 151). It is intertwined with an individual's perception and life preferences. Their position is that trying to assess this for someone else is, therefore, inherently difficult, and possibly fatally ethically flawed.

Quality-of-life measurement and quality-adjusted life years (QALY) are measures of life expectancy, adjusted for disability and pain. They reduce complex social and wellbeing factors to a single score. Increasingly, narrative has been suggested as a better way of understanding such complex qualitative concepts (Edgar, 1997). The narrative approach to ethics examines stories told by patients or professionals, or experiences recorded in published material, to understand what issues are prominent from those particular perspectives.

When QALYs are used to point to the relative successes of some treatments—and to justify funding certain health programs at the expense of others—this generates debates about ethics. The use of QALYs was one highly controversial aspect of the Oregon cost program, discussed in Chapter 10 'Regulation and availability of health and community services'. There is also concern that formulas developed for determining increases in QALYs in relation to a particular condition may lead to a false expectation of real benefit for all sufferers of that condition (Fryback & Lawrence, 1997). A significant issue is that the experiences of some patients are then generalised to others, so it is an average experience that is used as a benchmark, rather than the opinion of each patient given their own context and experiences.

Quality-of-life discussions highlight the practical and pragmatic aspects of negotiation of realistic care on an individual basis with each client. Some professions work more with quality-of-life dilemmas than others. For example, rehabilitation counsellors engage a client in constructive discussion and organise social, emotional and physical management plans to maximise the client's quality of life following an accident, illness or physically demanding experience—such as drug addiction. What they are aiming for is to maximise the health and the life choices of their client. Quality of life is a value-laden term. It prompts reflection on what you should aim for with your patients—what you could allow or facilitate your clients to aim for.

When the outlook for a client is poor, there may, at some point, be a debate as to whether treatment should continue. When children are involved, this debate can be particularly heart wrenching. The pain and suffering inherent in the child's condition, as key features of their quality of life, and in the proposed treatment, should be weighed against their expected life span. The extent of the potential benefit is ethically crucial in deciding whether to continue with aggressive treatment—for example, treatment that involves painful invasive surgery or other procedures causing pain and disruption to a child's life. The benefits should be weighed against the risks. For instance, prolonging life for a short time may not be a benefit that justifies as much risk as would the benefit of providing a potential cure (Leiken, 1989, p. 19). Adults may choose a time when, for them, engagement in active health care just doesn't seem worthwhile.

Given the emphasis of an indivdual's perspective remains central to assessment of wellbeing, quality-of-life measures are used and have continued to evolve. A Health-related Quality of Life (HRQL) measure was used by the Australian Government when gauging the disability related impact of health issues on individuals' lives, from their own perspective (Australian Government, 2000).

Preferences for involvement in decision making

Each treatment decision you contribute to is tinged with the ongoing debate about defining care, doing good and the extent to which the views of health care workers and clients should be taken into account in coming to decisions about treatment. The process of making treatment decisions is, therefore, dynamic. The same balance is not necessarily achieved in all decisions.

REFLECTION: TREATMENT PROCESS AND DECISIONS

In clinical situations, ethics issues centre on a real patient. Describe a case in which a decision of some sort needs to be made, and in which there are different views on what should be decided. If you or your fellow students have access to a clinical setting, try this exercise with the decision faced by a real patient, being careful not to identify the patient. You could also construct a case as a group, using a hypothetical patient.

You could concentrate on the structure of care. For instance, you might like to consider the choice of receiving and managing care for a chronic and serious condition at home or in hospital, or the choice of labouring and delivering a baby at home or in hospital. You could focus on a care objective choice, such as pursuing active treatment for an old injury, or continuing to manage it conservatively.

Gather as much information on the issue from the perspective of the patient and the family as you can. Analyse and interpret this to help in defining the dilemma. Then list possible alternatives for actions, checking these with colleagues, supervisors and a doctor on the team. Identify the most likely solution to the dilemma, and the advantages and disadvantages of each option. Try to keep your own views separate from the analysis of what the parties think. In a clinical setting, the next step would be to consult each party to see if a consensual decision can be reached, or if there is one course of action with the most agreement.

The Western cultural context is crucial in striking an acceptable Western balance between promoting client choice and choosing the best care on offer—in principlist terms, this is a balance between beneficence and autonomy. Health care workers from a Western background and context should be aware that striking this balance is not considered as important in some cultures: doctors and health professionals simply do the best they can for the client, and the client makes very few real decisions about their own care.

In some cultures, informed consent is not seriously pursued. It is not that health care workers are intentionally trying to limit autonomy or cause harm to clients, but simply that the health care workers do not think full information and choice will be most beneficial for the client. At a time of great vulnerability for patients, health professionals most want to care for the client; they want to take the burden of decision making so that the client can feel secure and gather their own resources for recovery. In some cultures, when a patient is terminally ill with few realistic treatment options available, professionals routinely would not disclose the prognosis, or even diagnosis, to the patient.

At the height of autonomy in Western health care contexts—and arguably far less favourable outcomes of cancer treatments—the custom of withholding certain information as an acceptable option was discussed, and noted to be a feature of health care in the past in some countries such as Japan (Hoshino, 1996). If judged acceptable by the standards of the context and culture and jurisdiction, health care professionals could inform the family—rather than the patient—of the bad news so that the family can ensure that they can make the patient comfortable (Brahams, 1989). Patients in these cultures may appear to be less self-determining—in a Western sense of autonomy—and may be reluctant to decide any serious matters without consulting their family (Hoshino, 1996, p. 12). Family consultation is uniformly and routinely included in many treatment settings nowadays, particularly in aged care and critical care settings.

Cultural preferences on physician disclosure of information—diagnosis, treatment options and prognosis—has been found to vary widely in a systematic review of available research literature in the USA. Despite great variation of views among minority groups—Hispanic Americans, Asian Americans, Eastern European Americans—when viewed as a group, more minority Americans prefer non-disclosure compared with individuals of white Western European background (Larkin & Searight, 2014).

That those in Western health care find a lack of information and lack of choice for the patient fundamentally unsatisfactory is a product of a preference for liberty (Berglund, 1997). A cultural emphasis on autonomy can also directly challenge a commitment to beneficence and non-maleficence. As you will discover in Chapter 7 'The limits of care', you must continually decide whether, as health professionals, you can collude in the facilitation of harm if clients want something that you regard as harmful. You must decide whether allowing and promoting autonomy is a good in itself, along the lines of libertarianism, or whether the good you value is something more derived, like health. Max Charlesworth supported the libertarian position in his classic text *Bioethics in a Liberal Society* (1993). The libertarian position is explored further in Chapter 7 'The limits of care'.

General standards and principles can help. Regulations and standards provide a practical limit to what is allowable, and may be helpful if you need to explain to clients why their care cannot be negotiated in exactly the way they are hoping. Regulations also provide a minimally essential position for the involvement and decision making of the patient in their care. You will explore informed decision making further in Chapter 8 'Lifelong practice in decision making'.

In deciding if someone can make an informed decision, the extent of their capacity and competence should be considered. Always keep in mind that exercising autonomy depends on the rational consciousness and reasoning capacity at any particular time.

Health care challenges and veracity

The health care worker and the client exchange and discuss information. Each continually takes stock of the situation facing them. This is where good notes can be invaluable. These medical records serve as a record of what happened and what has been explored, as well as thoughts on what might be useful to pursue. Information is so central to the assessment of conditions and options that it assumes key ethical significance. Information disclosure on both sides becomes a key dynamic in negotiating treatment. The health care worker often holds significant pieces of health information as a result of their knowledge of health sciences, their ability to interpret test results, and their conversations with other health professionals.

Information disclosure from a health professional to a client is probably best understood in a consultation context. A role situation such as described by Beauchamp and Childress entitled 'Non disclosure of prostate cancer' is useful as a starting point (Beauchamp & Childress, 2001, pp. 418–19). In this situation, a retired man has just had tests done as part of a routine physical check-up. His doctor knows that these tests indicate 'inoperable, incurable carcinoma'. The man has recently lost his wife, and is planning a trip overseas. The man, who is as yet unaware of the test results, visits the doctor who says nothing of the indications. After leaving the doctor's office, the man returns to ask, 'I don't have cancer, do I?' The doctor answers, 'You are as good as you were 10 years ago'.

This type of scenario illustrates weak paternalism in action. The doctor's response to the man's question is not the only possible response. It was the response chosen by the professional, for the moment, perhaps to put off telling the patient until a later date, perhaps because the professional wished to avoid imparting bad news. Telling bad news is part of health care, and it is dealt with later in this chapter.

The essential part of the dilemma is that the doctor had access to information that could have affected a patient's decision about treatment or management plans and also life plans. Should the health professional have told the man about his condition when he asked 'I don't have cancer, do I?' Weak paternalism in a trusting treatment relationship can be seen in many situations, such as in the classic ethics scenario, when providing fuller information was delayed. It has particular significance because joint input is needed for treatment decisions to be made. **Paternalism** can be at odds with **veracity**. Bear in mind the science and best practice information can constantly change, and the acceptable information to disclose will

paternalism
Decision-making framework in which care and control of another is undertaken.

veracity
Truthfulness, accuracy and completeness in information relied on by others.

change all the time, so every time a scenario such as this is considered, it is best considered with the most up-to-date clinical practice and scientific information.

You will remember reading about the tort of negligence in Chapter 3. In any treatment decision that is made, relevant information is needed from a professional so that the decision is informed. This is part of what makes consent to treatment valid. If a professional should have—according to the standard of information disclosure applied by the courts—disclosed certain material information, and did not, they could be found negligent.

Three information disclosure standards have emerged in recent debates about disclosure in the health professions:

- *The professional practice standard*—information given to patients by professionals that is that normally disclosed to other patients, and as disclosed to other patients by peers undertaking similar procedures.
- *The reasonable person standard*—information given to patients that a reasonable hypothetical person (in legal terms this person is referred to colloquially as the person 'on the Bondi tram', or in a British setting, 'the person on the Clapham omnibus') would want to know before considering the options and making an informed decision and consenting to the procedure.
- *The subjective person standard*—information given to patients that is normally disclosed by the health professional, or reasonably desired by the client, but tailored by the professional to suit the individual client's situation or specific concerns.

REFLECTION POINT

Standards of information disclosure

Returning to the Beauchamp and Childress scenario, try to think of the response that the doctor would have given under each of the three outlined standards.

Here are some possibilities, based on responses from other groups in the past.

- The *professional practice* group often has the doctor talking to colleagues to hear their view on what to do. The central notion here is that peer practice in similar situations determines acceptable disclosure.
- The *reasonable person* group often speaks in terms of what people usually want to know to make x, y or z decision. A fairly common approach in disclosing information is then taken.
- The *subjective person* group usually advocates entering into a conversation with the patient to find out whether the person really wants to know (or if they are asking not to be told). If the patient does want to know, the doctor then needs to find out how much the person would want to know before disclosing further information. This group requires an atmosphere of negotiation between patient and doctor.

The information disclosure part of the consent process can be contentious, with the type and amount of information on material risks—that is, material to the patient—at issue. This is an example of testing appropriate and feasible autonomy. Of course, standard information is more efficient to deliver than tailored information. A balance between the two approaches is sought.

How much information clients should have before they make decisions depends on the philosophical framework that clients, carers and our society are prepared to support. For instance, under a libertarian framework—in which each person decides what is best for them, and pursues their own best interests and happiness—the maximum information, and therefore the maximum corresponding choice, would be available to them. Max Charlesworth writes that under a liberal society, restrictions on autonomy would be limited. Governments could still discourage excessive individualism, and could promote 'altruistic concern for others' and 'a recognition of community values', but the basic autonomous agent must have the opportunity to make real choices (Charlesworth, 1993, pp. 3, 5, 6). On the other hand, under a paternalistic framework, lesser information and choice could be supported if such restriction was for the client's good. Strong paternalism, in which a client's expressed wish is overridden, is less common than weak paternalism, as Pellegrino and Thomasma write. Weak paternalism occurs when someone cannot give full informed consent or is not given the full range of options, and the physician decides in advance what might be in their best interests. Limited or sole options that correspond with this are then presented (Pellegrino & Thomasma, 1988, p. 7).

It is the reason for the lack of full information disclosure that is ethically critical here. The time available in consultation, knowledge of medical jargon, and so on could be presented as reasons for the presentation of limited information by a physician. Should any of these reasons be enough to impinge on the client's interest in full and informed decision making? You could reflect on why you presented fuller information for one client, or one procedure, and not for another.

The following dilemma is an exercise in using the principles to aid ethical reflection. The vignette is drawn from a study on ethics in the general practice setting in the mid-1990s: the author and a group of multidisciplinary researchers asked GPs and consumers of the services of GPs to nominate their ethics concerns. Vignettes were written to reflect these concerns, and the general practitioners and consumers were then convened to discuss possible solutions to the dilemmas contained in the vignettes (Berglund et al., 1997).

A 22-year-old man, Mr Y, had been very active until experiencing some unsettling symptoms. He saw his GP, had a lot of tests, and was eventually diagnosed with early-stage multiple sclerosis (MS). His GP said nothing much could be done at this stage, but advised Mr Y to stay active, and gave him something to help with that. The GP said that the medication was called dexamethasone, and explained the dosage required without giving further instructions. Mr Y was worried about the medication and was surprised to find out six months later, when he read the pharmacist's instructions, that he had been taking steroids.

In discussing the dilemma, many consumers focused on the responsibility they thought each patient should take to inform him or herself about the treatment being offered—this translates, in terms of the ethical principles discussed above, into the principle of autonomy. Consequently, they focused on the fact that Mr Y did not seek more information about the medication and did not read the pharmacy details until six months after purchasing the drug. However, the GPs wondered at the apparent paternalism of the doctor, who had decided that acting beneficently did not include allowing the patient to make an informed decision.

The balance between the possible long-term effects of steroids and the benefit in prescribing something to stave off early degeneration in MS could also be raised. If these steroids are thought to be beneficial, then under the principle of justice such drugs should be made equitably available to all those who might benefit. You could apply the same discussion to more recent drug treatments for MS. How then should the care be delivered?

There is a caution to be made here: justice is about the distribution of a good. This is different from the legal sense of justice. In other words, in ethics, justice is a resource issue, as is explained further in Chapter 10 'Regulation and availability of health and community services'. A further caution is that the autonomy at issue is the client's autonomy, not the professional's. (Autonomy is discussed in Chapter 4 'An ongoing dialogue relying on ethics traditions' and Chapter 7 'The limits of care'.) It is clear that, having summarised possible concerns, using the principles as an aid, further discussion needs to take place on the issues raised in the vignette. Neither the principles nor the summarising process alone solve the dilemma.

In a treatment relationship there will be points of progress and points of decline. There will be good news to tell in relation to progress, and bad news to tell if the prognosis or diagnosis is grim or is not what was hoped for. Some health care workers are better than others at being frank with their clients, just as some clients are better at hearing the truth than others. The willingness to relay bad news—for instance, to discuss imminent death with a patient, and the emotional preparation for it—is increasingly regarded as part of professional skill. If you choose to have an open and frank relationship with your client or patient, and this is a culturally influenced decision—as discussed earlier in this chapter—you are upholding veracity. Upholding veracity does not necessarily mean telling a client all the bad news in one sitting. When unfavourable results become available, it is common to have a number of meetings with the patient so that the information and its implications can be discussed, and future management can be planned as the patient gradually comes to terms with the bad news. Breaking bad news is a skill that can be learnt.

Any bad news told to a client needs to be relevant to the client and must be information that is used in the further treatment or management of the client's condition. How risk or information is conveyed can dramatically alter the dynamics of the client's recovery process. It is important not to destroy a client's hope, as hope is essential for recovery and for achieving the best quality of life possible (Surbone, 1997).

REFLECTION: ADMINISTRATIVE INFORMATION AND DECISIONS

Consider an administrative decision to close one-third of the 12 intensive care beds available in a tertiary care hospital over an upcoming holiday break. As a small group, discuss the ethical elements of that decision. Then decide what information should:

- be given to health care personnel working in the hospital
- be passed on to acutely ill patients
- be given to patients planning elective procedures.

In an ethics study on this topic, perceptions of clinicians and managers on the consequences of bed-closure decisions were analysed. Concerns were raised over fairness, accountability of the decision, and poor prior publicity of the decisions to key staff (Rocker et al., 2003).

Thinking about your local health institution context, how would you develop this analysis further?

You may want to concentrate on entitlements and access to resources, which is discussed in Chapter 10. You may consider the amount of information that should be available as part of ethically robust and legally valid informed decision making, as in Chapter 8, and if this sort of information is important to the consent that will be documented for any upcoming elective procedures. You may like to consider whether this decision is reviewable as would be consistent with the principles of fair administrative decision making, as in Chapter 3. You may think about the community's trust in a health care system, and the ethical importance of such system level decisions being checked with the community, as was discussed in Chapter 2.

There is some concern that professionals are not trained to uphold veracity, or be truthful, with sufficient vigour. This has been particularly noted in competitive training settings, such as medical school. While senior researchers have, with some surprise, discovered instances of cheating and lying by students, students themselves do not register the same level of surprise at these findings. Students reported doing what they can to get through. In her prize-winning essay on ethics, a medical student reflected on the way in which some of her fellow students lied and presented a false picture of their ambitions when trying to secure training placements in particular fields of medical practice (Young, 1997).

Young (1997) observed the discrepancy between this behaviour and the centrality, to medicine, of honesty in dealings with colleagues and patients, quoting the then current American Medical Association's code of ethics: 'a physician shall deal honestly with patients and colleagues, and strive to expose those physicians deficient in character or competence, or who engage in fraud or deception'. Veracity with colleagues and clients is part of the trust-forming relationship between society and professionals, and between individual practitioners and health care workers and their clients.

People are increasingly asking: If veracity is routinely degraded in personal lives, how can it be upheld with clients? Attention is now being given to reinforcing veracity in all dealings between those involved in health care—students, professional peers, educators, clients, and the general public—as a first step towards veracity in health care relationships. In the context of health care education, we should encourage students to say if they don't know something, rather than having them pretend that they know (and try to bluff). There is a danger, as there is for all professionals, that in pretending to know something, you may overstep the bounds of your own skill and make a mistake: a client may be given the wrong information, or a procedure may be conducted incorrectly. It is ethically responsible to acknowledge that you don't know something. Such an acknowledgment is an active reflection on the limits of your skill, similar to the skill-limit exercise you did in Chapter 2. When this happens, it is your professional responsibility to ask for help, but then also to remedy the deficit in your knowledge, to apply your new-found knowledge to the problem at hand, and to implement proper treatment once you know what to do. In short, it is acceptable not to know, and to admit it; but having done so, it would be ethically irresponsible if you then failed to remedy the gap in your knowledge or skill.

This discussion has focused on the disclosure of important information by the professional to the client. Some of the information disclosed could be test results, the client's physical status, and what treatment options were available and their concomitant risks and benefits. Recently, ethics and law has also focused on whether clients are entitled to see their own medical records for themselves, and whether they have a right to access those records. It is generally acknowledged that the client does not 'own' the record, as it was made in the course of treatment by a professional, for the purposes of professional assessment and management. The record includes *aide-mémoires* (French for 'memory aids' or 'triggers'), as well as personal information about the patient. Yet, as it is primarily about the patient, shouldn't the client be able to see it? Shouldn't there be frankness and veracity about its contents?

While the National Health Service in the UK supports patient access and control over electronic distribution of their own data, the British Medical Association expressed concern that if patients share their information 'online', they will have lost control over sensitive information, and also that narrative *aide-memoires* noted by the doctor may not be easily interpreted nor be appropriate for a wider audience (British Medical Association, 2011).

There is concern that some information could be harmful or distressing to clients, and that the information should only be available if professional explanation and counselling are also available. This concern amounts to a belief that any disclosure of information in health records should really be done in the context of normal consultative disclosure processes, and is less about veracity than about healthy and full communication between professionals and client. The main exceptions to a health agency providing access to records when requested by the individual about whom they are written are:

- if the record contains private information about someone else
- if having access to the record could affect the person's physical or mental health or wellbeing
- if there is an overwhelming public interest in lack of disclosure.

The interests in privacy and disclosure need to be weighed before such a decision is made. As you will read in the next chapter, holding something in confidence has a similar public interest importance, and breaching that confidence requires a consideration of competing interests.

The end of treatment

The ending of a health care relationship is a natural consequence of the beginning of that relationship. While the process of ending a health care relationship is studied by many—such as rehabilitation workers, acute care workers and counsellors—it is sadly neglected by others (Burnard, 1994, p. 103).

You may feel unable to offer care, and the end of your part in treatment may in fact be very early. There clearly is a difference between condoning an action and providing compassionate care for people affected by—or at risk from—that action. This is similar to the difference between, on the one hand, the obligation to provide care, and on the other, the obligation—in cases where clients have done something that we find abhorrent, or where we have ethical objections to the treatment they desire—to pass the responsibility for care on to others.

Health care workers occasionally come face to face with this difference. For instance, at the time of the 1996 Port Arthur massacre in Tasmania, the injured victims and the alleged gunman were brought for hospital treatment to the same emergency department. Workers dealt with the injured victims as well as the alleged perpetrator, all of whom were entitled to the best available care on offer. Those who felt that, if confronted with the responsibility of dealing with the alleged gunman, they could not place the best interests of the patient first, excluded themselves from the job of caring for the alleged perpetrator. A challenge to your willingness to care may be posed at any time by your cultural and moral sense of good, as is discussed by Olsen in relation to nursing (Olsen, 1993).

More routinely, when you have already become engaged in a caring role, once a task has been completed and the objectives of the relationship have been met, it may be time to move on to a new set of objectives. Of course, there can be reference points for reassessment. You can nevertheless stay in this cycle of defining objectives and monitoring progress repeatedly, as new objectives are set and health is monitored over a long period of time, if your role is to be available long term or if the process of treatment and management is a long-term process. Each phase of treatment and its objectives are therefore distinct.

Your level of satisfaction with the completion of a phase of treatment or the termination stage of a treatment relationship probably depends on the clarity of the goals identified early in the relationship.

Consider this case from the UK, in the context of reorganisation of aged care and home standards, public assistance for fees for residents, and allocation of subsidised care placements in designated homes. In the context of the start of this reorganisation, an elderly woman was required to move from the aged care home she had been in for some years. Her doctor opposed her move from the care home, believing that the 90-year-old's best interests were to remain in what she knew to be her home. Five days after the move, she died, and the GP reportedly entered the cause of death as 'acute stress reaction to the move', refusing to list natural causes of old age on the death certificate. He championed her care, and continued to champion her interests in opposing the authorities' decision, despite the public interest in imposing financial constraints of public monies for each individual's care provision. An inquiry ensued. The media coverage of the case extended over many months, and became a public petition for further government attention to the needs of old-age pensioners, and, specifically, individuals in aged care (*Gloucester Echo*, 2003; McVeigh, 2003). The commitment by the local doctor illustrates the nature of the strong responsibility the health professional feels to the individual patient. It is above the constraints of justice and imperatives to reallocate resources. The commitment continued after the patient had passed away.

If you, as a health care worker, are asked to do something you cannot or will not do, this may signal that your aims are incompatible with your client's aims, that the end (at least in part) of your treatment relationship is imminent, and that your client should be transferred to another health care worker. It may be useful to ensure that the client understands the full implications of what they seek, and why you feel you cannot be involved as their health care worker. When nothing more can be achieved by active treatment, the focus can properly shift to care and comfort. Health professionals find this particularly difficult when dealing with young patients, but it can be difficult with many other patients as well (Sorlier et al., 2001). Team support in recognising the decision to shift the focus of care is helpful not only for the patient but also the health carers.

If the treatment relationship deteriorates for any reason, the patient may need to be referred to another health carer. So, a treatment relationship can end even though treatment is not yet complete. A transfer can be effected with professionalism, and without apportioning blame. The issue is determining the best way to proceed with care for the patient—and that takes precedence over individual feelings of disappointment.

To have a client return time and again when there is really no need, other than force of habit, could be viewed as overservicing. The health care worker may be taken to task by their peers—overservicing implies that the service is not being provided to meet a clear and reasonable objective. It may still be financially rewarding for the provider, but may not be providing any real or relevant service to the client. This dilemma highlights the importance of re-examining the good that is intended in any treatment relationship, and the fundamental assumption that care is relevant and appropriate if it is to be lawfully funded under the public health system, as you will read in Chapter 10.

Medicare has a compliance program to identify fraud and billing at rates higher than are justified. Providers are liable to repay the full amount of the service (Australian Government, 2016). Under the *Health Insurance Act 1973* (Cth) at section 3, a professional service that attracts a Medicare benefit is defined as a 'clinically relevant service', and breaches of the provisions of the Act can be the subject of Professional Services Review. The Australian Government Professional Services Review was established to combat over-servicing and inappropriate practice. (See <www.legislation.gov.au> for the legislation and <www.psr.gov.au> for details on the Professional Services Review.)

Summary

You have learnt that by focusing on the individual client or patient's journey, you can reflect on practical aspects of health care standards, which are intended to support a safe and acceptable health care journey for every person. You have learnt about the practical aspect of upholding patient rights and respect for each patient's integrity in every health service encounter, as each encounter is part of a patient's health care journey. You will now be able to identify the legal and ethics underpinnings of these fundamental standards.

STUDY QUESTIONS

1 Thinking about a health care patient who has embarked on their health care journey and is midway through their treatment, explain the theoretical importance of respect for that patient.
2 Illustrate how you can uphold a patient's dignity, and give reasons for why you should or would uphold a patient's dignity.
3 Describe the information disclosure standards and explain in your own words what they mean for practice. Illustrate your explanation with your own hypothetical case situation.
4 Referring to statutory legal standards in Chapter 2 and Chapter 3, highlight two examples of unacceptable conduct and two examples of prohibited conduct.

SAMPLE ESSAY QUESTION

1 Give three reasons why good quality communication is important in health care. Support your statements with ethics, law and regulation examples.

REFERENCES

[ ]. (2003, 29 July). We're improving our care services, *Gloucestershire Echo*, p. 9.

Appelbaum, P.S., & Grisso, T. (1997). Capacities of Hospitalized, Medically Ill Patients to Consent to Treatment. *Psychosomatics*, *38*(2), 119–25.

Australian Commission on Safety and Quality in Health Care [ACSQH]. (2018). *Australian Charter of Healthcare Rights*. Retrieved from www.safetyandquality.gov.au

Australian Government, Department of Health. (2000). *National Survey of mental health and wellbeing, health-related quality of life, mental health of young people in Australia, 2000*. Retrieved from www.health.gov.au

Australian Government, Department of Health. (2016). *Fraud prevention and compliance: Increased billing assurance for the Medicare Benefits Schedule*. Canberra: Australian Government.

Australian Healthcare and Hospitals Association. (2011). *Policy paper on oral health*. Deakin, ACT.

Beauchamp, T.L. & Childress, J.F. (2001). *Principles of biomedical ethics* (5th edn). New York: Oxford University Press.

Berglund, C.A. (1997). Bioethics: A balancing of concerns in context. *Australian Health Review*, *20*(1), 43–52.

Berglund, C.A., Pond, C.D., Harris, M.F., McNeill, P.M., Gietzelt, D., Comino, E., Traynor, V., Meldrum, E., & Boland, C. (1997). The formation of professional and consumer solutions: Ethics in the general practice setting. *Health Care Analysis*, *(5)*2, 164–7.

Bernat J.L., & Peterson, L.M. (2006). Patient-centered informed consent in surgical practice. *Archives of Surgery*, *141*(1), 86–92.

Brahams, D. (1989). Right to know in Japan [letter]. *Lancet*, *2*, 173.

British Medical Association. (2011, 11 January). Information revolution could mean patients have more access to records. Retrieved from www.bma.org.uk

Burnard, P. (1994). *Counselling skills for health professionals* (2nd edn). London: Chapman & Hall.

Charlesworth, M. (1993). *Bioethics in a liberal society*. Cambridge: Cambridge University Press.

Consumers Health Forum of Australia. (2018). *Out of pocket pain: The $10,000 issue*. Deakin, ACT: Consumers Health Forum. Retrieved from www.chf.org.au

Deber, R.B., Kraetschmer, N., & Irvine, J. (1996). What role do patients wish to play in treatment decision making? *Archives of Internal Medicine*, *156*, 1414–20.

de Ridder, D., Depla, M., Severens, P., & Malsch, M. (1997). Beliefs on coping with illness: A consumer's perspective. *Social Science & Medicine*, *44*(5), 553–9.

Edgar, A. (1997). A discourse ethics approach to quality of life measurement. In A. Surbone & M. Zwitter (Eds), *Communication with the cancer patient: Information & truth*, *Annals of the New York Academy of Sciences*, 809, 30–9.

Fryback, D.G., & Lawrence, W.F. (1997). Dollars may not buy as many QALYs as we think: A problem with defining quality-of-life adjustments. *Medical Decision Making*, 17(3) 277–84.

Henry, D., Keys, C., Balcazar, F., & Jopp, D. (1996). Attitudes of community-living staff members towards persons with mental retardation, mental illness, and dual diagnosis. *Mental Retardation*, *34*(6), 367–79.

Honderich, T. (Ed.) (1995). *The Oxford Companion to philosophy*. New York: Oxford University Press.

Hoshino, K. (1996). Information and self-determination. *World Health*, *5*, 12.

Larkin, C., & Searight, H.R. (2014). A systematic review of cultural preferences for receiving medical "bad news" in the United States. *Health*, *6*, 2162–73.

Jennett, B. (1989). Quality of care and cost containment in the U.S. and the U.K. *Theoretical Medicine*, *10*(3), 207–15.

Jonsen, A.R., Siegler, M., & Winslade, W.J. (1998). *Clinical ethics: A practical approach to ethical decisions in clinical medicine* (4th edn). New York: McGraw Hill.

Leiken, S.A. (1989). A proposal concerning decisions to forgo life-sustaining treatment for young people. *Journal of Pediatrics*, *115*(1), 17–22.

McVeigh, A. (2003, 22 July). Violet Townsend inquiry reaction. *Citizen*, pp. 12–13.

Newton, J.S., Ard, W.R., Horner, R.H., & Toews, J.D. (1996). Focusing on values and lifestyle outcomes in an effort to improve the quality of residential services in Oregon. *Mental Retardation*, *34*(1), 1–12.

Olsen, P. (1993). Populations vulnerable to the ethics of caring. *Journal of Advanced Nursing*, *18*, 1696–1700.

Pellegrino, E.D., & Thomasma, D.C. (1988). *For the patient's good*. New York: Oxford University Press.

Rocker, G.M., Cook, D.J., Martin, D.K., & Singer, P.A. (2003). Seasonal bed closures in an intensive care unit: A qualitative study. *Journal of Critical Care*, *18*(1), 25–30.

Royal Children's Hospital Melbourne. (2017). *Clinical guidelines (nursing) nursing assessment*. Melbourne: Royal Children's Hospital. Retrieved from www.rch.org.au

Sorlier, V., Forde, R., Lindseth, A., & Norberg, A. (2001). Male physicians' narratives about being in ethically difficult care situations in paediatrics. *Social Science & Medicine*, *53*(5), 657–67.

Surbone, A. (1997). Truth-telling, risk, and hope. In A. Surbone & M. Zwitter, *Communication with the cancer patient: Information & truth (Annals of the New York Academy of Sciences)*, *809*, 72–9.

Surbone, A., & Zwitter, M. (Eds). (1997). *Communication with the cancer patient: Information and truth (Annals of the New York Academy of Sciences)*, *809*, 72–9.

Young, T. (1997). Teaching medical students to lie. *Canadian Medical Association Journal*, *156*(2), 219–22.

LEGISLATION

Health Insurance Act 1973 (Cth)

CHAPTER 6

Personal information privacy and public interests

LEARNING OBJECTIVES

- To appreciate legal and professional obligations to safeguard health information.
- To appreciate overriding obligations in matters of public interest.
- To appreciate public interest considerations in the conduct of health research.

KEY TERMS

compulsory	privacy
confidentiality	private interest
conflict of interest	public health
liberty	public interest
mandatory	

Privacy, confidentiality and public interests

You have read about the patient's journey through health care. For a patient, some parts of their health care are intensely private matters. Only they know how significant and personal a piece of information is for them. They may choose to discuss certain issues with family and friends who are close to them—but then again, they may not.

The following Reflection challenges you to reflect again on the objectives of care that you have considered in Chapter 5 'Respect for a patient's journey'.

REFLECTION: CAN A WISH ALWAYS BE ACTIONED?

Sometimes clients choose to limit how many people know about their medical condition, even when they are quite ill, as in the following scenario.

An ambulance is called to a house where a woman in her late 50s has had a cardiac arrest. Many of her relatives are visiting for a family gathering, and most of them are highly emotional about the situation and unsure what to do. The ambulance crew starts basic resuscitation measures, working through a routine protocol, when the local GP, who has also been called, comes rushing around the corner and says, 'Stop'. The family look totally startled, as do the paramedics.

Can you guess why the GP might have said 'Stop'? Perhaps the GP knew something that the ambulance officers didn't know—and even something that the family didn't know. What the GP knew was that the woman did not want active treatment in the event of a life-threatening situation. She did not want active treatment because she wanted to die quickly rather than linger, and she was greatly influenced by the fact that she had terminal cancer, which she had not disclosed to her family. She had chosen to keep that a secret so she could enjoy whatever time she had left without her family and friends worrying unduly about her. That was her choice and, as it happened, she suffered a heart attack prior to the expected rapid deterioration in her health. The GP's knowledge of this was the reason he called out to the ambulance crew to stop active resuscitation. Unlike the family, the GP knew the woman's secret—and he also knew her wishes. She had been unable to inform the ambulance officers of her wishes because, by the time they had arrived, she was almost clinically dead.

Whether the GP is able to action the secretive wish and ask the ambulance officers to stop depends partly on the question of when health care workers should stop active care. The standard operating procedures of the ambulance officers begins when they are called to attend. Some of these regulations and guidelines are available on the services' websites, such as <http://www.ambulance.gov.nsw.au> for the Ambulance Service of New South Wales, which notes the guidelines are publically available due to legislative requirements in the *GIPA Act (Government Information [Public Access] Act 2009 [NSW])*. The presumption is that paramedicine regulations require the implementation of protocols of care, in the absence of clear authority otherwise. The ethical choices available in the next steps in care were partly discussed in Chapter 4 'An ongoing dialogue relying on ethics traditions', and you will also read more on the difference

+ continued

between care and comfort on one hand, and active restorative treatment on the other—provided appropriately documented decisions have been made in other chapters.

The GP's role and relationship with the woman was quite different. This made it feasible that a different priority for immediate care could be confidently identified. You may like to consider if the wishes were documented, and whether they were clear to the standard expected in advance care directives. You can read more about contemporary developments in advance care planning in Chapter 8 'Lifelong practice in decision making', and the specific regulations that would apply if the scenario was considered in the presence or absence of an advance care directive.

You know that you are in a private domain as health care workers because you hear personal details and see personal things that are not routinely disclosed or seen. You are in this privileged position so you can help.

Imagine a friend tells you a secret, which you know is quite personal and has been difficult for your friend to discuss. Soon after, you and your friend have a falling out. When chatting with some mutual friends a few weeks later, you use your old friend's situation as a humorous example of the problems people can get themselves into. Everyone has a laugh, but you feel terrible afterwards, convinced that what you did wasn't 'right'. So, what is the problem with that type of gossiping and breach of earlier confidence? Perhaps you can express it in terms of potential harms, or in terms of previously agreed obligations.

We can and do choose to keep some secrets in our social interactions. Yet we also know that some information needs to be disclosed in the course of everyday life. We seem to accept this in relation to dealings with many institutions, such as when we disclose details to our bank, the taxation department, our employers, and so on. Some health information needs to be disclosed for treatment to be selected and provided. Some of this information is private, but that does not mean that clients need to tell everybody everything, or that health care workers should expect to know everything about their clients. You need to know as much as is necessary to provide proper care, and no more. Your respect for your client's individual integrity is demonstrated by allowing the client to make a decision about what is too private—or unnecessary or unacceptable—to disclose.

Whenever we have disclosed information that is private and personal—personal even if only because it has our name on it—we do so with an understanding of why it was asked for, and what it will be used for. Personal and private information includes:

• verbal information
• information about one's body
• disclosing one's body to view.

It is when that personal information potentially becomes available to a wider audience that we become worried about privacy and confidentiality. We are worried because we have lost some control over how and what the information is used for. Once information is potentially available to a broader audience, we further trust that those who seek access to it are authorised to have this access—and that they will respect it.

REFLECTION: PREFERENCES FOR PRIVACY

In a group, turn to the person next to you and tell them a secret about yourself. Tell them something that you don't necessarily want everyone to know. Before you tell them, alert them to the sensitivity of the information by asking them not to tell anyone else. If you think of something but decide you really don't want to tell anyone, let them know you'd rather not say anything. Then, count how many people had a secret that they decided to tell, and that they therefore entrusted to their neighbour. Make a note about how you feel having decided to disclose a secret, or having chosen not to—at least for the moment.

You may prefer not to take part in the exercise. Either way, the feeling of vulnerability or potential vulnerability, is as close as you can come to the hypothetical situation of a patient who is faced with a decision about whether to disclose something private. Remember the feeling, and also note that everybody has made their own personal choice on disclosure given their own reaction to the opportunity to disclose something private.

Those people who chose not to tell their neighbours anything in the information disclosure in the Reflection exercised their right to privacy, and we might think of those people as being inherently private. Those people who told a secret now have to trust that their neighbour will not tell anyone else, and that the confidentiality of that secret will be upheld.

INTEGRATED LEARNING AND PRACTICE

Are you staying in or opting out of My Health Record?

It is a matter of intense public debate whether centralised electronically available health records for a patient's own care can be available across treatment settings and providers—and also managed so that privacy is protected. In Australia in late 2018, individuals were asked to consider whether they would prefer to opt out of a centralised My Health Record system. This system was ready to roll out nationally after a lengthy trial.

You could find a media commentary on this issue, or look at the Parliament of Australia website for information on a Senate Committee inquiry that was initiated in 2018: <www.aph.gov.au>.

The additional mechanisms that are being debated to further safeguard the system involve ethics and human rights debate, along with legal and regulatory standards. Privacy safeguards are central in this discussion, prompting the *My Health Records Amendment (Strengthening Privacy) Bill 2018* (Cth). Keep this contemporary debate in mind as you read more about personal information privacy. The debate highlights the public interest in maintaining information privacy, and guarding against unwarranted disclosure, and a different public interest in allowing reasonable access to information for certain purposes.

privacy
State of secrecy or concealment.

confidentiality
Limited distribution of another's personal information, due to respect for privacy.

Privacy and **confidentiality** have re-emerged as a prominent ethics issue in the modern electronic information era. Privacy and confidentiality have always been an ethics concern. They are integral to maintaining human dignity and are concerns derived from the principle of 'respect for persons' (Flaherty, 1989, p. 9)—otherwise known as autonomy. You may remember that respect for persons is essential in ethical dealings with clients and patients. The challenge in modern societies and health care institutions is to balance the commitment to respect, privacy and confidentiality with the need for information about individuals. Access to personal information is increasingly regulated. Laws have been strengthened to protect privacy. There is an integrated effect of law, ethics and regulation on privacy on all aspects of personal information that is collected, stored, accessed and distributed in health care contexts.

The issue common to both privacy and confidentiality is respect for an individual's control over their own personal information. Information privacy issues centre on control of access to personal information. Confidentiality issues are derived from privacy; confidentiality relates to control over the use or further disclosure of that information.

In practice, privacy relates to what personal information should be collected or stored, while confidentiality is concerned with the storage, security and use of personal data that has already been stored (Westin, 1970, pp. 6, 7). It is important to understand the difference between privacy and confidentiality because so many debates and guidelines rely on the distinction. Consider a 'Private & confidential' notice on an envelope. The word 'private' implies that there is no public right of access to the information inside—only authorised persons should open the envelope and read its contents. To comply with this instruction is to recognise the interest that individuals have in being able to limit access to information—in other words, their rights to privacy. The word *confidential* implies that those persons who are granted permission to read the contents have an obligation to guard against further lessening of individual privacy—for instance, by preventing non-authorised persons from reading the contents of the document. It also means that their use of the information should take into account its confidential nature—its substance should not be revealed to others (Berglund, 1990).

This explanation illustrates the limited direct control that individuals have over their private information, beyond the initial disclosure. Individuals rely on their confidants to maintain desired levels of privacy and to use the information in the expected manner. They also rely on those who are not granted access to the information to respect that situation.

Think about what you might do if you received a letter that was not intended for you. You could return it to the sender, or pass it on to the person who is the rightful recipient—if you knew that person—without opening it. To open the letter would be to pry. That feeling of prying is what you get when you invade someone's privacy. The rule that you should not open or read other people's private correspondence is fairly straightforward. However, you might receive correspondence where the name on the envelope is very similar to your name and to the name of a colleague. What would you do then? One solution would be to open the letter together, and together read one line at a time until you identify whom it really belongs to. That way, neither person would read more private information than was needed to identify the proper recipient.

Some simple safeguards with regard to privacy and confidentiality can be undertaken at your work.

You might be asked to sign a confidentiality undertaking that you will not knowingly access any personal information—such as in health records or electronic medical records—that you do not need to access in order to carry out your work responsibilities properly and efficiently. This includes a declaration that you are aware of your obligations under the relevant privacy legislation, such as the *Privacy and Personal Information Protection Act 1998* (NSW) and the health privacy principles contained in the *Health Records and Information Privacy Act 2002* (NSW). Comparable privacy legislation is in place in other states and territories.

Routine audits of electronic access to patient files are conducted in institutions, as part of their institutional governance safeguards. When well known people attend a service, it is highly likely that an audit of who accessed their records will be undertaken. This highlights members of staff who have not been involved in their care and who may have breached their obligations to only access relevant information. Further disciplinary action is then probably implemented, as this is potentially a serious breach of acceptable processes and procedures within an institution. (For more about the process of investigating departures from acceptable conduct, see Chapter 2.)

INTEGRATED LEARNING AND PRACTICE

Why is guarding against a data breach so important?

Ethics reminds you that the information and control over it is centrally important to respecting a person's integrity.

The law expresses the community's support for being proactively careful in how personal information is collected and stored.

Recent regulations make data storage everyone's priority in health services. The mandatory notification of data breaches mean that data storage is taken very seriously, just like a mandatory notification of a health practitioner if you have a reasonable belief they may pose an unacceptable risk to the public.

The Australian privacy principles are called Australian Privacy Principles. They are set out in Schedule 1 of the *Privacy Act 1988* (Cth), and deal with:

- open and transparent management
- compliance
- collection, dealing, integrity and storage
- access to and correction of personal information.

The Notifiable Data Breaches Scheme is provided under Part IIIC of the *Privacy Act 1988* (Cth). The establishment of the provisions, in amendments to the *Privacy Act 1988* (Cth), with the *Privacy Amendment (Notifiable Data Breaches) Act 2017* (Cth), established the Notifiable Data Breaches (NDB) scheme in Australia. From 22 February 2018, certain data breaches must be self-reported by agencies and organisations with existing personal information security obligations under the Act. Legally binding guidelines and rules are issued by the Australian

Information Commissioner, and these are legally binding as legislative instruments, under the *Legislative Instruments Act 2003* (Cth).

The mandatory data breach notification requirements are explained in supporting documents issued by the Office of the Australian Information Commissioner (OAIC) (2018). Personal information in relation to health is termed 'sensitive information', and is subject to the most stringent obligations, one of which is that the OAIC is notified of any breach. Unauthorised access or disclosure of personal information, or loss of information held by an entity—which is likely to result in serious harm, when the entity is not able to prevent that harm—must be notified. For example, an employee browsing sensitive information without legitimate purpose, or leaving hard copy or an unsecured computer behind on public transport.

The provisions reflect a renewed public emphasis on privacy. Privacy breach concerns relate to:

- unauthorised paper records
- verbal disclosures
- mislaid or unsecured records
- cybersecurity.

You will need to think old school as well as modern times in safeguarding information in your health care work.

Being aware of the strict requirements as you start to work with private and confidential information helps you to appreciate the value of safeguarding privacy at all times.

Some information needs to be written down during the provision of health care. Notes based on the information gathered about the client are called medical records, or health records. Those records are stored for further reference. The notes should be accurate and complete so that they provide a good basis for following a client's progress and making future treatment decisions. There is little ethical debate about that.

It is when those notes are not safely stored—or when they are made available for a wider purpose than treatment of the individual—that ethical concerns are most prominent. Professional associations for medical records personnel are acutely aware of this responsibility. In large institutions, organising files and computerised records for easy access and protecting unauthorised access to them are the primary roles of medical records personnel or health information management professionals. Their codes of ethics have long acknowledged their responsibility for safeguarding confidentiality.

That responsibility is usually expressed in terms of a duty to respect and secure the information, within legal and regulatory limits. As adapted from principle III of the American Health Information Management Association (AHIMA) *Code of Ethics*: 'Preserve, protect, and secure personal information in any form or medium and hold it in the highest regard the contents of the records and other information of a confidential nature, taking into account the applicable statutes and regulations.' (AHIMA, 2017). The AHIMA *Code of Ethics* has also stated in the past: 'Both handwritten and computerized medical records contain many sacred stories—stories that must be protected on behalf of the individual and the aggregate community of persons served in the healthcare system' (AHIMA, 2017). This wording explains the sensitive personal nature of the information that you are responsible for.

REFLECTION: MOVEMENT OF INFORMATION

Identify a piece of personal health information in your professional work and track its progress. Take a blank page and draw a box labelled 'information'. Draw a circle for each place that this information moved to, using arrows to denote the movement of the information. On your diagram, note who collected the information, who knows about it, who accessed it, and how it was used for the client's treatment. Then, look back through your trail and note the potential points at which information could be leaked or used for an unapproved purpose. Those leakage points may be at handover, at moments of minimal security, and so on.

Discuss whether the following situation—or a similar one—would be likely to occur at your health care workplace. This vignette was developed in a GP ethics project, in which GPs and consumers nominated their concerns, and then met to discuss vignettes such as this one (Berglund et al., 1997).

A GP walked into the staff coffee room of his group practice surgery and found the staff discussing, with a great deal of amusement, the diagnosis and circumstances of a patient of his who was a well-known television personality. Members of the staff were passing around a fax containing a report about the patient from a specialist consultant. The doctor remonstrated with his staff about confidentiality.

The real danger of each potential leakage point in the information trail you constructed for the last exercise is that while each person may genuinely need access to the information for the primary reason of client care, they may not understand the importance of privacy and confidentiality—in other words, they may not understand how important such ethical obligations are in a large institution, or society.

Privacy and confidentiality

PRACTICE EXAMPLE

Jennifer Haines

Jennifer has been a Registered Nurse for 40 years and spent most of those years practising in critical care areas, ICU, CCU, Neurosurgery ICU and Emergency Department.

A young clinician has just interviewed a patient about his attempted suicide for all sorts of personal, emotional and sexual reasons. After the interview the clinician sits at the lunch table in the tearoom and tells the nurses present everything that had been said to her by the patient in that interview. When challenged by one nurse that she should not be revealing information given to her in confidence in a professional interview, two other nurses wanted to continue to hear more as 'they could read it all in the notes anyway'.

+ continued

1   Was the patient's confidentiality breached?
2   What obligations do our professional codes and standards place on nurses to protect patient privacy and confidentiality?

Next time you are in a public area, think about how common it is to hear sensitive information discussed by other people in places such as lifts, walkways, theatres, etc. It is amazing that such sensitive information is discussed loudly in public places; the participants in these conversation seem to be oblivious to the crowds of people around them, many of whom are only too pleased to have something to listen to as they wait for the lift to get to their floor, or for the concert to begin. It is a useful guiding rule not to discuss work outside the workplace, and especially not to name patients or clients as you discuss their background or particular treatment scenario, unless you are discussing the case with health workers who are part of the treatment team and need to know who the person is, and you are in a secure environment.

Within the work context, there are also things that constantly alert us to the presence of private and confidential information. When messages are delivered in a way that can be viewed by others, they are essentially opened letters. Only as much of the message should be read as identifies the recipient; the message should then be kept securely for that person. Some institutions used a folder, like a large envelope, so that faxes were not left lying on desks or in pigeonholes for others to see. You will find that there are standard operating procedures for guarding privacy and confidentiality of personal health information that are specially written for the form of the documentation and storage that is used in your health institution. To act on information contained in a message destined for somebody else is a breach of respect. Of course, this also applies to when you hear private or confidential information that was not intended for your ears. The same applies to shared email addresses.

Using electronic locks and passwords on computers and other electronic devices is one safeguard. Keep lockable filing cabinets locked so that only authorised persons can open the cabinet and read files. If you are working with confidential material on your desk, cover it up when you have meetings with other people around your desk, unless the information is relevant to their work role. Other people do not routinely need to see the contents of all the confidential files in your office. If you happen to be opposite someone else's desk and a confidential letter is in your line of vision, turn it over and say something like, 'I probably shouldn't see that and it is difficult not to notice it as I talk to you'. If you are discussing clients, you should do so in a private and secure area.

Once information is disclosed and written down or distributed, you need to guard against the lessening of privacy and confidentiality. Concerns about privacy, and understanding when it is ethically acceptable to breach privacy, tend to focus on the notes taken by health care professionals. It is the information in these notes that will be made available to others, if justified in the public interest.

REFLECTION: REGULATED INFORMATION

Different privacy protection applies in different contexts, but there is a trend in most jurisdictions to protect the privacy of an individual's information, and to improve security to ensure this. The information should not be transmitted further unless the individual consents to specific further use of the information, or there is explicit outweighing of public interests in this privacy to justify the transmission and use. Review the explanations about the privacy principles and recent regulatory developments in this chapter. Then read the example of privacy provisions outlined in one jurisdiction's privacy legislation.

Each jurisdiction uses its own variation on the privacy terminology, so you will see privacy principles with various names in different legislation and guidelines. A portion of the Health Privacy Principles, which New South Wales government agencies must adhere to unless an exemption circumstance arises, are reproduced here as an example of the detailed requirements that apply to the privacy and confidentiality of personal health information. This is a small section of the legislative provisions, on collection and security in retaining the information. There are also further detailed provisions that include accuracy and access, disclosure and linkage.

Schedule 1 Health Privacy Principles

1   Purposes of collection of health information

(1) An organisation must not collect health information unless:

(a) the information is collected for a lawful purpose that is directly related to a function or activity of the organisation, and

(b) the collection of the information is reasonably necessary for that purpose.

(2) An organisation must not collect health information by any unlawful means.

2   Information must be relevant, not excessive, accurate and not intrusive

An organisation that collects health information from an individual must take such steps as are reasonable in the circumstances (having regard to the purposes for which the information is collected) to ensure that:

(a) the information collected is relevant to that purpose, is not excessive and is accurate, up to date and complete, and

(b) the collection of the information does not intrude to an unreasonable extent on the personal affairs of the individual to whom the information relates.

3   Collection to be from individual concerned

(1) An organisation must collect health information about an individual only from that individual, unless it is unreasonable or impractical to do so.

(2) Health information is to be collected in accordance with any guidelines issued by the Privacy Commissioner for the purposes of this clause.

+ continued

4   Individual to be made aware of certain matters

(1) An organisation that collects health information about an individual from the individual must, at or before the time that it collects the information (or if that is not practicable, as soon as practicable after that time), take steps that are reasonable in the circumstances to ensure that the individual is aware of the following:

(a) the identity of the organisation and how to contact it,

(b) the fact that the individual is able to request access to the information,

(c) the purposes for which the information is collected,

(d) the persons to whom (or the types of persons to whom) the organisation usually discloses information of that kind,

(e) any law that requires the particular information to be collected,

(f) the main consequences (if any) for the individual if all or part of the information is not provided.

(2) If an organisation collects health information about an individual from someone else, it must take any steps that are reasonable in the circumstances to ensure that the individual is generally aware of the matters listed in subclause (1) except to the extent that:

(a) making the individual aware of the matters would pose a serious threat to the life or health of any individual, or

(b) the collection is made in accordance with guidelines issued under subclause (3).

(3) The Privacy Commissioner may issue guidelines setting out circumstances in which an organisation is not required to comply with subclause (2).

(4) An organisation is not required to comply with a requirement of this clause if:

(a) the individual to whom the information relates has expressly consented to the organisation not complying with it, or

(b) the organisation is lawfully authorised or required not to comply with it, or

(c) non-compliance is otherwise permitted (or is necessarily implied or reasonably contemplated) under an Act or any other law (including the *State Records Act 1998* [NSW]), or

(d) compliance by the organisation would, in the circumstances, prejudice the interests of the individual to whom the information relates, or

(e) the information concerned is collected for law enforcement purposes, or

(f) the organisation is an investigative agency and compliance might detrimentally affect (or prevent the proper exercise of) its complaint handling functions or any of its investigative functions.

(5) If the organisation reasonably believes that the individual is incapable of understanding the general nature of the matters listed in subclause (1), the

organisation must take steps that are reasonable in the circumstances to ensure that any authorised representative of the individual is aware of those matters.

(6) Subclause (4) (e) does not remove any protection provided by any other law in relation to the rights of accused persons or persons suspected of having committed an offence.

(7) The exemption provided by subclause (4) (f) extends to any public sector agency, or public sector official, who is investigating or otherwise handling a complaint or other matter that could be referred or made to an investigative agency, or that has been referred from or made by an investigative agency.

5   Retention and security

(1) An organisation that holds health information must ensure that:

(a) the information is kept for no longer than is necessary for the purposes for which the information may lawfully be used, and

(b) the information is disposed of securely and in accordance with any requirements for the retention and disposal of health information, and

(c) the information is protected, by taking such security safeguards as are reasonable in the circumstances, against loss, unauthorised access, use, modification or disclosure, and against all other misuse, and

(d) if it is necessary for the information to be given to a person in connection with the provision of a service to the organisation, everything reasonably within the power of the organisation is done to prevent unauthorised use or disclosure of the information.

Note. Division 2 (Retention of health information) of Part 4 contains provisions applicable to private sector persons in connection with the matters dealt with in this clause.

(2) An organisation is not required to comply with a requirement of this clause if:

(a) the organisation is lawfully authorised or required not to comply with it, or

(b) non-compliance is otherwise permitted (or is necessarily implied or reasonably contemplated) under an Act or any other law (including the *State Records Act 1998* [NSW]).

(3) An investigative agency is not required to comply with subclause (1) (a).

(Health Records and Information Privacy Act 2002 (NSW)*)*

Similar legislation is provided in other states and territories. At federal level it is provided in the *Privacy Act 1988* (Cth), and *Privacy Amendment (Private Sector) Act 2000* (Cth).

It is important to realise that individuals could suffer harm if a promise of confidentiality of personal information is not upheld. A separate philosophical decision has informed the guidelines on whether any disclosure, harm or embarrassment is justified, as will be discussed soon. The key point is that there is potential harm in any breach of confidentiality.

On a broader level, the disclosure of personal information could also threaten the public's trust in the confidentiality of certain relationships, such as banking, employment and health care relationships. Health care relationships, in particular, are based on trust in the confidentiality of the information provided. A threat to an individual harms not only that person, but also others because it erodes their trust in similar relationships (Beauchamp & Childress, 1983, p. 232).

The essence of privacy and confidentiality is that information is disclosed under certain conditions; these conditions consist of particular promises of confidentiality and particular expectations as to how the information will be used. Truthful information is given in exchange for that trust. The professional's obligation to maintain the confidentiality of the information continues until the informants give consent to the further distribution of the information (Westin, 1970, p. 374).

The lack of individual control over personal information, and the demand for this information by others, is of particular concern when information is collected in institutional settings, and when it is centralised and stored in computerised data banks. The danger is that if stored personal information can be used for another purpose, privacy interests will be overridden without adequate consideration of the importance of that further use, or in spite of professional concerns that confidentiality should be maintained (Westin, 1970, p. 383; Flaherty, 1989, p. 5). We rely on others, usually professionals or administrators, to use their discretion in deciding whether or not our information privacy interests should be overridden. In health care, clients rely on health care workers and records administrators to protect their privacy interests and treat their personal information with respect.

However, the conflict is that interests in privacy and confidentiality, just like interests in autonomy, are not absolute. The problem for all health care workers is in deciding when obligations to maintain privacy and confidentiality can be overridden by other obligations. These obligations have long been recognised as able to be overridden by competing interests (Australian Law Reform Commission, 1983, p. 20). Following are some examples of public interests (Czecowoski, 1984, pp. 1–3):

- Society has an interest in the release of information that will assist in preventing other members of society from suffering harm. Societies need some personal information to assess the welfare of their members and to protect others from harm caused by infectious diseases.
- Health care systems need access to personal information in order to assess their own effectiveness and efficiency, and to improve so that others may be better served. Access to information is justified if research is directed towards preventing harm to others in the future (this would be the kind of argument put forth by research organisations to support their access to information).

You can probably think of some more examples from other professional spheres.

There are some general rules for health care workers to consider in relation to the confidentiality of their health records or medical records:

- Confidentiality should be maintained, and consent sought for further use or disclosure of information, unless there is an overriding public interest. (This interest is generally mandated by another body, not just by the health care worker.) Thus, when public interest overrides the duty of confidentiality, it is legitimate to breach confidentiality. These interests include the reporting of infectious diseases and the provision of evidence in criminal trials in response to a subpoena (and at the discretion of the court).
- Confidentiality should be maintained because otherwise there is the potential for harm to be done to the client, which would contravene the health care worker's duty of care to the client.

It is difficult to specify the precise circumstances that would justify an infringement of privacy and confidentiality, apart from the sorts of extreme public interest provisions mentioned above. The primary question in relation to the release of information in the ordinary course of health care is: 'Does the information disclosure serve the purpose of the treatment that the patient originally agreed to?' Each jurisdiction makes its own decision on whether legislation should precisely set such circumstances. If you read further over the provisions in privacy legislation, find the disclosure principle provisions, and bear them in mind as you read further.

Whenever there is a request for the disclosure of information, professionals need to identify the full extent of their obligations both to keep information confidential and to disclose it. Consideration of the distinction between public and private interests may be a useful part of this process of identifying the extent of these obligations.

Weighing public interests in access and in privacy is part of an ethics committee's consideration when researchers wish to access health records for their research.

The distinction between public and **private interests** in privacy is similar to philosopher J.S. Mill's distinction between social and personal morality, which is discussed in more detail later in this chapter. Generally, **public interests** affect groups of people as a whole, whereas individual interests affect individuals in particular circumstances. Individual interests in privacy are generally upheld, except where there is a substantially greater public interest that cannot be achieved if that private interest in privacy is allowed. An example of a public interest in privacy is the need for trust to be maintained in confidential health care relationships so that members of society are not dissuaded from seeking health care for fear that the information they give to health carers will be disclosed to all and sundry. This is a public interest because this safeguard is needed in order to maintain a healthy society. An example of a private interest is the need for information to be guarded carefully because individuals may be harmed, socially, if their information is disclosed.

J.S. Mill said, 'as soon as any person's conduct affects prejudicially the interests of others, society has jurisdiction over it, and the question whether the general welfare will or will not be promoted by interfering with it, becomes open to discussion'. However, Mill also states that if a person's actions affect only themselves, and they are of 'full age' and an 'ordinary', meaning average, 'understanding', there should be 'perfect freedom, legal and social, to do the action and stand the consequences' (Mill, 1975, pp. 92–3).

private interest
Issues of importance and significance to an individual, defined on an individual basis to be in that person's best interest.

public interest
Issues of importance and significance to the structure of a community, and to the general benefit of a significant group of a community's members.

The importance of maintaining privacy and confidentiality of personal information, such as health information or other details of a person's life, can be protected by law. Equally, defining limits of obligations to maintain privacy and confidentiality obligations can be found in legislation and case law. The terminology used in the debates on the application of laws and guidelines often mimics the language of philosophers, such as J.S. Mill. Libertarianism places the personal freedom of the individual at the centre of analysis. That freedom is claimed as a right, unless there is sufficient reason to limit it. In J.S. Mill's thesis, *On Liberty* (Mill, 1975), the importance of **liberty**—and the limited circumstances when a person's liberty can be infringed—are reasoned. The only acceptable reasons for limiting liberty are if a serious and imminent risk is posed to another individual, or if the fabric of society is threatened. Mill described different types of liberties, of thought and action, and claimed that all people had a right to exercise these as they wished, and they should only be 'interfered' with if others were at risk. So if the conduct concerned only themselves, the following approach should prevail: 'Over himself, over his own body and mind, the individual is sovereign' (Mill, 1975, pp. 92–3).

liberty
Freedom of will, as expressed in choice of thought or action.

The legislative provides for consent requirements for the collection, use, storage and further disclosure of personal information. The legislation demonstrates a societal commitment to personal integrity and autonomy that should not be overridden lightly. The regulations build in accountability, in that another person or entity decides if access or use is justified.

Safety and notification processes and public law

Similar wording to privacy legislation also appears regularly in safety and notification laws, regulations and guidelines, which provide the authority to restrict liberty and to restrict an individual's particular freedoms. For individuals trying to decide whether action is warranted, the reasoning is also useful, as active reflection and use of discretion is the preferable course for any professional of integrity.

In privacy legislation, the circumstances when the requirement for consent to release and use personal information can be waived are generally limited to times when a related purpose warrants the further use, or circumstances of public importance, in that it can and likely does affect others. For example, consent can be waived if:

- it will 'prevent or lessen a serious and imminent threat to the life or health of the individual concerned or another person'
- it is required or authorised under law
- it is necessary for the enforcement of a criminal law (or the payment of a penalty in the criminal justice system)
- it is to protect the public revenue.

So, while the duty to maintain confidentiality is strong, it is not absolute: it can be breached when serious imminent risk to others exists. In some situations of significant and imminent risk of serious danger to a known person, there can even be a duty to disclose confidential information. This duty was tested in the famous legal case *Tarasoff v Regents of University of California*, in which a patient told a psychiatrist that he (the patient) was planning to harm someone. The psychiatrist was found to have a duty to disclose this so that the person the patient was planning to harm could be protected (*Tarasoff v Regents of University of California* [1976], as discussed in Devereux, 1997, pp. 220–1). This duty was said to depend on whether the potential victims are identifiable and whether other protective mechanisms are available (Coverdale, 1996, p. 67).

Health practitioners have a legal obligation to notify the relevant authorities if they hold a reasonable belief that any person or persons pose a risk to a child. Under child protection laws in Western Australia, *Children and Community Services Act 2004* (WA), it is a mandatory legal requirement for doctors, nurses, midwives, teachers, police officers and boarding supervisors to report all reasonable beliefs about child sexual abuse to the Department of Communities—Child Protection and Family Support. A reasonable belief can be based on 'professional judgment and objective observation which identifies warning signs or possible indicators of child sexual abuse', and can include circumstances of:

- bribery threat
- exploitation or violence, or the child has less power than the person involved
- significant disparity in the developmental function or maturity of the child and the person involved (Government of Western Australia, 2008, pp. 10–11).

Similar guidelines are being developed for the notification of possible elder abuse, or abuse of other people in circumstances of heightened vulnerability, as may be the case for people with disability (Australian Government, 2017).

The health professional does not need to have the proof of improper or dangerous conduct. Investigating the issue and deciding whether an allegation is proven is up to other authorities. The health professional's obligation is to notify a reasonable belief in a timely way so that investigation and any protective action can be put in place in a timely and effective way.

The codes of ethics of conduct, or codes of ethics for health care professionals generally offer the advice that privacy is not absolute and can be overridden. For example, the Pharmacy Board of Australia's *Pharmacy Code of Conduct for registered health practitioners* states that 'Patients or clients have a right to expect that practitioners and their staff will hold information about them in confidence, unless information is required to be released by law or public interest considerations' (Pharmacy Board of Australia, 2011).

The codes provide guidance rather than precise answers about which interest should take precedence in specific situations. This means that further professional discussion and advice is essential.

Competing interests to privacy interests are acknowledged in broader policy discussions. Some public interests rely on the flow of information, such as in human rights protection, for social interests, and for business interests. Individual liberty and, in this case, privacy, are supported, but social limitations are placed on both due to public concerns over the welfare of other members of society, and given the need to protect the structure or 'fabric' of society.

A judgment regarding the relative merits of different interests is tested in court from time to time. For instance, a court was asked to decide if the Red Cross should be granted immunity from disclosing the identities of blood donors to persons subsequently infected by blood donation. The court considered survey results—the survey having been done for the court hearing—that showed that many people would not donate blood without assurances of confidentiality. The court ruled that the public interest in assuring confidentiality, so that people would continue to donate blood, outweighed the interests that those infected had in the disclosure of the identities of blood donors (*PD v Australian Red Cross* [1992]).

Note also that for public release of government information, there is a reverse test, as the public interest in providing transparent and open accountable fair and objective government is only restricted if there is an overriding public interest against disclosure, such as involving the protection of an individual's personal information (*Government Information (Public Access) Act 2009* (NSW), section 3(1), section 14).

When health issues pose a public health risk to others more generally, the information can become 'notifiable', which means that it is mandatory to release to a relevant public health authority. Australia has a surveillance mechanism for notifiable diseases, and surveillance case definitions are provided by the Department of Health. A few of the recently added notifiable diseases listed for the start of alphabet are:

* avian influenza in humans (AIH)
* Barmah Forest virus infection
* brucellosis
* chlamydial infection
* dengue virus infection
* diphtheria
* flavivirus infection (unspecified, including Zika virus infection case definition) (Department of Health, 2017).

You could look up more on the Department of Health website. The National Health Security Agreement is in place between the Commonwealth and all states and territories so that information can be shared to support a coordinated national response to public health emergencies, and between Australian governments and WHO or other countries when required, supporting the *National Health Security Act 2007* (Cth). The National Health Security Agreement notes as part of its 'recitals' of objectives:

> Australia's accession to the *International Health Regulations (2005)* requiring Australia to develop multi-level capacities in the health sector to effectively manage public health threats and to develop, strengthen and maintain the capacity to detect, report and respond to public health events.
>
> *Australian Government (2011)*

This demonstrates a country and world perspective on significant public health risks, and the corresponding overriding public interest in sharing such health information.

Cryptosporidium

Kath Weston

Kath has worked as a senior infectious diseases surveillance officer with New South Wales Health at the Public Health Unit in Western Sydney, predominantly in the sphere of 'health protection' which includes providing advice to health practitioners and the community about vaccination and infectious diseases, organising responses to urgent public health issues, as well as disaster management during outbreaks.

Public health threats from infectious agents such as waterborne parasites are part of the usual workload of a Public Health Unit. The emergence of new disease threats, such as avian influenza and Ebola, bring additional challenges. Public health orders can be used to quarantine individuals or to require mandatory testing or treatment of cases or contacts, or to close premises that constitute a risk.

A common application of the *Public Health Act 2010* (NSW) is the power to close public premises on public health grounds. A good example is ordering the closure of a public swimming pool where there is evidence of cryptosporidium in the water. Cryptosporidium is a parasite transmitted via faeces, which contains the spores of the parasite. It is the most common cause of diarrheal illness and outbreaks linked to swimming pools and other water recreation venues. The Public Health Unit is usually alerted to a cryptosporidium outbreak when there is an increase in laboratory notifications of the disease. Interviews with cases can reveal a common source such as the local swimming pool or water playground. Urgent action is needed to reduce risk of further cases, and the pool can be ordered to close until it has been disinfected. A notice indicating the public health order to close the pool must be displayed at the facility.

Managing risks from serious diseases such as avian influenza, tuberculosis, Ebola or typhoid requires an urgent response. Most members of the public who are infected or who have been in contact with a case of one of the above diseases are responsible and will comply with Public Health recommendations for testing, treatment and quarantine as required.

However, when these voluntary measures are not adopted, public health orders can be given if there is a risk to the public. Such orders can be used to require testing or treatment, or to require a case to provide a list of susceptible contacts. These orders are in line with the Australian *Biosecurity Act 2015* (Cth), which recognises the public health risk involved if cases or contacts do not voluntarily agree to quarantine recommendations.

What information might public health authorities give to people taking infants and small children to public swimming pools?

A media release can be helpful in educating the public about the importance of hygiene at public swimming pools. Parents should be informed not to allow children with diarrhoea to swim in a pool for at least two weeks after having diarrhoea. They should ensure young

+ continued

children are taken frequently to the toilet, and should use waterproof tight-fitting pants over swimmers for children who are not toilet-trained.

How else can you get cryptosporidium infection?

Cryptosporidium is present in the faeces of infected humans and animals. People become infected when the parasite is ingested, such as through drinking contaminated water or through person-to-person contact, particularly among small children, such as in a childcare setting. For this reason it's important for public health staff to do a thorough interview of cases to find a common link, such as a swimming pool or childcare setting. It's critical to keep an open mind when interviewing cases, and not to assume the source will always be a swimming pool.

Why does the laboratory tell the Public Health Unit about different diseases?

The Australian National Notifiable Diseases Surveillance System (NNDSS) collects laboratory confirmed notifiable data from states and territories of Australia in accordance with the *National Health Security Act 2007* (Cth) and the *National Health Security Agreement 2008*. This data collection allows public health authorities to have a better understanding of community significant diseases, or to monitor patterns of antibiotic resistance. The data can help to determine when to develop health promotion activities or to send out public health alerts to health care providers. Notifiable diseases include:

- vaccine-preventable diseases—such as measles
- diseases transmitted through insects—such as malaria
- diseases transmitted through livestock—such as Q Fever
- sexually transmitted diseases—such as gonorrhoea.

Practice example references

www.legislation.nsw.gov.au
www.health.nsw.gov.au
www.legislation.gov.au

PRACTICE EXAMPLE

Measles

Kath Weston

The *Public Health Act 2010* (NSW) aims to prevent, control and manage the spread of disease. While aspects of the Act relate to managing a single individual with a contagious disease, it's also important to recognise the role of the Act in managing other people who may be at risk from that infectious individual.

A good example is measles, a serious disease with risk of complications and often requiring hospitalisation. In the early stages of measles there is no rash, but the person may have a high fever, cough and flu-like symptoms. Someone with these early symptoms is highly infectious. Simply being in the same room as this person can cause an unvaccinated person to become infected.

Here is a case to consider. Jay, a 35-year-old man with no history of vaccination, has recently returned from a trip to Asia. He develops measles symptoms three days after his return home. Jim visits his local medical surgery and sits in the waiting room for about 30 minutes before he gets to see the GP.

The GP organises testing for Jim and rings the local Public Health Unit to notify a suspected case of measles. Jim is isolated at home, but a major issue for Public Health staff is the GP's waiting room. All of the people who were in the waiting room during the 30-minute period when Jim was waiting need to be assessed for risk. Moreover, people who enter the waiting room for the next two hours are also at risk, as the measles virus can survive and be transmitted for up to two hours after the infected person has left the room.

The Public Health Unit staff ask the GP reception staff for a list of people in the waiting room for the two-and-a-half-hour window from the time Jim first entered the waiting room. They want names, dates of birth and telephone contact details. This raises questions of privacy and patient consent for release of personal details held by the practice.

The objectives of the *Public Health Act* state, 'The protection of the health and safety of the public is to be the paramount consideration in the exercise of functions under this Act' (*Public Health Act 2010* (NSW) No 127, section 3).

3(1)   The objects of this Act are as follows:

   a   to promote, protect and improve public health,

   b   to control the risks to public health,

   c   to promote the control of infectious diseases,

   d   to prevent the spread of infectious diseases,

   e   to recognise the role of local government in protecting public health.

   f   to monitor diseases and conditions affecting public health.

3(2)   The protection of the health and safety of the public is to be the paramount consideration in the exercise of functions under this Act.

www.legislation.nsw.gov.au

In Jim's case, the GP practice is allowed to release the details of the other patients in the waiting room so that they can be contacted by Public Health staff in a timely manner, assessed for risk and, if necessary, given measles vaccine or immunoglobulin to prevent development of the disease. This immediate action is critical to minimising further spread of measles.

Are there any other people who may be at risk?

Public Health staff would need to find out:

- the vaccination status of the GP practice staff
- the vaccination status of people who live at home with Jim

+ continued

- whether Jim has been in contact with infants under 12 months of age—too young to have received measles vaccination
- other places that Jim might have visited—such as his work, cinemas, shopping centres, hospitals, churches, friends and family.

The number of 'contacts' associated with one case can often be in the hundreds.

What issues might arise among unvaccinated health care staff in GP surgeries and hospitals?

Apart from their personal risk of contracting a disease from a patient, staff may not be aware they have a contagious disease when they attend work. A neonatal-care nurse with a cough may not be aware that their mild cough is pertussis—whooping cough—which can be life threatening for unvaccinated infants. A health care worker with early measles symptoms might think they can work through their flu-like symptoms—but may actually be in a position to transmit measles to immunocompromised patients in their facility.

For these reasons, state health policies have been developed that require all staff to be vaccinated against diseases like pertussis and measles.

What sort of details about Jim should be released to the media?

A media release can be very helpful in raising awareness of a case of measles so that people who may be at risk can be on the lookout for symptoms. Information that can be released about the case—Jim himself—should be limited to the places Jim visited while infectious, and should not contain any identifying information.

Consider the limits placed on the choices that an individual can make in relation to a public-health issue, such as immunisation. In Australia, Commonwealth welfare benefits such as childcare benefits and family assistance benefits can no longer be received by parents if their children are not fully immunised with recommended vaccinations even if they have conscientious objections to their children being immunised. Under the policy, which was revised in 2016, objection can still be made on certain limited medical or religious grounds. It was debated in the House of Representatives as part of the *Social Services Legislation Amendment (No Jab, No Pay) Bill 2015* (Cth) (Parliament of Australia, 2015). Such limits are justified with the argument that there is a community necessity to ensure herd immunity is maintained.

Your own actions as a health professional in minimising risks to others could also be examined. Do you have a choice about whether to be fully immunised before working in a health context? You will likely find that your employment is conditional on you demonstrating that you are fully immunised, with a list provided to you. This is an aspect of governance that was mandatory for you—a condition that you must fulfil if you accepted the offer of employment. Placing yourself in a health role means that your immunisation status as an adult is no longer a routine personal morality matter. You can explore the concepts of personal morality and social morality further in Chapter 7 'The limits of care'.

The principles of balancing interests can be found in international examples of public health crises due to serious epidemics, and action may be needed before a condition is well defined. Information is gathered rapidly as the threat to the public unfolds, and as the scale of the potential threat to the public becomes known or able to be estimated.

Notice how jurisdiction—legal authority and power—is important to each country's policy. In previous threats of severe acute respiratory syndrome (SARS) and bird flu, countries were able to implement border controls at airports because that was the first practical point that their jurisdiction began.

The SARS outbreak, which began in November 2002 and reached the most serious epidemic proportions in China by mid-2003, was legislated as a notifiable condition in many countries. Quarantine provisions—that is, limiting the movement of people affected, or people in contact with those affected—were also made on public interest grounds. The WHO requested international cooperation and central reporting of SARS cases and infection patterns. Health outcomes were made available routinely on a public website as soon as they became available to the WHO (World Health Organization, 2003).

The WHO also became involved in issuing descriptions of symptoms to be vigilant for, travel warnings and containment advice, as it tracked the epidemic in countries worldwide. In ethics terms, the measures were justified on grounds of serious and imminent risk if the information were to remain private.

REFLECTION POINT

Organisational regulation

Find out what one organisation's policy was on SARS. You could use your university, workplace or local school as examples. See if there were travel restrictions, limitations on attendance after travel, exclusion based on symptoms, and so on. Find out how the policy was argued in terms of ethics, and take particular note of any wording on risk and interests.

If you had the opportunity to rewrite this policy, what would you suggest? Take into account the symptoms and health consequences—including the mortality and spread of SARS. You will find crucial facts to consider on the WHO website <www.who.int>, or in local health authority warning or alert documents.

Can you think of any other identifiable—and potentially catastrophic—transmissible diseases that also had an international dimension? How about bird flu? In particular, one form of avian influenza, named H5N1? Priorities for care provision and research into bird flu were championed by society, to protect the communities. This serves as an example that the public, through their governments and international alliances, can express active social support for research directions, especially in the face of threats or risks, and when current care and knowledge is insufficient to deal with a major perceived risk. For instance, an unprecedented sum of money—around US$2 billion—was made available to the United Nations by member nations to investigate and contain H5N1 (Parry, 2006).

Avian flu (H5N1 strain) raised similar issues to SARS in terms of the importance of identification and containment of risks, and the need for rapid response. An epidemic in birds, affecting large wild bird populations worldwide and many domesticated flocks, poses a potential risk not just to further birds, but also to humans. Bird handlers have predominantly been at risk of infection, with serious life-threatening infections reported in some people. So far, these have largely been in the developing world. Avian flu is potentially a large-scale threat to the human population if it mutates into a virus that is easily transmissible between humans. Mass culling of birds has been undertaken in areas where the bird flu has been identified. Quarantine provisions apply to affected areas in terms of trading in birds. Infected people are ideally treated in quarantine conditions.

Some flu drugs (e.g. oseltamivir) could be used for the rapid onset of symptoms, once bird flu was identified, but the worldwide stocks were limited, and governments tried to stockpile certain amounts for frontline health and emergency workers. Prescriptions from individuals without symptoms, who tried to stockpile some in case they might need it quickly, became near impossible to fill. Vaccine trials were underway in 2006, but had not promised high enough effectiveness to be relied on for protection from H5N1 bird flu (Robotham, 2006).

There was also concern that as vaccines became available, they should be equitably available (Gostin, 2006). As a transmissible mutated virus that could initiate a pandemic has not yet occurred, the exact mutated virus that needs to be countered by a vaccine has not yet been developed. The WHO's advice was that a precise vaccine would not be readily available early in a pandemic in any case, and to supply vaccine for the whole world of 6.7 billion people over a six-month period would not be feasible (World Health Organization, 2006, 2007).

Given that background, try the following exercise on risk and assessment of risk from a private (personal) or public perspective.

Bear in mind that best practice is to be aware of not only authority to act and coerce through laws designed to protect the health of the public, and of the power or possibly duty to do so, but also the importance of exercising restraint so that the powers to act are tempered by only using as many of those powers as are necessary. Discretion is exercised by selecting the least restrictive means to achieve the necessary good for the public, as described in the seminal work on power and discretion by Gostin (2016).

CASE EXAMPLE

Risk and assessment

Imagine you are a small farmer in a developing country. You rely on the meagre income from your chickens to feed your children. One chicken has recently become sick. List your concerns.

Now you are a medical response team on an international goodwill mission. While overseas, there is a policy that Australian laws apply to the team members, as well as the local jurisdiction laws—with local laws prevailing if in conflict. You decide to see if you can treat those affected. The farmer refuses you entry to their property. The children are nowhere in sight, but a neighbour says they are too weak and too ill to be outside. What are your concerns?

Now imagine you are a public health official with the WHO, and you hear the rumour about a small farmer with a sick chicken in a remote village. List your concerns.

Compare your listed concerns. Should any concerns outweigh or take precedence over the others? Why or why not? Try to justify your position, and make use of the law and ethics theory you have learnt in this and previous chapters.

Take one of the official roles a little further, and prepare an email about what you think should happen next, and back your advice with your reasons. Make sure your reasons are legally informed.

Note that **public health** practice is compatible with assessing individual and community risk, and setting and imposing limits in the public interest. This broad notion of care, and taking responsibility for deciding what is in individuals' best interests, is a form of paternalism. The notion of paternalism underlies much of public health practice in instances of serious risk. Factors are identified and acted upon for the good of a community—independent of individual preferences. As risks decrease in magnitude and probability, more individual choice is offered.

> **public health**
> Field of health care concerned with assessing and improving health and preventing illness or disease on a population basis.

Quarantine wards attempt to balance the aim of treatment with the aim of protecting others in society from diseases. Looking back into the history of quarantine, we can see instances where it was applied too widely—for instance, the practice of isolating people with developmental or mental disabilities. The balance—between treatment and protection—of risk that society is prepared to accept determines the laws and regulations that health care workers then implement. These historical approaches would be out of step with the definition of false imprisonment that is applied today, as well as the principles of lawful detention. Private interests have, at heart, an individual's freedom to determine their own interests—and therefore their own actions. This balance of public versus private interest is a social issue of ethical importance. As eminent scholars have noted, public health is in effect a paternalistic position, which seeks to impose 'good' for the community as a whole, within certain limits that are socially determined. The private sphere is intruded upon in the interest of the health and safety of the community (Beauchamp, 1999, p. 59).

In essence, posing risk to others is a public health issue. Debate can centre on whether there actually is a risk, and in what circumstances. It is dubious whether many bloodborne diseases should be described and treated as a significant routine health risk if there is no contagion risk in the course of normal population contact, such as airborne contact. However, tuberculosis and influenza are both airborne and clearly pose significant public-health risks. This assessment of risk is crucial. Unless the level of risk is established, the infringement on one person's rights in the interests of the rights of others is very difficult to justify ethically.

Ensuring that an individual remains informed about their own personal health information is a further safety measure. A client who is informed of an imminent serious risk that they could pose to others could act to minimise risk to others. For instance, after a person gives blood to a blood bank, their blood is tested for a range of hepatitis conditions. If there are positive results for any of these conditions, the person is informed and counselled to pursue health care for their own benefit, and they are advised about behaviours that pose risks to others. Their blood is discarded from the donor pool. There is a large degree of trust placed in the individual to minimise their risk to others so that the infection can be contained.

It is likely that we will always have to live and work with the reality of both the duty of confidentiality and the demand for access to personal health information given potential health risk. This will continue to pose challenges.

REFLECTION: MANDATORY INFORMATION GATHERING

Concentrate on a contemporary potential public health concern. For instance, you could find out a little more about yellow fever, or Ebola or immunisation schemes that are implemented with children. Identify a helpful initiative. Then, thinking about the health concern and context, construct a suggested argument for voluntary, mandatory or compulsory health implementation of the initiative.

A *voluntary action* is one that can be suggested, and then each person is free to decide whether or not to participate.

A **compulsory** *action* is that which is required of everyone, and is enforceable. So, for instance, it might be compulsory for all citizens to register the birth of a new baby with a central registry. No exceptions are granted, and the action is enforceable under criminal law.

A **mandatory** *action* is one that is only required on certain choices and obligations. Dress rules in some clubs and restaurants are one example. The dress requirements apply to people who wish to dine or socialise there. The requirements do not become 'compulsory' for everyone, nor do they apply in other places apart from those establishments. Yet if you wish to go in, you can expect to be checked according to the mandatory dress rules, and turned away if you do not comply. Another mandatory requirement is seeking entry to certain territories, by asking permission to cross a border into another country.

In the health care context, the call for mandatory testing is an expression of possible rules to apply to those who choose to make use of the services of health care.

Gather a few facts about your chosen example, and then try constructing a few points in argument for and against a mandatory, compulsory or voluntary approach to your initiative. You could take the writings of J.S. Mill as a starting point. Mill wrote about the philosophical importance of liberty and of not putting others at risk. Some examples of voluntary, mandatory and compulsory initiatives are shown in Table 6.1.

compulsory Required action for all, with enforcement provisions.

mandatory Required action, contingent on being under certain command and corresponding enforceable obligations.

TABLE 6.1 VOLUNTARY, MANDATORY AND COMPULSORY INITIATIVES

Health objective	*Voluntary*	*Mandatory*	*Compulsory*
Improved efficiency and effectiveness of patient care through availability of centralised individual health records to health carers	Individuals may opt out of inclusion of their records, and access and use of centralised health record system for their future care needs	Development of infrastructure for centralised information management of health records, to include existing care records of instances of publicly supported health care	
Improved health of the population through improved community herd immunity	Recommended vaccination schedules for children made available for parent information and decision	With limited medical and religious grounds exemptions, immunisation requirements imposed for children of parents receiving certain government benefit support Exclusion of children from school in case of outbreak, for their safety	
Safeguard the public through management of notifiable disease outbreaks	Testing and treatment recommendations for individuals at risk Quarantine recommendations for individuals likely infected	Notification to authorities of positive test results for those who have presented for testing	Public health orders for individuals to comply with testing, treatment and quarantine requirements as warranted, if lack voluntary implementation of recommendations

The exercise prompts assessment of the relationship between the particular liberty and the particular potential harm or risk that is posed. For instance, it may be that what is required is an improvement of the care or community practices to prevent spread or cross-infection, rather than intervention or collection of personal information. This exercise illustrates that, in order to construct arguments about ethics, it is necessary to have a good grasp of the facts—in this case, clear information on risk and the benefits of mandatory testing. The exercise also highlights that the factual context can change over time, as clinical practices and standard treatment evolves. For instance, has the procedural risk been managed by safer equipment or procedures? Ethical arguments are perhaps best constructed in conjunction with fellow professionals who can provide this crucial factual information. If you can alter the level of risk posed, your ethical analysis would also change.

As an example, you could refer to a published tutorial exercise on proposed mandatory HIV testing of patients and professionals (Berglund, 1995). At the time of writing the tutorial, undergraduate and postgraduate health students were beginning their training in the early days of HIV (human immunodeficiency virus) and AIDS (acquired immunodeficiency syndrome). It is now manageable, but early on, was recognised as a long-term disease that posed serious and life-threatening risks to sufferers (Centers for Disease Control, 1987; Bacchettis & Moss, 1989).

The context was that, in the early years, health carers and health care institutions were very concerned about HIV/AIDS issues and the implications for clinical practice. The concern centred on the fact that HIV is a bloodborne virus. Exposure to blood or other bodily fluids that contain the virus could pose a risk to others. Transmission could occur from patients to other patients or professionals, or from professionals to patients. Fear of contagion was a primary concern of health professionals dealing with AIDS into the 1990s, as evidenced by a Canadian survey (Taerk et al., 1993). Internationally, there was extensive ethical debate over whether health carers were obliged to care for people with HIV or AIDS, given the potential risk to their own health (Tegtmeier, 1990). Now, it is a routine part of practice, and professionals expect to encounter patients with bloodborne viruses, much more so in some countries and communities. Infection control and universal precautions have improved considerably.

Health care is, by its very nature, a risky business. As a health care worker, you will be in contact with people who are ill, injured, or both. You will sometimes be exposed to dangerous situations and you will also expose your clients to some risk. Actively doing good and intervening often entails some risk. Your skill and care can minimise that risk. Institutional factors also influence how risky a procedure may be. Managing a risk can involve limitations to each individual's autonomy, and philosophical tools help you to weigh up whether infringements on autonomy are reasonable.

Research using personal information

You might like to jump forward to Chapter 7 'The limits of care' to read the section on the conduct of research, as you consider the use of personal information for research purposes, and the integrated standards that guide that use. The use of personal information is just one issue in research ethics. The ethical significance of the disclosure of personal information, and the regulation of access, storage, disclosure and use of information, with supporting legal standards, is highlighted here, as you consider the challenging concepts of access to potentially valuable personal information for the wider community.

Control over personal information is a fundamental extension of the principle of 'respect for persons'. It means giving an individual control over information about themself—not just control over their own physical self, which is often protected by consent. Confidentiality of information implies that personal information should be held in confidence, and should not be included in any further research or made available for other purposes unless the individual whom the information is about gives consent. Confidentiality obligations are tested in research that uses information that is already stored for another purpose—such as medical records—and in research that involves collecting information that may be useful for another purpose.

The use of personal information for purposes other than those consented to requires sufficient public interest in those further purposes—and this decision often falls to the ethics committees in the case of research. Under the *Privacy Act 1988* (Cth), guidelines under section 95 serve as a legislative instrument that requires ethics committee consideration of the public interest in research relative to the public interest in privacy.

The human research ethics committee system is explained here, as it is central to this discretionary decision making. Keep the information on ethics committees in mind when you read the more general section on research conduct in Chapter 7 'The limits of care'.

There can be some confusion about how to refer to ethics committees that consider the ethical acceptability of research protocols before they are allowed to proceed. The committees have different names depending on their jurisdiction:

- UK—research ethics committees
- New Zealand—health and disability ethics committees (HDECs) or institutional ethics committees (IECs)
- USA—institutional review boards (IRBs)
- Australia—human research ethics committees (HRECs).

In Australia prior to 1999, committees that consider research ethics were called 'institutional ethics committees' (IECs). In Australia, committees that consider clinical treatment ethics are called clinical ethics committees, but they are called IECs in the USA. This generic term 'research ethics committees' denotes the function of the committees.

In Australia, research of more than low risk must be reviewed by a HREC, using the National Statement in its deliberations. HRECs are composed of at least eight members, with a required minimum composition of:

- a chairperson
- two laypersons—one man and one woman
- one person who performs a pastoral care role in the community—such as an Aboriginal elder or a minister
- one lawyer—who is not engaged to advise the institution
- at least two members with knowledge of and experience in the types of research considered—who may be drawn from a pool of suitable researcher members depending on proposals to be considered
- at least one member who has knowledge and experience in the professional care, counselling or treatment of people.

Research involving a 'low or negligible risk' to participants may be delegated to a different panel for review. Strictly speaking, HRECs do not express institutional standards, because they remain independent from the institution, and their members are not, for the most part, employees of the institution. At least one-third of the members should be from outside the institution. HRECs do not often monitor research directly, and monitoring is more broadly an institutional responsibility. However, they do receive regular reports from researchers on their projects, and on any adverse events that have accompanied this research. The committee can inspect research sites or records, or interview participants if they wish, either randomly or in response to concerns about research process or risks (National Health and Medical Research Council, Australian Research Council & Universities Australia, 2007, updated 2018, Section 5, pp. 84, 87).

The documentation of ethics consideration and approval by a properly constituted research ethics committee is a practical and important safeguard for researchers and institutions, demonstrating a willingness to comply with obligations and responsibilities in the ethical conduct of research.

Very similar systems operate in many countries. In the UK, research ethics committees (RECs) are the committees that review research at an institutional level. The committees are overseen by a health department authority and there are required governance arrangements, including the composition of committees: 'A REC should contain a mixture of people who reflect the currency of public opinion ('lay' members), as well as people who have relevant formal qualifications or professional experience that can help the REC understand particular aspects of research proposals ('expert' members)' (Department of Health, 2012, p. 20). The procedures are increasingly streamlined, including standard application forms, information sheets for participants, and committee decision-making and documentation processes. There are additional guidelines available, issued by research councils, to assist research ethics reflection by researchers and deliberations undertaken by committees (Economic & Social Research Council [ESRC], 2010).

In New Zealand, Health and Disability Ethics Committees (HDECs) consider if research meets the requirements of Ethical Guidelines for Observational Studies and Ethical Guidelines for Intervention Studies. Membership should include those with diverse perspectives, including 'a recognised awareness of te reo Māori and the understanding of tikanga Māori, ethical and moral reasoning, law, the perspectives of wider community (e.g. the perspectives of consumers of health and disability services, ethnic community), the design and conduct of intervention studies, the design and conduct of observational studies, the provision of health and disability services, reviewing either qualitative or quantitative research, and the perspectives of student community' (Health Research Council of New Zealand, 2012, p. 5). The New Zealand system of streamlining ethics considerations was in large part initiated 20 years or so ago, after an inquiry into cervical cancer research.

The common requirement for committees to include community members, laypeople not affiliated with the institution, nor involved with research or health care, is to increase openness, transparency and accountability. These members provide an independent point of view. It is also routine for committee members to declare conflict about certain matters that are before a committee. For instance, that they are employed by the institution that seeks x, y, or z, or that, as a researcher, they are affiliated with the research team seeking approval. In that instance, a member would remove themself from making a decision about that particular proposal. The perception of potential conflict of interest attracts as much criticism as actual **conflict of interest**, so it is something that is guarded against quite strictly.

conflict of interest
A situation in which two potentially opposing and incompatible interests exist.

It is vital that any balancing of interests is undertaken in a proper manner.

Determining if ethics standards are maintained in any proposed research protocol is potentially complex, given the regulatory and legal and ethical considerations. National funding bodies and professional associations generate their own guidelines and discussion papers about the balance between the public interest in access for research practice purposes and the public interest in privacy, bearing in mind the requirements that apply in particular jurisdictions under law.

Generally, there is guidance on the circumstance in which the use of personal data for research may constitute a specific exception to the general requirement for a consent process, including that:

- involvement in the research carries no more than low risk
- gaining consent would be impracticable
- a mechanism exists for future participants to opt out of participating
- public interest in the proposed research or activity substantially outweighs the public interest in the protection of privacy (National Health and Medical Research Council, Australian Research Council & Universities Australia, 2007, at 2.3.6; *Privacy Act 1988* [Cth]).

The exception to consent is not granted lightly. Ethics committees are required—as the only decision makers who are entitled to do so—to decide this and, in doing so, to consider if the public interest in the promotion of the research 'outweighs to a substantial degree the public interest in adhering to that Information Privacy Principle' under Commonwealth privacy provisions (see section 95, *Privacy Act 1988* (Cth); National Health and Medical Research Council, 2014). Generally, people other than the health care worker make the judgment as to whether one public interest outweighs another. The health care worker still needs to consider any request for confidential information and should refer it to the appropriate authorities if the request is clearly not consistent with the purpose of treatment.

Research that is directed to the improvement of a health service is often able to be conducted without seeking the consent of individuals to the use of their information. (See if you can find the section and clause that allows this in privacy legislation.) Quality improvement (QI) or quality assurance (QA) research is usually understood as research that has low or negligible impact on individuals. Ethics approval is needed for this research. There remains an ethical imperative to deidentify a person's information as soon as is practical after accessing it for the data collection. This is to minimise any unauthorised further access, use or disclosure in an identified form, which would pose a significant risk to a person's privacy.

The debate on appropriate use of information is a worldwide, long-running concern, which peaks with heightened community concern. Two recent projects stand out in discussions: a Swedish project linking 1500 individuals' medical, educational and financial records; and an Icelandic study holding detailed genetic information in a database. Both projects were frequently debated, as was whether such large collections and linkages of data would be acceptable to other communities (Andersen & Aranson, 1999).

In the 1970s in the USA, a number of commissions into research participation collected instances of embarrassing situations that were caused by clinical information being disclosed in other contexts. The following extract is from the report of one of these commissions. As one witness told the Commission: 'a researcher was doing a follow-up study of people who had been enrolled in a methadone maintenance program ... The contractor had the name and address of one particular individual who had been enrolled in the program several years previously, and the contractor went to the individual's residence. It was a Saturday night and the person was having a party and the contractor said, 'Hi, I am so-and-so from such-and-such an organisation, and we are doing a follow-up study of patients who had been enrolled in the methadone maintenance program.' A similar incident that came to the Commission's attention involved the recontact of patients who had received treatment at an abortion clinic. On both instances the recontacts were unwelcome, resented and extremely embarrassing to the persons contacted (National Commission for the Protection of Subjects of Biomedical and Behavioral Research, 1978, p. 309).

The sensitivity of personal information has been a feature of guidelines for modern research practice, and this incident led to tightening of US privacy rules.

In the USA, the professionals need to keep in mind the federal regulations, particularly the latest Department of Health and Human Services Privacy Rules, which came into effect in April 2003. The rules support patient privacy in the context of a sufficient flow of information for quality medical care. This regulation has had implications for the way organisations store their information, further refined due to the Security Rules for standards for confidentiality, integrity and availability of electronic health information, in force from April 2005. The Privacy and Security Rules are enforced and administered by the US Department of Health and Human Services Office for Civil Rights. Their implementation has prompted the generation of standard consent forms for potential further use of the information, which health care professionals can provide to the patient to sign if further use is anticipated. It can be very difficult to recontact all patients at a later date to seek their permission, so it is now sought upfront.

REFLECTION POINT

Keeping up with regulations

As an exercise in keeping up to date on regulations in different jurisdictions, look up the summary Privacy Rules and Security Rule, under the US Department of Health and Human Services at <www.hhs.gov>. Search for the web address under the department name, or go through the US government link (Department of Health and Human Services, HIPAA Administrative Simplification Regulation Text 2013). Then, look up one profession's response to the regulations, such as comment in reaction to the HIPAA (Flores & Dodier, 2005). Journals are a vital discussion forum, as professionals share their views on how to comply with the regulations in professional practice, and what difficulties they face as professionals dealing with confidential information.

Summary

You have learnt that privacy and confidentiality are more than shorthand terms. You can appreciate that so much effort is necessarily directed by society to define and highlight the fundamental importance of personal integrity, and that integrity extends to personal information concerns as well as physical integrity concerns. You now recognise that considerable integrated legal, ethics and regulatory work has already been undertaken in important issues such as information privacy, and that it is ongoing. You have also learnt about the balancing of public interests, and that law and resulting regulation seeks to balance those interests in a way that is ethical and acceptable to the community.

STUDY QUESTIONS

1   Explain the legal, regulatory and ethical importance of privacy principles.
2   Describe an instance in which privacy can be breached. Support your reasoning with relevant law, ethics and regulation.

SAMPLE ESSAY QUESTIONS

1   List the relevant Privacy Principles from one Australian jurisdiction.
2   Explain the legal significance of legislation on privacy.
3   Explain the ethical significance of at least five Privacy Principles.
4   Source and outline two regulations or policies that give effect to the principles in a health setting.

REFERENCES

American Health Information Management Association. (2017). *AHIMA code of ethics*. Retrieved from http://www.ahima.org

Andersen, B., & Aranson, E. (1999). Iceland's database is ethically questionable. *British Medical Journal, 318*(7197), 156.

Australian Government, Department of Health. (2011). *National Health Security Agreement*. Retrieved from http://www.health.gov.au

Australian Government, National Disability Insurance Scheme. *NDIS quality and safeguarding framework*. Retrieved from http://dss.gov.au

Australian Law Reform Commission. (1983). *Privacy*. Background Report No. 22, Vol. 1, Canberra: AGPS.

Bacchetti, P., & Moss, A.R. (1989). Incubation period of AIDS in San Francisco. *Nature, 338*, 251–3.

Beauchamp, D.E. (1999). Community: The neglected tradition of public health. In D.E. Beauchamp & B. Steinbock, *New ethics for the public's health* (pp. 57–67). Sydney: Oxford University Press.

Beauchamp T.L., & Childress, J.F. *Principles of biomedical ethics* (2nd edn). New York: Oxford University Press.

Berglund, C.A. (1990). Australian standards for privacy and confidentiality of health records in research: Implications of the Commonwealth Privacy Act. *Medical Journal of Australia, 152*, 664–9.

Berglund, C.A. (1995). Mandatory HIV testing of patients and professionals: Bringing ethics into practice. *Medical Education, 29*, 360–3.

Berglund, C.A., Pond, D.C., Traynor, V., Gietzelt, D., McNeill, P.M., Harris, M.F., & Comino, E. (1997, April). *General practice and ethics: Listening and understanding concerns raised by general practitioners and consumers*. Paper presented at the Fifth National Conference of the Australian Bioethics Association, Melbourne, 3–6 April 1997.

Centers for Disease Control. (1987). Revision of the CDC surveillance case definition for acquired immunodeficiency syndrome. *Morbidity and Mortality Weekly Report, 36*(supp. 1S).

Coverdale, J. (1996). Ethics in forensic psychiatry. In W. Brookbanks (Ed.), *Psychiatry and the law: Clinical and legal issues* (pp. 59–70). Wellington: Brookers.

Czecowoski, B.J.A. (1984). *Privacy and confidentiality of health care information*. Chicago, Illinois: American Hospital Association.

Department of Health. (2012). *Governance arrangements for research ethics committees: A harmonised edition*. Retrieved from www.gov.uk

Department of Health. (2017). *Surveillance case definitions for the Australian National Notifiable Diseases Surveillance System*. Australian Government. Retrieved from http://health.gov.au

Department of Health and Human Services. *HIPAA administrative simplification regulation text*. (2013). 45 CFR Parts 160, 162, & 164. Retrieved from www.hhs.gov

Devereux, J. (1997). *Medical law: Text, cases and materials*. Sydney: Cavendish.

Economic & Social Research Council [ESRC]. (2010). *Framework for research ethics* [FRE]. Retrieved from www.esrc.ac.uk

Flaherty, D.H. (1989). *Protecting privacy in surveillance societies*. Chapel Hill: University of North Carolina Press.

Flores, J.A., & Dodier, A. (2005). HIPAA: Past, present and future implications for nurses. *Online Journal of Issues in Nursing, 10*(2), 5.

Gostin, L.O. (2006). Medical countermeasures for pandemic influenza: Ethics and the law. *Journal of the American Medical Association, 295*(5), 554–6.

Gostin, L.O. (2016). *Public health law: Power, duty, restraint* (3rd edn). Oakland: University of California Press.

Government of Western Australia, Department of Communities Child Protection and Family Support. (2008). *Mandatory reporting of child sexual abuse in Western Australia: A guide for mandatory reporters*. Retrieved from http://dcp.wa.gov.au

Health Research Council of New Zealand. (2012, November). *HRC Guidelines for Ethics Committee Accreditation*. Retrieved from www.hrc.govt.nz

Mill, J.S. (1975). On liberty. In *Three Essays* (pp. 92–114). London: Oxford University Press.

National Commission for the Protection of Subjects of Biomedical and Behavioral Research. (1978). *Report and Recommendations: Institutional Review Boards.* Also *Appendix to Report and Recommendations: Institutional Review Boards.* Department of Health, Education, and Welfare Pub. No. (OS) 78–0008. US Government Printing Office, Washington DC.

National Health and Medical Research Council. (2014). *Guidelines under Section 95 of the Privacy Act 1988.* Retrieved from http://nhmrc.gov.au

National Health and Medical Research Council, Australian Research Council & Universities Australia. (2007). *National statement on ethical conduct in human research.* (Updated May 2015 & July 2018). Retrieved from www.nhmrc.gov.au

Office of the Australian Information Commissioner. (2018). *Notifiable data breaches scheme.* Australian Government. Retrieved from www.oaic.gov.au

Parliament of Australia Bills and Legislation. (2015, 22 October). *Social Services Legislation Amendment (No Jab, No Pay) Bill 2015, Bills Digest, 36, 2015–16.* Retrieved from http://aph.gov.au

Parry, J. (2006). Funding of bird flu initiative exceeds expectations. *British Medical Journal, 332*(7535), 198.

Pharmacy Board of Australia. (2011). *Pharmacy Code of Conduct for registered health practitioners.* Retrieved from www.ahpra.gov.au

Robotham, J. (2006, 18–19 February). High-dose bird flu vaccine trial fails. *Sydney Morning Herald*, 3.

Taerk, G., Gallop, R.M., Lancee, W.J., Coates, R.A., & Fanning, M. (1993). Recurrent themes of concern in groups for health care professionals. *AIDS Care, 5*(2), 215–22.

Tegtmeier, J.W. (1990). Ethics and AIDS: A summary of the law and critical analysis of the individual physician's ethical duty to treat. *American Journal of Law & Medicine, 16*(1–2), 249–65.

Westin, A.F. (1970). *Privacy and freedom.* New York: Atheneum.

World Health Organization. (2003). *Alert, verification and public health management of SARS in the post-outbreak period.* Retrieved 14 August 2003 from www.who.int/csr/sars

World Health Organization. (2006). WHO News: Pandemic flu—communicating the risks. *Bulletin of the World Health Organization, 84*(1), 9–11.

World Health Organization. (2007, 23 October). Projected supply of pandemic influenza vaccine sharply increases. [Press release]. Retrieved from www.who.int

LEGISLATION

Children and Community Services Act 2004 (WA)

Government Information (Public Access) Act 2009 (NSW)

Health Records and Information Privacy Act 2002 (NSW)

Legislative Instruments Act 2003 (Cth)

My Health Records Amendment (Strengthening Privacy) Bill 2018 (Cth)

National Health Security Act 2007 (Cth)

Privacy Act 1988 (Cth)

Privacy Amendment (Notifiable Data Breaches) Act 2017 (Cth)

Privacy Amendment (Private Sector) Act 2000 (Cth)

Privacy and Personal Information Protection Act 1998 (NSW)

Social Services Legislation Amendment (No Jab, No Pay) Bill 2015 (Cth)

CASES

PD v Australian Red Cross, New South Wales Supreme Court, unreported, December 1992.

Tarasoff v Regents of University of California 17 Cal. 3d 425 (Cal. 1976).

CHAPTER 7

The limits of care

LEARNING OBJECTIVES

- To appreciate the integrated and practical contributions of law, regulation and ethics in defining the limits of care.
- To further explore best interests and autonomy.
- To understand that both personal and social limits impact on health care.
- To learn about the integration of law, ethics and regulation in research and development of new treatments.
- To practise applying principlist frameworks in research ethics.

KEY TERMS

benefit

best interests

consent

personal morality

risk

social morality

transparency

Personal and social morality, best interests and autonomy

The choices of an individual are made within a social context. Such decisions are therefore potentially subject to social limits, but this needs to be carefully reasoned given the widespread support for autonomy in ethics reasoning frameworks.

To start with one ethics reasoning framework as an example, the famous early libertarian John Stuart Mill thought that individual liberty should be allowed—within certain limits. This applied to the different liberties of:

- consciousness
- thought and feeling
- expressing and publishing opinions
- tastes and pursuits
- being able to unite with others for any purpose.

The limits to liberty proposed by Mill were, broadly, limits upon:

- causing serious and imminent harm to others
- threatening other's similar liberties
- threatening the fabric of society.

risk
Likelihood of negative effect or outcome; possibility of significant negative outcome.

personal morality
Significant lessons prompting reflection to identify a virtuous, right or acceptable course of conduct of an individual, largely affecting that individual.

social morality
Significant lessons prompting reflection to identify a virtuous, right, or acceptable course of conduct of individuals, with significant implications for the choices then available to others in society.

These limits take into account the respect that we should afford others—as well as expect ourselves—and the need for all to live in a society that has established structures and boundaries. Interestingly, Mill did not think that liberty should be limited on the sole grounds that the person's choice would harm themselves. He thought that competent adults should be free to **risk** their own health and wellbeing without interference. If you take the view that society should not take primary responsibility for defining what a good is—as nobody can really define the good to aim for except the client—you would be an extreme libertarian. As J.S. Mill writes, each person can and should decide for themselves what is in their best interest; having decided what is in their best interest, that person has a right to it, unless it conflicts with similar rights of others, or threatens the fabric of society (Mill, 1975).

The libertarian position places autonomy first, unless it can be argued, under fairly limited circumstances, that autonomy cannot be granted. The extreme libertarian position would place client choice first, rather than the current or available professional view of what is the best treatment. Whether or not autonomy and the client's wish, or choice, should override the professional's ideal view of beneficence—or even what they think is reasonable care, or the best care to provide—may depend on your preferred ethical reasoning framework. The mainstream view is that the client's wish should not override the professional's view of appropriate care, but a strongly committed libertarian may well argue it should, unless the choice threatened others' choices or the way society was structured to care for all in some way.

Mill's essay *On Liberty* supports a difference between **personal morality** and **social morality**. That is, if something affects no other person, it should be in the realm of their own choice. However, if it affects others—by threatening the fabric of society, or by threatening other people—then it is a social issue, and the liberty can be legitimately constrained by social decision.

By definition, most health care systems do not respond only to what each individual wants. Governments and administrators try to decide what is a good, thereby anticipating what people will want and need, and make resource allocation decisions on the basis of providing that defined good. Most systems are, therefore, not strictly libertarian.

However, the limits that Mill identifies as reasonable limits to autonomy are useful, as they help to define rights that we are prepared to acknowledge within an existing health care system and in routine health care decisions. The institution may only offer a limited range of treatment options. In setting up institutions, we show our concern for the health of all people in society, and most limitations imposed by institutions are intended to protect the integrity and health of all people rather than any one individual. These limitations may be interpreted as social limitations protecting the social structure of the health care institution.

Under our health system, a public patient in hospital may not be able to choose their own doctor, while a private patient can. If individual public patients wanted to choose their own doctors, but could not pay for the doctors' services, we may feel justified in denying them that choice on the grounds that the system, as our society has set it up, can stretch to allowing them treatment options, but not their choice of doctor. We may accept that it is more important to protect the social system than to promote autonomy.

In Mill's terms, this means that we are prepared to limit personal choices in relation to the allocation of resources because the question is one of social morality. In a less strict sense, we have decided that people cannot have unlimited choice of health care and, consequently, unlimited spending on this health care, because this would affect other people in society to an unacceptable degree. The key to this is that autonomy and client preferences—or wishes—are not absolute. They must be weighed against competing liberties and interests.

We are used to limiting autonomy in an institutional context. If you think of our society, we have rules that tacitly limit autonomy on a number of grounds. For instance, a person who likes to drive will be allowed to do so, but only on the road. You read about driving restrictions as an example of societal regulation in Chapter 1. If the person likes to drive fast, we might say that that type of driving should be done on freeways, and not in suburban streets. Why? One explanation is that we have judged it too dangerous to others if these limits to driving are not imposed. So that person's wish or preference for fast driving should not be to the detriment of others. Another example is the person who likes to drive but also likes to drink. We say yes to each of that person's wishes, but stipulate that these things should not be undertaken together, as we judge drink-driving to be too dangerous to both the driver and others.

Public health Act provisions now ban smoking on public premises, including public hospitals. For instance, in Victoria, smoking was banned in public hospitals and community health services from April 2014, and fines for breaches can be applied, as established under the *Tobacco Amendment Act 2014* (Vic). The bans are justified, given the harm caused to people from smoking, and in the interests of ensuring patients are not subjected to second-hand smoke, as the Minister for Health, Jill Hennessy explained (Premier of Victoria, 2015). This is similar to a parking fine, as an administrative level fine. Local hospital settings may have designated smoking areas that are set apart from the off limits areas—you will find these areas are outside, away from public access ways and ventilation ducts. In Queensland, where smoking has been banned at all times in all staff and patient areas of health care and residential aged facilities and five metres beyond their boundaries under the *Tobacco and Other Smoking Products Act 1998* (Qld), and *Tobacco and Other Smoking Products (Smoke-free Places) Amendment Bill 2015* (Qld), which applied from 1 September 2016, a 'nominated smoking place' can be designated in residential aged facilities, as part of their outdoor area.

If you decide to turn up for work when you are sick—what is the potential effect of this decision on others? Is it a personal morality decision? What if you work in a ward for people with compromised immunity?

If you do not follow routine protocols such as infection control and handwashing, what risks are others exposed to? Is that risk yours to take?

Is not washing your hands your decision to make freely? When you read the regulations excerpt below, consider if the regulations represent a collective statement consistent with a social morality stance that has been debated and arrived at for the professional health context. Hand hygiene policy is commonly set out as the five moments of hand hygiene, and it is a piece of regulation that you will have learnt very early in your clinical setting.

Infection control and handwashing might seem like simple matters, but the fact that there is a policy demonstrates the need for it and the reasoned justification for it. It is a matter of safety and governance and professional integrity that once a policy is set, each professional has a personal and professional responsibility to heed the requirements.

As stated in Hand Hygiene Australia's hand hygiene policy, personal vigilance and institutional implementation of the policy is essential (Hand Hygiene Australia, 2018). The objective is stated in the introduction:

> There is convincing evidence that improved hand hygiene can reduce infection rates. More than 20 hospital based studies (including systematic reviews) of the impact of hand hygiene on the risk of healthcare associated infection have been published between 1977 and 2011 … Despite study limitations almost all reports showed an association between improved hand hygiene practices and reduced infection and cross transmission rates.

The manual explains the Five Moments for Hand Hygiene as follows:

> The 5 Moments for Hand Hygiene are a theoretical model of how infectious agents can be transferred between a healthcare worker and patients. It is inclusive of all occasions where a patient's safety can be endangered by the care given by a healthcare worker; where opportunity exists for transfer of infectious agents between healthcare worker, patient and the healthcare environment.
>
> Moment 1:   Before touching a patient
> Moment 2:   Before a procedure
> Moment 3:   After a procedure or body fluid exposure risk
> Moment 4:   After touching a patient
> Moment 5:   After touching a patient's surroundings.

The policy goes on to outline the barriers that must be addressed to implement a hand hygiene policy consistently:

> Poor hand hygiene practice among HCWs is strongly associated with healthcare associated infection transmission and is a major factor in the spread of antibiotic-resistant organisms within hospitals ... Despite this, efforts to improve the rate of hand hygiene compliance have generally been ineffective or their efficacy poorly sustained. Numerous barriers to appropriate hand hygiene have been reported ... including:
>
> - hand hygiene agents causing skin irritation and dryness
> - The perception that patient needs take priority over hand hygiene
> - Hand washing sinks/basins inconveniently located and/or not available
> - The perception that glove use dispenses with the need for additional hand hygiene
> - Insufficient time for hand hygiene, due to high workload and understaffing
> - Inadequate knowledge of guidelines, protocols or technique for hand hygiene
> - Lack of positive role models and social norms
> - Lack of recognition of the risk of cross-transmission of microbial pathogens
> - Until recently, lack of scientific information showing a definitive impact of improved hand hygiene on healthcare associated infection rates
> - Simple forgetfulness.

REFLECTION POINT

Practical safety steps

Find a reminder sign in your workplace about washing hands or infection control. Is it on the reception desk, to remind people with flu symptoms not to come into the health facility? Is it in the toilet, to remind everyone to play their part in limiting the spread of germs and bacteria? Is it over a hand sanitiser station? Consider what language is used in that reminder about risks, limits and best interests, and choices that individuals can be encouraged to make, or boundaries that are set on behalf of the institutional residents or community.

Design a new sign of your own. Remember that your audiences may be different. Be sure to include the purpose of the reminder, the reminder message, and the authority you have in issuing the reminder. You can use pictures, symbols or text—or other forms of communication.

REFLECTION POINT

Social morality limits

Think of a situation in which a client's autonomy was limited, not by you but by the institution or resources.

Justify the limit imposed according to Mill's guidance or another ethics reasoning framework from Chapter 4.

Thinking more broadly, you could make a list of other personal morality decisions and social morality decisions in a health and medical context.

In our health care system, treatment choices that are made by clients are usually interpreted as questions of personal morality. In practice, under many regulations, we allow autonomy that is consistent with Mill's position. People can choose what type of treatment they would prefer, given a reasonable choice that has been afforded to them by their (public or private health) community, and they can even choose not to be treated at all. Provided they are not harming other people too greatly—by for instance spreading an infectious disease—their choice about treatment is their own, and their reasons for making that decision must be respected.

An individual perspective on risk and benefit

benefit
Positive effect or
outcome.

Some clients are risk takers—others are not. There is a difference between how much risk people are prepared to undertake for a perceived likely **benefit**. For instance, cautious people might not want to go parachuting on their days off, but risk takers might, because for them the thrill of the activity and the sensation of being airborne are worth the possibility of physical injury. How people approach their everyday health, health risks and treatment when they become clients varies in just the same way. The likely positive and negative effects or outcomes of different treatment or management plans are weighed up by individuals. This is a weighing of risks and benefits.

INTEGRATED LEARNING AND PRACTICE

Acceptance of advice

Imagine you are working in a rehabilitation team. As you make a start on this chapter, consider what issues you want to focus on, and what assistance you would like so that you feel able to make progress in the following case.

A young man, Mr Y, aged 19 years, has come to see you. Mr Y's health record shows that he has multiple health issues. He left school early, and had a slight learning difficulty as well as behavioural challenges that made getting along with authority figures tricky. He is on anti-epileptic medication, and has occasional rage outbursts. Recently, he was in a car with three friends, and was involved in an accident. At the time of the accident, one of his friends was riding on the roof of the car, and another was on the boot. The car was speeding on a dirt road, and rolled. Mr Y was inside the car in the front passenger seat. He broke his leg so badly that he needed surgery to have plates inserted. He is still on crutches. Mr Y's parents have rung you before the appointment. Apart from the lack of Mr Y's compliance with the physiotherapy suggested, they are worried about his risky behaviours, and want you to convince Mr Y to find new friends.

In identifying the issues, take the time to flick back through past chapters and perhaps the issues coming up in the next chapters to refresh your memory on professional skill, resources and allocation, meeting and working with patients, developing and diminishing capacities, and so on. The scenario is quite a bit more complex than it seems on the surface.

Non-judgmental harm reduction or minimisation approaches are quite well accepted in health care when patients pose a risk to themselves—such as with illicit drug use. Gaining trust is important, so that truthful disclosure is made on the substances being taken. Appropriate strategies to reduce substance use can then be trialled, while also monitoring a person's health adequately. One physician's advice was that in treating sports people who use performance-enhancing drugs, the first step is encouraging disclosure of dangerous practices, and understanding why that person has chosen to use them. If the sports people are elite and using drugs as a tool towards performance goals, they may only be engaged in reducing their usage over time. Recent gym users can be amenable to information about effective diet and training that can achieve the results hoped for more safely. For recreational users, other illicit drug use can be common, so different strategies may be needed. One physician's practice was to first of all acknowledge the illicit or dangerous drug use, and then start working collaboratively towards keeping each patient as safe as possible (Dawson, 2001). Can you work out which philosophical stance this harm minimisation approach is compatible with?

Australian nurses have been found to support harm reduction strategies such as needle and syringe programs for illicit drug users, which seek to reduce associated risk such as infections from shared needles (Ford, 2010). Harm reduction policy approaches to drugs, including cannabis, are supported by certain political parties such as The Greens in Australia, as noted on their website <www.greens.org.au>. The policies of many parties can change from time to time, so policy statements should be checked for currency before being relied on.

So far, we have established that autonomy is important, but it is not absolute, and there may be circumstances in which you are not obliged to promote it—and even some circumstances when it should be curtailed. In any situation in which you are deciding to promote, allow or limit autonomy, you need to consider the accepted standards relating to the extent of client choice. Sometimes there are clear standards to refer to, sometimes not.

Legal and administrative limits can help, but as professional ethics is about reflection, these standards must always be assessed from an ethics stance.

Professionals have their own threshold for allowing individual autonomy before they begin drawing boundaries to this autonomy. Philosophical stances can guide us as to where to place those bounds. Libertarianism is at one extreme, and even it acknowledges some limits on liberty. Paternalism is at the other extreme. And there are choices in between.

There is a debate in ethics about which principle—autonomy or beneficence—should take priority. There is really only a need to consider this when these two principles come into conflict: when the professional definition of caring and the client definition of what care they would like to receive diverge. Most beneficence models either give way to autonomy when the client's idea of good is very different to the professional's, or include autonomy as an integral part of the principle of beneficence.

If you were a paternalist, you would believe that your idea of good—and therefore your interpretation of the principle of beneficence—was applicable to everyone. There would be no need to change your view on good or your interpretation of beneficence, no matter how different your client's views were from yours. That means beneficence could always override autonomy. In extreme paternalistic stances, there may be little need to ask clients for their **consent** before doing something that you believe is good for them, nor would there be a need to tell them all the options before asking them to agree to something that you think is good for them. Many people associate this with the old style of health care, particularly the old way of conducting medical practice.

The paternalism associated with medicine, as practised in the past, cannot be entirely attributed to professionals: patients also abrogated responsibility and autonomy. This attitude is captured in the phrase: 'Doctor knows best'. The move away from this position has involved a developing sense of shared responsibility and the development of the model of a dynamic relationship between health care worker and patient. The modern rejection of paternalism amounts to a belief that the patient has a responsibility to double-check that the good being aimed at by the professional is compatible with their definition of a good.

The model of beneficence that builds-in autonomy still has something of that paternalistic attitude because it lets the professional define what the good is that they will offer. Ultimately, it is up to the client to make decisions within the limits set by the professionals, but the basic good that the professional is willing to help their client towards doesn't change. Pellegrino and Thomasma (1988) argue for 'autonomy within beneficence', as a model that is distinct from paternalism. This model acknowledges the complexity of the client's illness, as well as the professional input in determining what could be beneficent. This approach emphasises **best interests**.

Many modern philosophers and ethicists maintain that beneficence and autonomy are separate principles that can outweigh each other, but in different circumstances. This depends on the type of decision being made and the broader philosophical framework you choose to work under. A dramatic example might be a person who is terminally ill, and who wants to be removed from life support. Autonomy may be upheld if that is done, but

consent
Agreement.

best interests
That which is judged to be to the maximal benefit of a person or persons in maintaining or furthering their health and welfare.

if you think that beneficence includes the concept of sanctity of life—regardless of quality of life—you may not be satisfied that turning off the life support is beneficent. If you are a deontologist, you will be less likely to switch off the life support because, under deontology, fundamental rules, such as observing sanctity of life, must be obeyed irrespective of the circumstances. On the other hand, if you were a utilitarian, you might decide that the present and future happiness of the person, their family, and even other members of society is best served by switching it off. So you solve the dilemma by placing autonomy above the importance of life preservation, and justify this prioritisation of values by arguing that, overall, everyone would be better off if the life support were to be turned off.

An alternative balance between autonomy and beneficence is found in the 'enhanced autonomy' model, which encourages both health worker and client to exchange views, information and their respective understandings of that information. This raises the issue of the interpretation and value judgment of medical facts. If this is instituted solely by professionals, it is paternalistic; the enhanced autonomy model has the client participating actively in the interpretation and judgment of medical facts (Quill & Brody, 1996). The negotiation of treatment options is discussed further in Chapter 8, as part of informed decision making.

Encountering patients who adopt a preference that is not in keeping with your best advice is part of routine health care work. You do your best to assess people, and then give them advice. If they don't follow your advice, they can reduce their chances of effective recovery or improvement in their health. They used to be called 'non-compliant' patients—meaning they were not willing or able to do as advised.

A skills-based approach for learning reflection techniques so they are 'able to work through emotional responses of anger, frustration, defensiveness and detachment towards patients and others' has been developed. The emphasis of the training is on being aware of one's own emotional reaction if patients 'did not seem to listen' to advice or 'apparently did not care about their health, and remaining ready to care when the patient was 'ready' to engage with the care they could offer' (Shapiro et al., 2006). Non-compliant patients test your commitment to putting further energy into their care. The following Integrated learning and practice exercise is based on this skills-based reflective approach.

INTEGRATED LEARNING AND PRACTICE

What can I do when patients don't heed my advice?

In routine matters, the law upholds a client's right to choose what treatment and advice to act on, if any.

Models of autonomy in ethics help the carer to understand the balance to be reached between the carer's advice and the client's choice.

Policy and procedures help to prepare staff to behave courteously in all circumstances, including anticipating that patients can make choices seemingly at odds with professional advice.

REFLECTION POINT

Respect and patience

Imagine that you are in the role of the health carer in the following situation.

A client regularly appears at the walk-in, no-appointment-necessary clinic, usually when unwell and wanting a medical certificate that states he is unfit for work that day. Frequent advice is documented in the notes about the need to eat more healthily and exercise, so as to build an immune system that is more resilient to common infections, and for a follow-up visit so that any underlying cause of illness can be looked into.

With each appointment, the client's common response is, 'I don't have the time' or 'I am only here for a certificate', sometimes said in a hostile manner.

What is your reaction to this? When you think about your emotional reaction a little more, can you think of a better reaction to express to the client? If you have already had some practise in this skill, you may have options at the ready, which will help you to avoid an immediately emotional response towards the client. Consider: are you comfortable with this approach? Or is it a skill that you need to practise?

CASE EXAMPLE

From case decisions to policy

Look back at Integrated learning and practice on p. 214, as you now have quite a bit of time to devote to the perplexing issues raised by Mr Y's case.

Try to solve a couple of the ethical issues that arise in working with this young adult, preferably with the benefit of group discussion. You could role-play a process of consultation between the relevant parties, and suggest a compromise between them. You could explain to one or more parties why they have—or have not—been included in the process of discussion.

Then take the time to think a little more broadly about other people like Mr Y—who likes to take risks—and his friends who also liked to ride around in cars.

Looking back at Mr Y's case, try to identify issues that could usefully be the subject of general policy.

1 How could your institution develop a guideline or standard operating procedure that would help health practitioners and health care workers facing similar cases in the future?

2 Draft a guiding principle or statement for what should be done, or the process that should be followed in working out what to do next. (Be sure to justify your guidance with appropriate ethics theory, and perhaps reference other helpful policies and procedures for care in your institution setting.)

As you have read, health departments can generate policy and procedural clinical guidelines and regulations. Governance departments in large institutions are responsible for the implementation of these procedural guidelines and regulations, and may on occasions develop their own standard operating procedures.

Remember why a standard operating procedure is developed.

Best interests considerations are part of the practical professional assessment of a care provider. Given your skill and knowledge, you are equipped to assess and advise on what would be in a person's best interests. Sometimes, given imminent risk to self or others, care is provided using a substitute decision-making model.

One illustration of this is the system of referral to other health care professionals and treatment services. Referral is the option for someone to follow up a direction in assessment or treatment, so the care can be received if the person wishes to avail themself of that opportunity.

A medical practitioner or an authorised mental health practitioner, such as a mental health nurse, can refer people to a psychiatrist under the relevant jurisdiction's provisions of a Mental Health Act. The informed consent of the person for assessment and treatment is required for voluntary patients, so it is up to them to decide if they wish to pursue the options available in mental health assessment and treatment. Respect for their autonomy is paramount, and they are not forced to go.

Respect for autonomy has limits, such as when the referral is made in the belief that a person may be in need of an involuntary treatment order. Treatment under the mental health provisions is:

> any psychiatric, medical, psychological or psychosocial intervention intended to alleviate or prevent the deterioration of a mental illness or a condition that is a consequence of mental illness. For example, psychiatric medication, electroconvulsive therapy, immediate medical treatment following deliberate self-harm, or the use of nasogastric intubation for a patient with an eating disorder.

> *(Government of Western Australia, Mental Health Commission, 2015, p. 6)*

Professional assessment is made, after observing the person and having regard to information provided by another person and also a person's medical records, that such referral is necessary. All restrictions to a person's own decision making is carefully weighed up, as is required under strict legislative provisions. If the appropriate procedures are followed, then the reasonable restriction does not amount to the tort of false imprisonment, which is the unlawful detention of a person, You read about false imprisonment in Chapter 1, as it is a fundamental regulatory issue in health care contexts.

The mental health practitioner's belief that assessment is necessary is documented in a form, as in Form 1A under the *Mental Health Act 2014* (WA). If detention is necessary for the psychiatric examination, a medical practitioner or an authorised mental health practitioner can make a detention order, using Form 3A, initially for up to 24 hours. The forms are an important aspect of the regulations as they document the reasoning behind the referral for assessment or detention for that purpose, as is required under the legislation. Detention or restriction is a serious infringement on a person's liberty or autonomy and must be carefully justified. The preliminary orders are carefully time limited, and application for an extension of the order is a different process. The examining psychiatrist can order that the person is no longer a detained person, and this decision and reason is similarly documented in a separate form—Form 3E.

You could compare this to scheduling provisions, in which the liberty of a person is to be restricted, to the extent necessary and sufficient to safeguard an imminent risk to self or others, while treatment is undertaken. Form 6B is used by a psychiatrist for an inpatient treatment order, and approval from the Chief Psychiatrist is required. Form 5A is used for a community treatment order (CTO). Community treatment orders are the lesser form of restrictions—they still require certain treatment be undertaken, but a residential care setting is not required.

As also set out in the legislation, any interested person can complain about a decision or treatment, and appeals can be lodged to seek a review of certain aspects of the treatment orders. All orders made under the Mental Health Act can be reviewed if an application is made to the Mental Health Tribunal. That tribunal's decision can be reviewed by the State Administrative Tribunal, and in turn reviewed by the Supreme Court. So the administrative decisions are reviewable, as a basic requirement for administrative matters, which is a principle of law that you read about in Chapter 3.

The requirement for proper documentation and justification is similar in all jurisdictions. As in the Victorian equivalent assessment form, which is completed by a registered medical practitioner or mental health practitioner, the date of examination is documented, and the reason why an opinion has been reached is documented, as set out in the *Mental Health Act 2014* (Vic), Section 30 MHA 101 Assessment Order:

> I am satisfied that all the following criteria in section 29 of the *Mental Health Act 2014* (Vic) apply to the person:
>
> a the person appears to have mental illness (mental illness is a medical condition that is characterised by a significant disturbance of thought, mood, perception or memory); and
>
> b because the person appears to have a mental illness, the person appears to need immediate treatment to prevent:
>
> i   serious deterioration in the person's mental or physical health; or
>
> ii Serious harm to the person or to another person; and
>
> c if the person is made subject to an Assessment Order, the person can be assessed; and
>
> d there is no less restrictive means reasonably available to enable the person to be assessed.

REFLECTION: PERSONAL CHOICES

As a revision of this section, try answering the following questions. They will prompt you to reflect on the way you value personal morality, and autonomy, and how autonomy is justifiably limited or promoted.

1   Think of a situation in which you have promoted someone's autonomy. How did you do that? Were you satisfied that you acted properly?

2   Now think of a situation in which it has been difficult for you to accept the autonomy of an individual patient or client. What did you do? Were you satisfied that you acted properly?

3   Brainstorm what regulations or standard protocols would support your conduct to limit or promote someone's autonomy in each situation, and what ethics reasoning frameworks you would suggest support this position.

REFLECTION: SPECIFIC REQUESTS

A 15-year-old girl, Karen, who is doing her Year 10 exams soon, comes to see a GP. She says she feels tired but can't sleep, and is very worried that she won't do well in her exams. Karen asks for sleeping tablets. She does not want her parents or her regular doctor to know that she is seeking medical treatment.

Make some notes on how you would develop this analysis.

The most common starting point for ethics analysis is the principlist model suggested by Beauchamp and Childress, which uses the principles of beneficence, non-maleficence, autonomy, and justice. Once you separate out the issues into these four categories, you will have made a good start to recognising the complexity of the case. (Alternatively, you could brainstorm what might be a concern in each of the four categories.)

The ethics theories and frameworks are very helpful in deciding how to resolve conflicts between the shorthand principles.

The Beauchamp and Childress model has appeal partly because of its simplicity, and partly because it can be realistically undertaken by any interested party. Professionals can readily use it. So can patients themselves, if they wish, or the patient's family. It is useful for policy makers and administrators too, as it includes big-picture issues of resources alongside the potential complexities of individual circumstances and situations. It is quite useful in 'macro' community-type decisions, as well as 'micro' individual issues.

For Karen, autonomy and the decision-making process will loom large. Once you have the issue tagged under autonomy, you can start to identify what is problematic about it. You might look to the sections on privacy and confidentiality later in this chapter, or the discussion on competency and decision making in Chapter 8 'Lifelong practice in

+ continued

decision making'. The purpose of care might be discussed, and you could consider the options that may be open to the professionals who see Karen. Just stating the existence of an issue does not solve it. You will need to explore each issue, and discuss if the issues are in conflict—such as if a patient's choice (autonomy) conflicts with the needs and resources available to others (justice).

The obvious legal issue is whether Karen as a 15-year-old is able to make her own health care decisions, and you can read about this further in Chapter 8. The gravity of the situation and her corresponding capacity to comprehend relevant information and then make a decision is part of the legal analysis. The specific legislation and regulations about S4D drugs is also relevant, as you read in Chapter 1.

Thinking about the practical casuistry approach, the general approach of the clinic towards this type of situation—where a teenager is asking to be treated, independent of her family or guardian, and seeking a specific short-term 'fix' to what may be a complex larger problem—may well largely determine how Karen's request is handled. An 'acceptable' course of action may have already been defined by other experienced team members, and even if the ethical reasons remain unarticulated, actions by team members in the past in similar situations could guide the person treating the 'Karen' who presents as a patient this time. Tearoom chats and team meetings provide a wealth of lessons learnt from past cases, and these stories are the material of casuistry.

The practice or local health service may have some regulations and procedures that assist when considering how to handle teenagers as patients, partly due to billing and administrative concerns, and partly building-in checking processes so that a legally robust decision is able to be made before treatment commences.

Autonomy

Jennifer Haines

Jennifer has been a Registered Nurse for 40 years and spent most of those years practising in critical care areas, ICU, CCU, Neurosurgery ICU and Emergency Department.

An elderly patient is informed of a poor prognosis after being given a diagnosis of terminal cancer. An experimental treatment is available that the oncologist would like to trial on this woman.

The patient considers her position and decides that she does not want to be part of such a trial—and in fact wants no further treatment. She prefers to enter a palliative care home-based program. The oncologist disagrees with the patient's decision, as he believes the experimental treatment may well prolong and improve the quality of her life.

1   To what extent may the oncologist continue to persuade this patient to enter the treatment program?

2   Patients have autonomy when making decisions about treatment—but autonomy is not always given the same recognition when a patient wishes to refuse treatment. Why is that? What does 'informed consent' mean when a patient refuses treatment?

3   Imagine that you are the nurse looking after this patient. She is troubled by the advice given by the oncologist and wavering about her decision to refuse further treatment. She seeks your advice. What would you say to her?

Research and experimental treatment

Patients and healthy volunteers can be asked to take part in research. As you will read, regulatory safeguards are in place to protect research participants through national and international declarations, codes, statements and guidelines. Each health professional has a compelling obligation to reflect on the complex ethics implications of conducting research, during both the planning and conduct of research, and in putting their own patients forward as possible research participants.

Professional colleagues can provide advice on appropriate professional conduct, and each health profession's code of conduct and code of ethics can also provide a useful reference on values and principles to keep in mind in the conduct of research. Human Research Ethics Committees (HRECs) approve or reject proposed research after considering its ethical acceptability. In addition, institutions consider institutional risk and acceptability of research processes and approve or reject proposed research on governance grounds. Institutions consider their legal obligations as part of the separate process of governance approval, and decide if the risk to participants, researchers and the institution is acceptable in that institutional and jurisdictional context.

The World Medical Association's *Declaration of Helsinki* is the base document from which many research ethics guidelines have been developed. This is routinely discussed and updated at assembly meetings, but is still known as the *Declaration of Helsinki*, as that was the city where delegates met in 1964 and approved the earliest version of the Declaration (World Medical Association, 2008).

The similarity between statements is not surprising, given their common purpose of protecting human subjects and maintaining the progress of understanding through medical research. The statements are designed to ensure that unethical research—such as that examined in the Nuremberg trials—does not occur again. The Nuremberg trials examined, among other war crimes, medical research conducted on prisoners of war held by the Nazis. Those responsible for the experiments were put on trial and were, ultimately, convicted of having committed crimes against humanity. The experiments included sterilisations, placing people in freezing conditions to observe the effect on their body, infecting people with typhus to observe the reaction, and even killing so that the body could be dissected as a specimen. The resulting Nuremberg Code, setting out principles of how to deal with research subjects with respect and preserve their dignity, forms a vivid historical backdrop to many subsequent discussions of the ethics of research with human participants (Picker et al., 1988).

Researchers and committees plan and decide under relevant national ethics guidelines. These guidelines are important as standards because all researchers and HRECs are obliged to consider research in the light of the principles it promotes—sometimes due to funding provisos, and otherwise due to institutional requirements or professional expectations. You can access the relevant guidelines on the research council websites, or as linked by your research office website at your base institution or professional association, and you should do so if you are planning to conduct any research. The guidelines reflect the basic values of respect for human beings, research merit and integrity—as well as justice, beneficence and respect—as central values and principles to uphold in the ethical conduct of research (National Health and Medical Research Council, Australian Research Council & Universities Australia, 2007, updated 2018, Section 1, pp. 10–11). For current guidelines, see the following:

- Australia: www.nhmrc.gov.au
- UK: www.dh.gov.uk
- US: www.hhs.gov/ohrp
- New Zealand: www.hrc.govt.nz.

Acting with integrity

Integrity is part of professionalism. The *National Statement on Ethical Conduct in Human Research* (known as the National Statement) considers research merit and integrity first. It is an essential preliminary safeguard in ethical research. If a researcher is not sufficiently skilled in the research methodology being used in the research—or if the methodology is not appropriate for the research, or if the research direction is frivolous or spurious for any reason—the research might not be ethical. If a researcher does not demonstrate integrity by a willingness to actively reflect on the appropriateness and acceptability of their research at all stages of design and conduct, then the research might not be ethical. Active reflection and willingness to abide by the regulations and approval processes is relied upon as part of the ethics safeguards.

Complying with laws and governance requirements

The National Statement concentrates on ethics, and acknowledges that there are considerable statutory and common law obligations in a research context that are not covered in the one set of guidelines (National Health and Medical Research Council, Australian Research Council

& Universities Australia, 2007, updated 2018, p. 7). Research governance requirements are set out separately in the *Australian Code for Responsible Conduct of Research*, which includes requirements relating to:

- minimum procedures for data and records management
- supervision of research staff and students involved in research
- complaints on research
- misconduct investigations.

Procedures for potential misconduct investigations are set out in an *Investigation Guide* (Australian Government National Health and Medical Research Council, Australian Research Council & Universities Australia, 2018a; 2018b).

Theoretical and practical discussions of acceptable limits in research practice and research in the specialised field of research ethics have informed the development of the regulatory guidelines. Some of this background is explained here so that you gain an insight and understanding into the amount of thought and reflection contained in the current guidelines, at the same time that you start to think about practical aspects of conducting ethical research.

When you conduct research with people, you are researching human participants. Some possible methods of researching health in human participants include:

- accessing health records
- asking questions in an interview or questionnaire
- doing a physical examination
- performing a blood test or taking a tissue sample
- giving an experimental treatment
- performing an experimental operation.

You may be able to think of more types of research. If you can, note them down. You may notice that the methods above are expressed in terms of what you do with the participants. That reflects the key ethics concern in research: what are research subjects being asked to do? This is where ethics reflection on research should start. You may also notice that as the list progresses, the level of invasiveness increases. Research subjects, health care workers and the community are particularly concerned with more invasive or intrusive research procedures.

Have you ever been asked to take part in research? A phone survey perhaps? A questionnaire at the doctor's practice? A focus group at university? What were you asked to do, and did you feel inclined to participate? Some people are generally more willing than others to take part in research. Everyone should be able to decline.

You may be surprised that all of these methods are thought of as involving human participants. Even looking at health records or analysing blood and tissue samples are thought of as researching people. Research still involves human participants—even if the people are not right in front of the researcher.

A guide to ethics reflection on research

A few general questions should guide your ethics reflection on research. If you participated, think about the research from the perspective of the researcher. You could answer these questions for any research project that you undertake in the future or that you have observed.

What is the research about? Is the researcher skilled enough to undertake it?

Research should have a purpose, a reason sufficient to justify the inconvenience or risk posed to the research participants. Researchers have a responsibility to care for research subjects, which includes being skilled enough to maximise care and minimise risk.

How are research subjects to be recruited? What are they being asked to do?

The recruitment of research subjects involves questions of acceptable burden, and free choice, on the part of subjects, in their decision to participate. What research subjects are asked to do can determine the ethics of the research: an ethical limit to the burden or risk to be borne by participants is always considered. However, this limit can change depending on the importance of the research, and the endemic risks faced by the potential participant.

How are the research subjects being asked to consent?

The consent of research subjects is paramount, particularly as research is by definition not necessarily for their benefit—there is little room to justify paternalism.

What purposes will the research be used for? Was the research worthwhile?

The likely use of the research determines both the importance of the research to the public, and the benefit for individual participants. Research can change how we think about the best available treatment or means of assessing health, or it can consolidate what we already know. Practical use of research indicates that putting research subjects through the research has been worth it. Only once the process is understood, and the results are known, can we really decide whether the research has been justified. The difficulty in terms of ethics is that this question has to be answered hypothetically before the research begins.

REFLECTION POINT

Ethics analysis of research

As a further exercise in applying these questions, take the time to look through a professional journal relevant to your profession and find a research article. A research article is one that explains the result of a research process, including the background of the research, the method of the research, what was found, and the researchers' interpretation of the findings. Then, discuss with a friend or colleague what you found and what ethics reflection the article prompted for you.

You can expect that the issues raised by the questions are interrelated. For instance, if a method is inappropriate because it does not fit the research purpose or produces erroneous results, the research could be seen as unethical, because—given that no advancement in knowledge will occur—the inconvenience to the subjects is for no purpose. If the subjects were drawn from a vulnerable or dependent population, and the research was used to improve health care for the affluent only, we may decide that the research is unethical because it is unjust. More connections between these issues are explored below, using a traditional research ethics principlist approach.

The Belmont principles

The Belmont principles—beneficence, respect for persons and justice—are used as tools here to identify and examine further key ethics concerns in research. As is suggested earlier in this book, the principles are useful as a shorthand way of checking that the relevant concerns are taken into account. The principle of respect for persons is a variation of the principle of autonomy, with a primary concern of ensuring free and uncoerced decisions to participate are made by participants. The principle of beneficence, when used as a Belmont principle, encompasses non-maleficence as well. It is about maximising benefit and care, and minimising harms or risks.

Issues can be categorised under the following Belmont principles:

- beneficence—issues involving the assessment of the risks and benefits to individuals
- respect for persons—issues surrounding personal autonomy
- justice—issues relating to the benefits and burdens to society in general.

This categorisation of issues is consistent with the suggestions in the *Belmont Report* for the use of these principles (United States Department of Health, Education, and Welfare, 1978). A comprehensive reflection on all of the principles is needed in every research situation. That is because some issues relate to more than one principle—there can be conflicting ethics concerns in research practice, as in any health practice. These principles frequently provide the foundation structure of research ethics guidelines, with the addition of the principles such as acting with integrity and compliance with local laws and institutional governance requirements.

Beneficence

The maxim 'do no harm', which is a major element of beneficence, is critical in research. This is because it is not always possible to achieve the other element of beneficence—the injunction to 'do good'—for each research participant. This is in spite of the future benefits to others—benefits that are frequently claimed as a justification for research.

An honest appraisal of what, and how much, benefit is likely from the research is needed. This benefit constitutes both the private and public interest in conducting the research, because some benefit may be to the individual participant, either during the course of the research or shortly thereafter, and some benefit may be to the community in the future. You can ask yourself the following question: What purpose does this research serve?

A risk assessment is a crucial first step in avoiding harm. The amount of risk that is acceptable—and by whom—and how that risk is assessed, is of ethical concern. Even though some studies suggest that the risk to research participants is low in most cases, any risk potentially violates the maxim 'do no harm' (Levine, 1986, p. 39). That means that all risk, even if minimal, should be explicitly acknowledged and documented.

After acknowledging risk, the next step is to assess whether that risk is acceptable. If the participant is already facing some sort of risk because—for example, he or she is suffering from an illness—this can make a difference to the ethical acceptability of research. If the proposal aims, ultimately, to reduce that risk, then this affects the risk–benefit assessment.

The risks participants are facing are crucial to the assessment of the ethics of including them in a research process:

- Is someone about to die if not treated?
- Is their condition worsening rapidly?
- Do they face endemic risks?

Facing endemic risks was a consideration in early vaccine research in which children in institutions were participants. In the infamous 1970s Willowbrook experiments, vaccine trials for hepatitis were conducted on developmentally disabled children living under care in an institution called Willowbrook, in the USA (Krugman & Giles, 1970, p. 1020). It was claimed that hepatitis was endemic there, and that, therefore, the children were likely to get it anyway. The side effects of the vaccine were therefore judged to be acceptable. This is a useful example for discussion of acceptable therapeutic boundaries, and recognising historical context before identifying appropriate standards. In my experience, the original research article, an account of a process that led to so much ethical and professional debate, fascinates health care students.

The primary importance of the obligation to care for and treat each patient was highlighted in the Tuskegee experiments in the mid-twentieth century, in which black American men were observed as their syphilis progressed—but were not treated. The observations continued even after treatment with penicillin became available (Jones, 1981). Similar cervical cancer observational protocols were discussed widely in the late 1980s (Coney, 1988). In that research, women in New Zealand presented regularly for what they believed were thorough check-ups. They believed that they would be treated for any gynaecological conditions diagnosed during the course of these check-ups. They assumed that if they were not treated, then nothing was wrong with them. However, the research was, in fact, to observe the development of pre-cancerous cervical cells. Many of the women progressed to cancer and died while they were participating in the research. The research prompted debate about the institutional review standards that were applied when the hospital was considering the ethics of the observational research. This debate also led to changes in the membership requirements of the New Zealand ethics committees (Gillett, 1989).

Risk is weighed against the potential foreseeable benefits to the participants and others. The benefits and harms of a potential therapeutic treatment are generally weighed against the benefits and harms of treatments that are already available (World Medical Association, 2008, Paragraph 32). The level of acceptable risk is lower in non-therapeutic research. Under the *Declaration of Helsinki*, research must be discontinued if harm may be caused to the participant (World Medical Association, 2008, Paragraph 20). An obligation to benefit and to do no harm is important in both therapeutic and non-therapeutic research. As the researcher's ability to fulfil the 'do good' maxim diminishes, their responsibility to fulfil the 'do no harm' maxim increases correspondingly. Ethics committees increasingly weigh up the 'value' of proposed research and the risk it entails (Cassaret et al., 2002).

Of course, risk can be difficult to assess, especially in procedures that have not been used before. In assessing risk in such situations, it may be useful to rely on similar research conducted previously on animals or very early approximations to human use—for example, in vitro examination of blood or tissue response. A high level of clinical and scientific judgment is needed to make this risk assessment. The acceptability of risk is necessarily a value judgment. As a researcher, you decide what you are prepared to ask people to undertake. Ethics committees make a similar judgment before research proceeds. Participants decide whether they are prepared to participate, and they take on those risks, for potential benefit to themselves or to others, or both.

The concern in all research is that some invasive procedure, whether physical or non-physical, may be performed on a participant. In medical research, this invasion is likely to be to the physical integrity of the person, but in non-medical research, this invasion is more likely to be to the psychological integrity of the person. Both physical and psychological integrity are essential to the wellbeing of the individual, and must be protected. Consistent with that concern is a commitment by the researcher to stop the research if the risk to this integrity becomes too great.

Health care workers are constantly striving to improve health care and the treatments they make available to patients. The belief that some good must be achieved is essential if a health care worker is to offer a potentially beneficial innovative treatment. Researchers can champion the research, as is illustrated by a British researcher commenting on a groundbreaking living-donor transplant, performed on a 21-month-old child: 'We presented it to a large ethics committee and convinced them, although there was hostility at first' (McBride, 1989).

There are occasions when patients themselves push the bounds of treatment to a point where it effectively becomes research. They might have heard about a new treatment that they want to try, or there might be no known cure or treatment for their illness and they are willing to try anything. This often happens when patients have a terminal condition, or a condition for which researchers and clinicians cannot offer an effective cure. For instance, there is well established evidence that HIV/AIDS patients consistently sought new and unproven treatments in the 1980s (Levine et al., 1991). In effect, they also forced their carers to become researchers. As there was a serious risk facing them, many people with HIV/AIDS might have decided that there was little distinction between research and treatment.

There is considerable responsibility placed on the individual health care worker in situations such as these. They still need to protect their patients from further harm, but when all available options have been tried, there is generally a willingness to let patients pursue more risky but as yet unproven treatments—such as using unlicensed drugs for 'blue babies' (Oliver & Webb,

2002, p. 1174). Occasionally, world attention is focused on patients who choose radically new treatments—for example, in the mid-1990s, the so-called 'Baboon man' asked for baboon-marrow transplants to be given to him as a possible immune system boost. He was suffering from HIV/AIDS. At the time, the health care professional involved said that the only surprise was that the experimental treatment went so well. It did not make him better, but it did not make him worse either. (Associated Press, 1996a, p. 11; Associated Press, 1996b, p. 9). When innovative therapeutic research involves patients of limited capacity—particularly children—there is unease among the community and the health professions. Community and ethics debate was heated when, in 1985, a newborn baby received a chimpanzee heart in an effort to keep her alive. She died shortly afterwards (Annas, 1995, p. 15). Treatments of 'last resort' can be allowed under exemptions provided in drug regulations, as you will read later in this chapter. A number of significant advances in cancer treatment have been developed as a result of aggressive treatments being tried by very ill people—for example, in melanoma treatments.

There is a long established ethical distinction between research that is for the benefit of the person or persons participating in the research (patients/clients) and that which is more for the general benefit of furthering knowledge. Therapeutic research is much more ethically acceptable than non-therapeutic research, although how therapeutic benefit is defined is itself a matter of debate. As a general rule, the crucial consideration for therapeutic benefit and possible harm is the individual's position, and the likely outcome for that individual of whatever procedure is being contemplated (Ramsey, 1976).

If the research is not therapeutic—that is, if it is not for the benefit of those participating—people with a diminished capacity, or those with developing capacity such as children, are generally less likely to be included (Berglund, 1995). People with limited capacity, such as children and young people, are protected by not including them unless the research is particularly relevant to them, or to people like them, and research on other groups cannot answer the question specific to them—that is, their participation is indispensable.

In the USA, the concept of minimal additional risk over the risks of daily life has traditionally been relied on when no direct research benefit to the child research participant is likely. A minor increase to this risk has been used as the acceptable standard only if those children have a disorder or condition, and the research is likely to benefit others from that group (Department of Health and Human Services, 1983, 1991; Department of Health and Human Services, Food and Drug Administration, 2001, 2013).

Respect for persons

The principle of 'respect for persons' seeks to ensure that an individual's wishes are respected, even if they differ from those of the researcher, or from those expected of the individual by the researcher. Each potential participant should be given the opportunity to express their wishes both before being included in the research, and throughout the research process itself. Broadly, the principle implies respect for the rights, wishes and individuality of the participant. Ensuring informed consent to research, and maintaining the confidentiality of the data, are both processes that uphold the dignity and individuality of research participants.

The fundamental ethical standard in research is that people should take part of their own free will. This is supported in several human rights statements, such as the *United Nations International Covenant on Civil and Political Rights* (United Nations, 1966) and in the United Nations Educational, Scientific and Cultural Organization's (UNESCO) *Universal Declaration on Bioethics and Human Rights* (UNESCO, 2005, Article 6[2]) which states: 'Scientific research should only be carried out with the prior, free, express and informed consent of the person concerned'. This is echoed in all research ethics codes. In order to uphold the integrity of the consent process, individuals who have the capacity to make decisions about research participation should be allowed to do so. They should also be free to withdraw at any time.

Apart from a persons' cognitive capacity to make decisions, the capacity for autonomous decision making also requires an environment that is free of coercion. If the environment is not free of coercion, a request for participation may not be ethical. This means that a refusal to consent should not lead to any detriment—other than the agreed-upon risks of the research—or loss of standing for the patient. Gaining informed consent as a routine part of any treatment procedure in which legal, ethical and regulatory requirements work together is examined in Chapter 8.

INTEGRATED LEARNING AND PRACTICE

Does everyone have to be in research if they are asked?

If it is research rather than QI or QA assessment, the law protects an individual's capacity to make a free and informed decision on participation, and international law is reflected in domestic laws to support consent as a basic right.

The priority of autonomy is maintained in all research ethics frameworks, and possible benefit to others does not override issues of potential risk to an individual.

Regulation supports this considered view, and ethics committees check that research is approved, including the use of ethically acceptable consent forms.

Ideally, research participants should be aware of the research process as it progresses from start to finish. This includes being informed of the results of the research, so that they may learn from it and can maximise the benefits or minimise the potential harm of the research for their own lives. To use people as subjects but not inform them of the results—if they wish to know the results—could seem exploitative.

Being a health carer and also involved in research is potentially ethically problematic, requiring a delicate balance between ensuring ongoing trust in care relationships, and not exposing clients to unnecessary risks. Carers may identify that their patient could be eligible to be involved in a new research protocol. The autonomous nature of the patient's decision is so important ethically that it is routine for another health care researcher to recruit subjects. That is because patients can feel obliged to be participants if asked by their own carers. This feeling of obligation is termed 'dependency'.

In one instance of apparent non-therapeutic research in the UK that received international attention—the storage of organs or tissues of children who had died, without specific consent from relatives—raised tremendous ethics concerns. Though stored, they were neither examined nor used, nor had consent for their removal or storage been given. The inquiry into the practice at a UK hospital centred on a particular doctor, but during the course of the inquiry the practice was found to be more widespread than one site or one doctor. Stricter guidelines were recommended for the retention of organs, and it was recommended that consent for examination be mandatory (Redfern et al., 2001). Regulations were subsequently refined to ensure acceptable protection of gaining consent, and maintaining integrity. Many commentaries were written on the process of grief and bereavement for families, on discovering there was more of their child to be buried. Public trust in the hospital system and in the veracity of treating doctors was also questioned. Nursing journals included rigorous ethical reflection and research on the issue, with paternalism identified as a problematic theme in the conduct that had been discovered (Coombes, 2001).

The question of how much to pay research subjects, if at all, is difficult to resolve, and ultimately depends on the population from which the research subjects will be chosen. Some compensation for participation is preferable, but it should not be so large as to amount to coercion to participate. Many researchers use a model of 'compensation for time'—in the form of issuing taxi vouchers and providing lunch vouchers for the day of the research—rather than monetary payment, which could induce low-income earners or unemployed people to take part in risky research for the money. This would effectively exploit that less affluent section of the population for the benefit of the whole population.

Justice

The principle of justice involves considering the fair distribution of the benefits and burdens of research within society. To achieve that, the duty of professionals to conduct research and to advance knowledge so that society may benefit needs to be acknowledged.

However, the advancement of knowledge cannot be at the expense of the individual patient or research subject, so concerns of beneficence and respect for persons take precedence. Research should not be regarded as ethical, no matter how great the community benefit, if individuals suffer too greatly in the conduct of that research. This concern over the suffering of research subjects is at the heart of criticisms in the Nuremberg trials of experiments conducted by the Nazis during World War II, and is a constant concern when underprivileged or institutionalised participants are used for research that is designed for the benefit of privileged or non-institutionalised persons.

In theoretical terms, you should note that placing beneficence and respect for persons over justice makes explicit the distinction between, on the one hand, the good for the individual and, on the other, the common good. It is important to remember the distinction when applying the principles. Economic writers may challenge the primacy of other principles over justice, preferring to set societal objectives—such as economic growth—which can be used to implement beneficence and respect for persons (Mooney et al., 1986, pp. 48, 49, 55). So, the distinction needs to be made clear when economic and practical resourcing discussions are held, so that the discussion is broadened into the ethical implications of choices that are made.

On a practical level, you need to assess:

- what the social benefits and burdens of the research will be
- who will bear the burden of research
- who will potentially benefit from the research.

Only after assessing these items can you make a decision on the acceptability of the research. The social assessment of the process and objectives of the research should be a consultative process with the relevant community. In early stages of research in specific communities, such as Aboriginal and Torres Strait Islander peoples' communities, it is a requirement that wide consultation be undertaken, as the research process itself is a collaboration and must be in tune with cultural and community values (National Health and Medical Research Council, 2018a, p. 2, 2018b).

Community support for potential advances should not be assumed, as eminent ethics commentators such as Hans Jonas have noted (1969). In early and ancient history, there is poignant evidence of community input into professional standards. For instance, the Roman public rejected most experimental treatment on people who were seriously ill, and publicly castigated health carers who undertook unacceptable experimental treatments, regardless of whether the experiments succeeded or failed (Ferngren, 1985). Contemporary Third World cultures may not necessarily share the notion of progress as it is understood in Western medicine (Dickens, 1991).

Western communities may also strongly disagree with new medical technologies and treatments on cultural or religious grounds. The German community opposed human-embryo experimentation, and public discussion of human-embryo experimentation and related issues—such as euthanasia and organ transplantation—was stifled in the 1990s when philosopher Peter Singer visited. According to one commentator on the heated community protests that accompanied Singer's tour, the community's distrust of such research may stem from the Nazi abuse of civilians during World War II in eugenically motivated experiments on humans (Nicholson, 1990). (Eugenics is the altering of the characteristics of a population through a wide variety of methods.) Research directions can be controversial. Community attitudes are divided on controversial research such as using embryonic stem cells (see Chapter 9), and also on whether such controversial research should be publicly funded (Weed, 2004). Community views can change, and such surveys quickly become historical data on what the community view was at a certain time.

The wishes of the community should be seriously considered by researchers if a social definition of justice is to be accepted. Under a social definition of justice, community advice must be sought so that the benefits and burdens—of specific advances in health care—to individuals and the community are acceptable. As Douglas stated, 'the public reception of any policy for risks will depend on standardized public ideas about justice' (1985, p. 5). Frankel similarly considered that limits to professional choices, particularly in research, should be provided through social policy so that individuals are better protected from harms that are regarded as unacceptable by society (Frankel, 1975, p. 46).

Chalmers and Silverman favoured 'public consideration' of formal and informal medical research as a type of risk assessment, not so much as a community judgment of acceptable risk but more because they believed that the community should take responsibility for the reality that progress involves some risk. They cautioned against the idealistic double standard of wanting the benefits of research without the inevitable risk of harm that accompanies research. They preferred the community to acknowledge that acceptable means for the ends of research must include risk (Chalmers & Silverman, 1987, p. 5).

The sharing of knowledge and the dissemination of information gained from research is an element of the duty to society to distribute the benefits and burdens more knowledgeably and fairly within that society. If you are conducting research, you should write up and present your results accurately, noting its pitfalls as well as its successes. Your findings and your description of the research should be made publicly available—for example, at conferences, in professional forums, or in professional journals. It is also advisable to make this information available in a form that can be accessed by the community.

The dissemination of knowledge saves the same burden of risk being placed on future prospective research participants needlessly. It maximises the potential benefits of research: disseminating the knowledge gained from the research allows others to move further on the basis of your results, instead of repeating the research (or failing to offer the best available treatment) because they are not aware of your results.

In summary, the key ethics considerations for researchers are:

- beneficence
- assessment of the benefits of the research
- assessment of the risks of the research
- weighing risks against benefits
- respect for persons
- informed consent from research subjects
- research subjects being free to withdraw from the research
- confidentiality
- informing research subjects of results
- paying or compensating research subjects
- justice
- advancement of knowledge for the benefit of society
- assessment of the distribution of benefits
- assessment of the distribution of burdens
- fair balance of benefit and burden
- sharing of knowledge and dissemination of results.

Ethics committees provide an opportunity for professional, institutional and community concerns about clinical and research practice to be discussed and decided upon. The committees are essential for researchers, who need their approval before they can conduct research, and they provide a useful referral processes for clinicians. Referring to professional codes, national guidelines and international standards should be routine for researchers who are planning research, in addition to seeking peer deliberation and discussion of issues.

These are designed to help researchers conduct research ethically and according to regulatory standards, and should be referred to by professionals. Ethics committees have an educative function, as well as a gate-keeping role. They can be asked for advice when researchers face difficult issues.

Now would be a good time to look back to Chapter 6 'Personal information privacy and public interests', to reread the description of the human research ethics committee (HREC) system.

If you are preparing to submit your research proposal, consider the logistics involved in tabling paperwork for a meeting and discussion. It is common practice for proposal deadlines to be one or two weeks before the meeting date. This allows time for agendas to be prepared; for the committee to identify and ask for any information missing from the proposal; and to make copies of the proposal and distribute these to the committee members. The members read the proposals before they meet, and they are expected to give each proposal due consideration.

As a researcher, you need to be aware of that review and reflection process, and give it the time it deserves. There may be administrative requirements particular to your ethics committee—for example, your committee may require you to submit multiple copies of the proposal. Find out these administrative details early on, preferably well ahead of the deadline for proposal submission, so that you do not miss the deadline for the meeting. Committees may only meet four times a year. You need to be careful that you do not unduly delay the granting of ethics committee approval.

REFLECTION: A PROPOSAL FOR CONSIDERATION

Try this group discussion exercise. Allocate roles to people along the lines of ethics committee composition. Australian committees have, as a minimum, a chairperson, two laypeople, a person with a pastoral care role in the community, a lawyer, two researchers in relevant fields, and a health carer from any of a variety of health professions. Various ages are commonly sought for this membership. You may prefer to construct a UK or NZ style committee to consider the proposal. When you have composed your 'committee' consider this proposal.

A community health fund has promised funding for a trial of a new treatment of eye infections, in a remote area. The researchers plan to provide refrigeration equipment for the duration of the trial, which is needed for the medicine and preparations, as this is routinely lacking in the area. The research will extend over a two-year period. People of all ages who attend the monthly community health clinic, and who are diagnosed by the community health nurse as having a particular type of eye infection, will be offered the chance to take part in the research. Half of the participants—randomly assigned on the basis of random numbers allocated for the sequence in which they attend—will be asked to follow the routine advice given, and the other half will be offered the new treatment regime. Researchers will follow up all patients at monthly

+ continued

intervals, and a serious deterioration in any participant will trigger a new assessment of treatment requirements. This assessment would take place in a community base hospital. Transportation for the assessment would be arranged by the research team. Any subsequent change in treatment advice and treatment arrangements, if they needed to withdraw from the research, would be the responsibility of the individual and community.

Working as a committee, be guided by a national statement on ethical conduct in human research, and by a general ethics guideline, such as your profession's code of conduct, code of ethics or population-specific guideline.

Once research is underway, the responsibility for monitoring the ethical conduct is shared: the researcher continues to reflect on the ethical dimensions of the process, as do their peers, the institution, the ethics committee, the funders, the participants, and the community.

Ethics committees can actively monitor and audit all research within their institutions, regardless of the funding source, and in some countries, government-funded offices undertake this responsibility for publicly funded research. For instance, public offices, such as the US Office of Research Integrity (ORI), set guidelines for research conduct and assess alleged research misconduct in publicly funded research, and supports institutions responding to allegations of misconduct by their members (Department of Health and Human Services, 2017). Information can be given to them by any complainant. Routine random audits can also be undertaken to check for study teams who disregard discrepant data, or data that does not 'fit' their hoped-for outcome, and they can generally check the integrity of data files and patient records. ORI publishes misconduct findings on their website.

REFLECTION: MONITORING AND INVESTIGATION

Imagine that you have to investigate an allegation about research misconduct made by Patient B, a research participant.

A new treatment is being trialled for the control of a chronic and debilitating condition, and Patient A is a close friend of Patient B. Although random allocations are meant to occur, Patient A apparently asked to be assigned to the treatment group after realising that the medication she had been assigned was no different from that which she had been taking for some time in the context of routine treatment. She had taken the medication she was given for the research trial to an independent lab and asked that it be analysed. It was three weeks after the trial had started, but she managed to change groups, and all of her data was allegedly transferred to the 'treatment' group for inclusion in that analysis. Patient B is disgruntled that she may be on the comparison group treatment, and has been told she cannot be informed which group she is in and, in any case, cannot change groups.

Alternatively, consider an allegation made by a junior member of a research team, in a large multi-institutional trial, that the published findings differ from that in the research records.

Consider what sort of evidence would need to be collected in order to investigate the allegations.

If proven, what action, if any, do you think should be taken against:

- the participants
- the investigators
- the institution.

Look up the ORI website <https://ori.hhs.gov>, to see if its summaries of investigations into allegations of scientific misconduct match your proposed process of investigation. The ORI 'evidence' records may help too. The basic process is to check facts, assuming there is a consent from research participants for the records to be available for audit, and then interpret the facts with the assistance of knowledgeable peers.

The reporting of research is an important step in ensuring that the results are known, and the effort and resources that went into the research have some tangible result. Knowledge is furthered—even if results are null, or not as expected—if you share what you have learnt by engaging in the research process.

The participants may also wish to know the results of the research, particularly if the findings are of personal relevance. In social research, it is common to expect to discuss the findings, as a courtesy to the participants and communities who made the research possible. When writing up results, there is an obligation to report the findings accurately, and be publicly accountable for those published findings. This is an issue of researcher integrity. Knowingly falsifying results is regarded as research misconduct.

Journal editors require authors to sign their explicit responsibility and public accountability for the research and the results as published. Authors must have made a substantial contribution to the design, data collection or analysis and interpretation, and drafting and approval of the final version of the reporting of results in the research process to be justified in claiming authorship (International Committee of Medical Journal Editors, 2016).

Journals will require documentation that a project has been approved by an ethics committee. This is to ensure that they do not publish research that has not been ethically reviewed.

Most journals now require conflicts of interests in the research—such as receiving sponsorship from commercial companies with an interest in the results—to be disclosed and published alongside the results in the interests of **transparency** and accountability. Readers can then judge the potential bias of the research report accordingly.

transparency Being candid and open to scrutiny.

You may have noticed research 'scandals' in the media from time to time. If you see an article about a research project that is portrayed as a scandal, think about whether the researcher's integrity or potential conflict of interests are at issue. Happily, most research is conducted without such ethical pitfalls, with most researchers being, in the large part, driven by a genuine desire to help others and make a difference to people's health and welfare, and maintaining the highest standards of professional integrity and accountability.

Drug regulation

When you treat people, you look at what you can do, and you look at what is available as a resource to use in that management or treatment process. Because new approaches and new treatments are constantly being developed, you need to keep up to date with professional literature to be able to make an informed assessment. This section considers the development of new drugs and the availability of pharmaceuticals. It is about the potential availability of a particular 'good', and could be read with the justice discussion in Chapter 10 'Regulation and availability of health and community services'.

The development and availability of new drugs is of tremendous ethical and social importance. It is fuelled by a need to find better ways of helping people with health problems, from niggling problems to minor episodic illnesses and chronic illnesses, right through to serious and life-threatening conditions. The development of new drugs involves a massive human-resources commitment and substantial financial investment. It relies on government policy to provide both incentives and restraints, in limiting risks posed to the public either as research participants or as end users of a drug that is released to market. Given the political, economic and social forces involved in drug development, it is not surprising that the policy objectives and guidelines surrounding this issue change from time to time.

The Australian drug regulation authorities consider pharmaceutical, chemical, animal, pharmacological and toxicological data—as well as clinical data—before a drug is approved. This data represents basic scientific information and information on the drug and its application in the clinical context. The Therapeutic Goods Administration (TGA), part of the Commonwealth Department of Health, relies heavily on skilled scientists and clinicians to assess the information. This system has developed gradually, taking shape from 1970 when Commonwealth legislation was revised to give the Minister for Health the power to issue permits for the importation of drugs based on an analysis of the drug's quality, efficacy and safety. Before the 1970s, the focus of the legislation was predominantly on the quality of manufacture of the drug, and on ruling out the likelihood that it posed severe and life-threatening risks (*Therapeutic Goods Act 1966–1973* (Cth), particularly section 29 (1), *Therapeutic Goods Amendment Act 1991* (Cth), section 4).

The realisation that thalidomide, an apparently harmless and effective morning-sickness drug, was linked to physical deformities in the children of mothers who took the drug resulted in tighter drug-evaluation systems in Australia and all around the world. However, in the quest for timely availability of new drugs, the drug evaluation system started to change again in the 1990s. Groups lobbying on behalf of AIDS patients conducted effective campaigns for a drug regulation system that 'maximises the safety and efficacy of treatments, while at the same time expedites access to those treatments' (Australian Federation of AIDS Organisations, 1991, p. 4).

Summary data to support the drug being registered is now permitted, and human research ethics committees (HRECs) are relied on for the assessment of the aspects of research proposals for drug trials in humans. In Australia, HRECs consider the ethics of the trialling of new drugs with healthy volunteers and in the clinical setting. They do so under the mandate of—but independently from—the institution in which the research is to be conducted, and they are guided by national guidelines, such as those you read earlier in this chapter. Ethics committees must ask: Does the proposed benefit justify the risk? And, if so, how much risk? Further, is it acceptable to expose human participants to this risk, and other potential risks, before it is known whether the treatment will in fact work?

As part of trial protocols, unapproved pharmaceutical substances and medical devices can be lawfully supplied under the Clinical Trials Notification (CTN) and Clinical Trials Exemption (CTX) schemes. In a CTN trial, the trial protocol is submitted to the HREC, and the HREC assesses the 'scientific validity of the trial design, the safety and efficacy of the medicine or device and the ethical acceptability of the trial process'. The TGA is then notified of the trial, after the sponsor and HREC and the Approving Authority have signed the form. Under the CTX Scheme, the TGA evaluates and comments on the application, relying on summary data on the pharmaceutical, including preclinical and clinical data (Therapeutic Goods Administration, 2004, pp. 12, 13).

It is recognised that where no proven treatments are available, all 'approved' goods have been found to be clinically unsuitable, or a drug has an established use but is not normally available in Australia, there is a place for the exercise of patient choice to undertake greater risk, and regulations allow for the import and supply of an unapproved therapeutic good to a patient, on a case-by-case basis, under the Special Access Scheme (SAS), or within a clinical trial.

There are three categories under the access scheme:

- *Category A* is only available for patients at risk of death or injury without treatment—that is, they have exhausted all available options, and only notifying the TGA is required.
- *Category B* is for goods with no established use, and there is an underlying limit to the amount of risk that people can choose to expose themselves to—and that limit is the willingness of professionals to help them. TGA approval is required. (It is increasingly recognised that there is a limit to the amount of resources that can be committed to trying unproven treatments.) Each application is considered on the grounds of appropriate choice, and appropriate risk.
- *Category C* is for medicines with established use elsewhere than Australia. Practitioners can supply these medicines, but must strictly comply with the rules set out for that Category (*Therapeutic Goods (Authorised Supply of Specified Medicines) Rules September 2017* (Cth)).

The government does not cover the cost of unapproved goods under the SAS, but sometimes sponsors do on compassionate grounds.

The emphasis in the Category C rules on informed consent and advising each patient of the unapproved nature of the medicine, and of potential risks involved, and maintaining principles of good medical practice, is as follows:

4 Authorisation to supply medicines

(1) A health practitioner of the class specified in column 5 in an item in table 1 is authorised to supply a medicine that:

(a) contains only the active ingredient or ingredients, in the strength or concentration (if any), specified in column 1 in the item; and

(b) is in the dosage form specified in column 2 in the item;

to a person if:

(c) the person is a patient of the health practitioner; and

(d) the medicine is to be administered through the route of administration specified in column 3 in the item; and

(e) the supply is for an indication specified in column 4 in the item; and

(f) the following conditions are satisfied:

(i) the health practitioner must inform the patient, or a parent or guardian of the patient, that the medicine is not registered or listed;

(ii) the health practitioner must ensure that the medicine is supplied only after receiving informed consent from the patient, or a parent or guardian of the patient;

(iii) the health practitioner must ensure that the medicine is supplied in accordance with good medical practice;

(iv) if the health practitioner becomes aware that the patient has suffered an adverse event in relation to the medicine, the health practitioner must notify the Therapeutic Goods Administration, and the sponsor of the medicine, about the adverse event, in accordance with subsection (3);

(v) if the health practitioner becomes aware of any defect in the medicine, the health practitioner must notify the Therapeutic Goods Administration, and the sponsor of the medicine, about the defect, in accordance with subsection (3).

(Therapeutic Goods (Authorised Supply of Specified Medicines) Rules September 2017, s4(1))

Clinical partners in research are needed in order to properly document and test the effectiveness of a new drug in human participants. One of the challenges for regulation and ethics in the applied research fields and the current age of globalisation is to transcend national and cultural boundaries, and to identify standards for research and development that are transparent, and acceptable to those affected by the research.

Pharmaceutical trials are an international endeavour. Regulatory, legal and contractual obligations are complex, particularly in multi-centre trials or with international funding partners. Harmonised standard operating procedures for research ethics and governance approval for multi-centre research—such as international drug trials—have been developed by some institutions. These procedures take into account the legal responsibilities of researchers and institutions and international *Good Clinical Practice* guidelines requirements for mutually accepted clinical data across jurisdictions.

Institutions can actively encourage research as part of innovative practice, and set out harmonised procedures for ethical and governance approval so that international partnership in clinical research is facilitated. The Royal Melbourne Hospital makes its streamlined standard operating procedures for approval of clinical trials publicly available on its website, and comments that: 'The Royal Melbourne Hospital (RMH) holds a strong philosophy that clinical trials are not supplementary or adjunct to patient care—they are patient care' (Royal Melbourne Hospital, 2018).

The International Conference on Harmonisation Good Clinical Practice (ICH GCP) guideline (1996), developed from the *Declaration of Helsinki*, is the international best practice standard on sponsor and researcher responsibilities. The Australian regulatory authority for drug trials, the Therapeutic Goods Administration (TGA), has adopted the European version of the GCP guidelines with some annotation so that the National Statement is applied in the case of conflicts between the documents, and local legal obligations also apply in the designing, conducting, recording and reporting of clinical trials:

> Good Clinical Practice is an international ethical and scientific quality standard for the designing, conducting, recording and reporting trials that involve the participation of human subjects. Compliance with this standard provides public assurance that the rights, safety and well-being of trial subjects are protected, consistent with the principles that have their origin in the Declaration of Helsinki, and that the clinical trial data are credible.
>
> *(Australian Government, Therapeutic Goods Administration, 2000, p. 6)*

Drug regulation illustrates how fluid the debate over acceptable risk and objective benefit is. The debate can swing depending on the context, perceived threat and available resources. Every now and then, a trial of a new medicine in humans brings about unexpected harm. When this happens, the need for protective mechanisms, and considered weighing of risks against benefits, is highlighted. Drugs are tested on healthy volunteers in the early phase of clinical trials. Catastrophic immune responses can and do occasionally occur in such trials, such as in one trial in the United Kingdom in 2006. Remarkably, all six of the volunteers survived, with one requiring months of hospitalisation and all of them facing serious long-term health issues. Predictably, calls for tighter restrictions on potential risks posed to participants followed—for instance, in a *Lancet* editorial piece, as well as with vigorous discussion of consent protocols for such trials (2006).

The conduct of research in different contexts, such as the developing world, was a topic under intense discussion over the last decade. Drug companies routinely conduct large research projects in developing countries, with treatment groups receiving treatments at no cost. The World Health Organisation (WHO) guidelines on drug research are updated from time to time, to apply across national boundaries so that research trials are of a high safety standard, even when countries do not have their own requirements. This approach is aimed at a basic protection, regardless of country, and is consistent with the WHO's universal view of health promotion.

The background to one of the more contentious issues was that when new treatments are being trialled, there is commonly a comparison group that does not receive the new treatment. This is so that the effects of the trial treatment on the research participants can be compared and evaluated against others with similar conditions, and not just against changes in the condition of the human participants who are receiving the treatment. This forms a more reliable comparison, and is the standard approach in quantitative research studies (Berglund, 2001). Traditionally, placebo groups were the comparison, and those in the placebo group did not receive treatment of any kind.

Now, however, the norm is that the best proven and available treatment is given to those in the comparison group, so they are no worse off than if they were not in a research trial. The effect of the new treatment can then also be compared to how people progress if they received the standard treatment of the day. In the developing world, the difficulty is that the best proven treatment simply may not be affordable or available to people. It is a difficult ethics quandary for researchers—who want to help and fulfil their duty to take part in improving medical care and treatment—to decide what their responsibilities are to research subjects in countries where the basic care is not as good or lacks many choices available to similar research subjects in the developed world.

The World Medical Association requirement was changed so that the best available treatment for the participants, both during and after the conclusion of the trial, needed to be identified for the ethics committee's consideration. There is ongoing discussion about the merits of this standard (Blackmer & Haddad, 2005). Comparison to a placebo when a current proven intervention exists is not acceptable.

The availability of pharmaceuticals, and their trialling, has attracted heated debate, particularly in the African context of high morbidity rates and the impoverishment of large affected communities (Lee, 2005). When trials were rapidly conducted during the Ebola crisis, there were concerns that many trials lacked sufficient and rigorous research controls, so conclusive evidence on which drugs had been effective would remain elusive (Burton, 2015).

Drug production is a business, conducted by companies that need to turn a profit to sustain their business and investment, and ongoing contribution to further research and development. Drugs developed and produced by pharmaceuticals are products, and must be paid for by consumers, or by the government or their insurer on their behalf. The government decides separately if an approved drug can be subsidised so that it is more readily available to the public in the Australian community at a reduced cost. This is done through the Pharmaceutical Benefit Scheme. Over 500 drug substances are included in the scheme, some in different dose forms and strengths and approximately $2 billion of Commonwealth taxpayer monies are used annually to fund the scheme.

The Schedule of Pharmaceutical Benefits is the list of subsided substances, and any restrictions that apply to the prescribing of them, such as the maximum quantities that can be prescribed or supplied, unless special circumstances apply and an authority is sought to vary from this, and the maximum number of repeat prescriptions on the script issued by the medical practitioner. These lists can be issued for particular treatment regimes—such as cancer treatments in hospitals. As one example, private hospital and public hospital supply of chemotherapy drugs lists are issued monthly (Australian Government, Department of Health, 2017). The price is agreed between the government and the sponsor, or drug company.

Making a list, checking it twice

Find a debate in current community or professional discussion forums about whether a drug should be listed. Notice what arguments are put forward in support or in opposition. Think about whether you agree or disagree and how your appreciation of the complexity of debates is developing.

There is tremendous pressure for drugs to be provided cheaply once they are proven effective. The regulatory limits to patent timeframes are one example of regulation that sets a reasonable limit to the profit phase for the commercial interests that contributed to the development of a new product. After that time, the public's interest in affordable access to the benefits outweighs the commercial interest. Once patents expire, the drugs can be produced in generic form, and potentially made more widely available. The potential relief for the public purse is recognised, as patients can be given a choice of generic or brand name drug when the medicine is supplied. The favourable impact on expenditure for the commonly prescribed statins attracted comment in the professional medical literature (Clarke & Fitzgerald, 2010).

Patents for the drugs are held by the pharmaceutical company, and intellectual property law protects those exclusive rights to manufacture the product. The balance of those rights can be altered by the government if it is considered to be in the public interest, and there has been considerable discussion over the wisdom of strengthening patents rights for pharmaceuticals, through patent extensions and trade agreements with other countries, partly given the barrier to competitor generic brands entering the market (Australian Government, Productivity Commission, 2016, p. 297).

Whether the pharmaceutical industry can be a medicine provider—particularly in less developed countries—is a matter of debate. The industry invests large amounts of money years in advance of any anticipated return on new drugs. It is a delicate balance for regulation to support innovation and also maintain safety and access to the best quality care that can be afforded within a community.

Summary

The way the fields of law, regulation and ethics combine or complement each other will have become familiar to you in earlier chapters. For, instance, in Chapter 6, you looked at public health issues, and the way different interests are balanced in reaching an acceptable rule or guideline that protects the community from undue harm caused by others. You have now built on that understanding by considering the limits of care. In thinking about balancing of best interests and autonomy in care provision limits for individual patients, some classic philosophical concepts of personal and social morality have also been revisited. You have also now had the opportunity to consider how regulatory standards in research and experimental treatment and the regulation of established drug therapies have been informed by principles derived from ethics and law.

STUDY QUESTIONS

1   Explain the difference between matters concerning personal morality and matters of social morality.

2   Describe a health carer's role in protecting and furthering the health of a patient or client. Support your opinion with relevant standards, sourced from law, regulation and ethics.

3   Outline key protections available for research participants, referencing international, national and relevant professional guidelines.

SAMPLE ESSAY QUESTIONS

1   Provide a reasoned ethics analysis of a research process that you sourced in a peer-reviewed professional journal.

2   Prepare a briefing paper for new staff on the process of research ethics and research governance considerations that apply to research conducted in a public health service in your jurisdiction, with a brief rationale explaining why these processes are in place.

REFERENCES

[ ]. (2006). Urgent changes needed for authorisation of phase I trials. Editorial. *Lancet*, *367*(9518), 1214.

Annas, G.L. (1985). Baby Fae: The 'Anything Goes' School of Human Experimentation. *Hastings Center Report*, *15*(1), 15–16.

Associated Press. (1996a, 6–7 January). Baboon man out of hospital. *Weekend Australian*, 11.

Associated Press. (1996b, 9 February). Baboon marrow fails to boost AIDS patient. *Australian*, 9.

Australian Federation of AIDS Organisations [AFAO]. (1991). *Submission to the Baume Review of the Drug Evaluation and Access Process in Australia, May 1991*. Sydney: AFAO.

Australian Government, Department of Health, PBS. (2017). *Schedule of Pharmaceutical Benefits: efficient funding of chemotherapy*, effective 1 August 2017. Retrieved from www2.health. vic.gov.au

Australian Government, National Health and Medical Research Council, Australian Research Council & Universities Australia. (2018a). *Australian Code for Responsible Conduct of Research*. Canberra: National Health and Medical Research Council.

Australian Government, National Health and Medical Research Council, Australian Research Council & Universities Australia. (2018b). *Guide to Managing and Investigating Potential Breaches of the Australian Code for the Responsible Conduct of Research, 2018*. Canberra: National Health and Medical Research Council.

Australian Government, Productivity Commission. (2016). *Intellectual Property Arrangements*. Productivity Commission Inquiry Report No. 78. Retrieved from http://pc.gov.au

Australian Government, Therapeutic Goods Administration. (2000, July). *Note for Guidance on Good Clinical Practice* (CPMP/ICH/135/95). Commonwealth Department of Health and Aged Care. Retrieved from http://tga.gov.au

Australian Government, Therapeutic Goods Administration [TGA]. (2004). *Access to unapproved therapeutic goods: Clinical trials in Australia.* Department of Health and Ageing. Canberra: Therapeutic Goods Administration.

Berglund, C.A. (1995). Children in medical research: Australian ethical standards. *Child: Care, Health and Development, 21*(2), 149–59.

Berglund, C.A. (Ed.). (2001). *Health Research.* Melbourne: Oxford University Press.

Blackmer, J., & Haddad, H. (2005). The Declaration of Helsinki: an update on paragraph 30. *Canadian Medical Association Journal, 173*(9), 1052–3.

Burton, T.M. (2015, 13 May). Disputes emerge on African Ebola Drug Trials. *Wall Street Journal.* Retrieved from www.wsj.com

Cassarett, D.J., Karlawish, J.H.T., & Moreno, J.D. (2002). A taxonomy of value in clinical research. *IRB: Ethics & Human Research, 24*(6), 1–6.

Chalmers, I., & Silverman, W.A. (1987). Professional and public double standards on clinical experimentation. *Controlled Clinical Trials, 8*(4), 390–1.

Clarke, P.M., & Fitzgerald, E.M. (2010). Expiry of patent protection on statins: Effects on pharmaceutical expenditure in Australia. *Medical Journal of Australia, 192*(11), 633–6.

Coney, S. (1988). *The unfortunate experiment: The full story behind the inquiry into cervical cancer treatment.* Auckland: Penguin.

Coombes, R. (2001). 'Paternalism' at the root of body parts nightmare. *Nursing Times, 97*(6), 10–11.

Dawson, R.T. (2001). Drugs in sport: The role of the physician. *Journal of Endocrinology, 170*(1), 55–61.

Department of Health and Human Services [DHHS]. (1983). Protections for children involved as subjects in research. *Federal Register, 48*, 9814–20.

Department of Health and Human Services [DHHS]. (1991). Protections for children involved as subjects in research. *Federal Register, 56*, 28032, 45 CFR Part 46, Subpart D.

Department of Health and Human Services, Food and Drug Administration. (2001). Additional safeguards for children in clinical investigations of FDA-regulated products. *Federal Register, 66*, 20589–600, 21 CFR Parts 50 and 56.

Department of Health and Human Services, Food and Drug Administration. (2013). Additional safeguards for children in clinical investigations of FDA-regulated products. *Federal Register, 78*, 2013, 12937–51.

Department of Health and Human Services [DHHS], Office of Research Integrity. (2017). *Sample policy and procedures for responding to allegations of research misconduct.* Retrieved from www.ori.hhs.gov

Dickens, B.M. (1991). Issues in preparing ethical guidelines for epidemiological studies. *Law, Medicine & Health Care, 19*(3–4), 183.

Douglas, M. (1985). Risk acceptability according to the social sciences. *Social research perspectives: Occasional reports on current topics.* New York: Russell Sage Foundation.

Ferngren, G.B. (1985). Roman lay attitudes towards medical experimentation. *Bulletin of the History of Medicine, 59*(4), 496.

Ford, R. (2010). An analysis of nurses' views of harm reduction measures and other treatments for the problems associated with illicit drug use. *Australian Journal of Advanced Nursing, 28*(1), 14–24.

Frankel, M.S. (1975). The development of policy guidelines governing human experimentation in the United States: A case study of public policy-making for science and technology. *Ethics in Science & Medicine, 2*, 43–59.

Gillett, G. (1989). The new ethical committees: Their nature and role. *New Zealand Medical Journal, 102*, 314–15.

Government of Western Australia, Mental Health Commission. (2015). *Mental Health Act 2014: Information for private psychiatric hostels.* Retrieved from http://mhc.wa.gov.au

Hand Hygiene Australia. (2018). *5 moments for hand hygiene.* Retrieved from https://www.hha.org.au/component/jdownloads/send/5-implementation/191-hha-manual

International Committee of Medical Journal Editors. (2016, December). *Recommendations for the conduct, reporting, editing and publication of scholarly work in medical journals.* Retrieved from www.icmje.org

Jonas, H. (1969). Philosophical reflections on experimenting with human subjects. *Daedalus, 98*(2), 245.

Jones, J.H. (1981). *Bad blood: The Tuskegee syphilis experiment.* New York: Free Press.

Krugman, S., & Giles, J.P. (1970). Viral hepatitis: New light on old disease. *Journal of the American Medical Association, 212*(6), 1019–29.

Lee, J.J. (2005). Comment: What is past is prologue: The International Conference on Harmonization and lessons learned from European drug regulations harmonization. *University of Pennsylvania Journal of International Economic Law, 26*, 151.

Levine, C., Dubler, N.N., & Levine, R.J. (1991). Building a new consensus: Ethical principles and policies for clinical research on HIV/AIDS. *IRB: A Review of Human Subjects Research, 13*(1–2), 1–17.

Levine, R.J. (1986). *Ethics and regulation of clinical research.* Baltimore and Munich: Urban & Schwarzenberg.

McBride, G. (1989). Living liver donor. *British Medical Journal, 299*, 1418.

Mill, J.S. (1975). On liberty. In *Three Essays*, pp. 92–114. London: Oxford University Press.

Mooney, G.H., Russell, E.M., & Weir, R.D. (1986). *Choices for health care: A practical introduction to the economics of health provision* (2nd edn). London: Macmillan.

National Health and Medical Research Council, Australian Research Council & Universities Australia. (2007). *National statement on ethical conduct in human research.* (Updated May 2015 & July 2018). Retrieved from www.nhmrc.gov.au

National Health and Medical Research Council. (2018a). *Ethical guidelines for research with Aboriginal and Torres Strait Islander Peoples and Communities: Guidelines for researchers and stakeholders.* Canberra: NHMRC. Retrieved from http://nhmrc.gov.au

Nicholson, R. (1990). Bioethics attacked in Germany [Editorial]. *Bulletin of Medical Ethics, 61*, 22.

Oliver, J., & Webb, D.J. (2002). Sildenafil for 'blue babies': Such unlicensed drug use might be justified as last resort. *British Medical Journal, 325*(7373), 1174.

Pellegrino, E.D., & Thomasma, D.C. (1988). *For the patient's good.* New York: Oxford University Press.

Premier of Victoria. (2015, 23 March). New smoking bans to start at hospitals and schools. [Media release]. Retrieved from http://premier.vic.gov.au

Quill, T.E., & Brody, H. (1996). Physician recommendations and patient autonomy: Finding a balance between physician power and patient choice. *Annals of Internal Medicine, 125*(9), 763–9.

Ramsey, P. (1976). The enforcement of morals: Non-therapeutic research on children. *Hastings Center Report, 6*(4), 21–30.

Redfern, M., Keeling, J.W., & Powell, E. (2001). *The Royal Liverpool Children's Inquiry: Summary & recommendations.* London: The Stationery Office.

Royal Melbourne Hospital. (2017). *Research.* Retrieved from http://thermh.org.au/research

Shapiro, J., Rucker, L., & Robitshek, D. (2006). Teaching the art of doctoring: An innovative medical student elective. *Medical Teacher, 28*(1), 30–5.

Spicker, S.F., Alon, I., de Vries, A., & Englehardt, H.T. (Eds). (1988). *The use of human beings in research: With special reference to clinical trials.* Boston: Kluwer Academic Publishers.

United Nations. (1966). *International Covenant on Civil and Political Rights* (entry into force 23 March 1976). New York: United Nations.

United Nations Educational, Scientific and Cultural Organization. (2005). *Universal Declaration on Bioethics and Human Rights.* Paris: Unesco.

United States Department of Health, Education, and Welfare. (1978). *Ethical principles and guidelines for the protection of human subjects of research.* [The Belmont report]. Publication No. OS 78–0012. Washington DC: US Department of Health, Education, and Welfare.

Victorian Government. *Mental Health Act 2014* (Vic), Section 30 MHA 101. Assessment Order. Retrieved from www2.health.vic.gov.au

Weed, M. (2004). Ethics, regulation, and biomedical research. *Kennedy Institute of Ethics Journal, 14*(4), 361–8.

World Medical Association. (2008). *Ethical principles for medical research involving human subjects.* [Declaration of Helsinki, 1964, as revised]. New York: World Medical Association. Retrieved from www.wma.net

LEGISLATION

Mental Health Act 2014 (Vic)

Mental Health Act 2014 (WA)

Therapeutic Goods Act 1966–1973 (Cth)

Therapeutic Goods Amendment Act 1991 (Cth)

Therapeutic Goods (Authorised Supply of Specified Medicines) Rules September 2017 (Cth)

Tobacco and Other Smoking Products Act 1998 (Qld)

Tobacco and Other Smoking Products (Smoke-free Places) Amendment Bill 2015 (Qld)

CHAPTER 8

Lifelong practice in decision making

LEARNING OBJECTIVES

- To understand the practical impact of standards in a person's treatment and care decisions.
- To appreciate the reasoning supporting each person's active part in decision making to the extent of their capacity.

KEY TERMS

advance directive	informed consent
capacity	informed decision making
comprehension	mental capacity
information	voluntariness

CASE EXAMPLE

Lifetimes of choices

When Leo started school, his teacher noticed him experiencing some difficulties in settling into routine, and following instructions, and that at times he showed some aggression or frustration towards other children. National Disability Insurance Scheme (NDIS) support offering early intervention was sourced with the help of the school and local community services. Throughout his primary school years, Leo attended a public clinic for health and behavioural management support. After he grew up, he had a few long-term partners and is now single again. He has a daughter in her 30s who sees him when she can.

Leo lives on his own, and is looking forward to his retirement, with more time for his hobbies and the community volunteer work at the local hospital that he loves to do.

1   As you read through this chapter, and you think about Leo's lifetime so far, list all of the hypothetical health-care related choices that were made along the way, and who made them.

2   Looking forward, what choices may lie ahead for Leo, and how will these choices likely be made?

Being ready to make decisions

Law, ethics and regulation are applied in a comprehensive way when treatment and care decisions are made. This is to protect the client's part in that decision-making process in a way that is consistent with their stage of development and capacity.

A decision to agree to a proposed treatment or care process is colloquially known as consent. This is a shorthand term. **Informed consent** refers to a process of consideration and decision making that demonstrates agreement. One way to express a lack of agreement—at least at the time an indication is sought—is to withhold consent. If agreement is not demonstrated, then by default permission or agreement to proceed has not yet been given. Dissent is an expressed disagreement with the proposed treatment or care process. Refusal of treatment is a clearly indicated decision to forgo an offered treatment or care process. **Informed decision making** is a more neutral term that includes both agreement and disagreement with a process of care and treatment that has been proposed, involving a process of consideration and reflection.

The basic elements of an informed decision apply to each treatment decision that is to be made. The health carer should consider if the individual decision maker:

- has capacity—in other words, is competent—to understand what they are being asked to consider
- has been provided with the relevant information

informed consent Agreement given based on information and understanding of the proposed process, significance of decision, and potential benefits or risks entailed.

informed decision making Alternative term for 'informed consent', also encompassing the active participation of both parties in determining options to be potentially agreed to, and in identifying significant material risks and benefits to be explored.

- comprehends that information
- makes a decision voluntarily
- has indicated a decision.

The health carer should then consider if this process of consideration and decision is supported in documentation, either as required or as advised, so that the process is evident to others in the future.

Autonomy and safety

Fiona Foxall

Fiona has been a Registered Nurse for almost 35 years and worked predominantly as an intensive care nurse in the UK and Australia.

Imagine that you are a senior nursing student working on a busy surgical ward on clinical placement. You have thoroughly enjoyed this ward and have received excellent feedback about your performance from the ward staff and your clinical facilitator.

You are returning a patient to bed after taking him to the bathroom and notice that Fred, the patient in the next bed, clearly requires your attention. Fred is a 73-year-old former barrister who underwent a laporotomy for acute bowel obstruction the previous day. His recovery so far, has been uneventful and all his vital signs have been within normal limits. Fred has received adequate pain relief, as he has not complained of pain and has slept well during the night.

However, throughout the morning, Fred has become confused and disorientated, which seems to be worsening. He has now soiled his bed and smeared faeces in his hair and over his abdominal wound. You approach him to attend to his hygiene needs, but he aggressively tells you that he does not want to be washed, as he is conducting a scientific experiment. When you gently persist, he becomes abusive and aggressive towards you. You gently explain that you need to clean his wound because it could become infected if you are not able to wash him. He becomes more abusive, pulls out his intravenous cannula and bleeds from the insertion site.

You are fully aware that you should always respect patient autonomy—but you are also aware that you need to maintain patient safety. You know that you need to act quickly to resolve this situation.

1   Does Fred have decision-making capacity?

2   What are the legal issues raised by this situation?

3   What are the ethical issues raised by this situation?

4   In view of these legal and ethical issues, what do you feel would be the best course of action to resolve this situation?

Competence is a general term relating to a person's capacity and readiness to perform certain specified skills or tasks. In the area of informed decision making, competence centres on cognitive capacity and the ability to analyse information and understand it meaningfully. Relevant information is essential to any consideration and decision process. The provision of relevant **information** may be facilitated by a health service and health carer. The next step is for that information to be understood by the decision maker. The two elements rely on each other. To be fully informed, you need to have access to good information, and also to appreciate its significance. The capability for understanding is competence. The capability is expressed in action by demonstrated understanding or **comprehension**.

information
Details specific to the issue under consideration.

You should ask whether your client is able to access relevant information, and then whether your client is able to understand it in the form it has been presented. You may be able to assist in that process by presenting the information in a readily understandable fashion. In some circumstances, you may have an obligation to do so.

comprehension
Understanding, specific to issues under consideration.

Voluntariness is the state of being free to decide a course of action with unconstrained will. A voluntary decision is also an informed decision when it is reached with the benefit of sufficient information, and the decision-making process is within a person's decision-making capacity at that time.

voluntariness
To decide own course of action with free and unconstrained will.

It is interesting to note that the elements of informed decision making and consent were explored and applied in an international law forum. The components were established in the 1949 international law case *US v Karl Brandt Nuremberg Code*. The joint tribunal was grappling with the atrocities committed during World War II. Individuals were held responsible for conduct that facilitated large-scale atrocities, such as a systematic program of medical 'research' on detained peoples. The motivation of the inquiry was partly to provide protection from such conduct into the future. The Chief Prosecutor is quoted as saying, 'The wrongs which we seek to condemn and punish have been so calculated, so malignant, and so devastating, that civilisation cannot tolerate their being ignored, because it cannot survive their being repeated.' There is a permanent memorial to the trials at the Palace of Justice in Nurnberg (Nuremberg), Germany, which includes a courtroom set out as it was when the trials were heard, to remind us of the gravity of what was considered and the ongoing relevance to modern society of what was decided (Museen der Stadt Nurnberg, 2013).

One of the lessons from these trials is that individuals remain responsible for cruel, inhumane treatment even if it is 'authorised' by a larger system, institution or state. You need to be constantly aware and take individual responsibility as a health practitioner or health care worker not to participate in or enable activities that are disrespectful to a person's right to decide what happens to their body themselves, or that are additionally cruel and inhumane.

Informed decision making is best achieved when someone has full autonomy, and is allowed to exercise that autonomy as they wish. To emphasise autonomy is to assume that people are able to set their own course in life, which includes decisions made in their own health care, in a reasoned way that suits them best. Autonomy, or self-rule, is then exercised. Ethically robust decisions are those that the decision maker has reached in a fully informed and carefully considered way—at least to the extent that the decision maker wishes to. As you read in earlier chapters, J.S. Mill, the famous early libertarian, thought that individual liberty should be allowed, within certain limits (Mill, 1975). Liberty, or autonomy, is important in many other ethics reasoning frameworks that you read about in Chapter 4.

Professions emphasise autonomy and informed decision making processes in their codes of behaviour.

For instance, the Medical Board of Australia's National Code for registered doctors in Australia states:

> Making decisions about healthcare is the shared responsibility of the doctor and the patient. Patients may wish to involve their family, carers or others (2.3) …
>
> A good doctor–patient partnership requires high standards of professional conduct. (Following this, issues are listed:) Treating each patient as an individual, and Encouraging and supporting patients to be well informed about their health and to use the information wisely when they are making decisions. (3.2)

And on decision making, which is also termed 'informed consent' in the National Code,

> Informed consent is a person's voluntary decision about medical care that is made with knowledge and understanding of the benefits and risks involved. The information doctors need to give to patients is detailed in guidelines issued by the National Health and Medical Research Council [NHMRC]. (3.5)

Notice that the National Code refers you to further guidelines, which means that these guidelines also have force in law, given that the Code has force under the National Law, which you read about in Chapter 1. So, reading the footnotes and the further guidelines from the National Health and Medical Research Council (NHMRC; 2004a, 2004b) is important so that you understand your obligations if you are a medical practitioner. The guidelines are also informative for other health care professionals, but they don't have the same legal force as standards to be upheld. You will read more about these guidelines later in this chapter.

The National Code offers further guidance:

> Good medical practice involves: Providing information to patients in a way that they can understand before asking their consent (3.5.1), and Obtaining informed consent or other valid authority before you undertake any examination, investigation or provide treatment [except in an emergency], or before involving patients in teaching or research (3.5.2), and Ensuring that your patients are informed about your fees and charges (3.5.3), and When referring a patient for investigation or treatment, advising the patient that there may be additional costs, which patients may wish to clarify before proceeding (3.5.4).

(Medical Board of Australia, 2014, pp. 6–9)

REFLECTION POINT

Informed decision making in standards

Read through one code of conduct, code of good practice or code of ethics and highlight all the issues that relate to autonomy, liberty and informed decision making and consent.

The formal components of informed decision making are supported by case law, including in:

- criminal law—particularly in offences of assault
- torts—particularly in negligence cases on provision of information before a valid informed decision is made (which you read about in Chapter 3).

As a health care professional, your record keeping of the informed decision-making process is essential. If there is no note or record about the decision-making process and the decision that has been made by the patient, it could be presumed it was lacking or insufficient—as you have no evidence for the process or the decision if the matter is brought before a court or administrative decision-making body, such as a standards or conduct committee.

The inadequate documentation and communication of an informed consent process can result in a finding of unsatisfactory professional performance, as listed in findings of National Boards by the Australian Health Practitioner Regulation Agency (AHPRA) (AHPRA, 2017). The term 'unsatisfactory professional performance' is used in Queensland for what may be termed 'unsatisfactory professional conduct' in other jurisdictions.

Failure to ensure appropriate and relevant or material information is available to the patient to enable them to make an informed decision can amount to unsatisfactory professional performance (AHPRA, 2016).

Gauging what level of detail to present to a patient, and how it should be presented, is not an easy task. Researchers constantly grapple with:

- the amount of information that clients in a health-care setting are able to understand
- the level of difficulty they can cope with
- the effect on their understanding of the way the information is presented.

As you will read later in this chapter, such issues are even more complex when dealing with people of limited capacity and competence. Regardless of what information you choose to make available, documenting a reasoned process for the level of information that has been given is part of the professional's responsibility.

This is one illustration of the way law and ethics work together in setting acceptable standards with a legal emphasis of a minimum standard. Everyone who works in health should be aware of the basic elements of such unlawful conduct or actions that are potentially harmful to clients. If these minimum standards are proven to have been breached, the worker and their institution could be exposed to administrative scrutiny of the conduct, as well as legal liability for the breach.

The public places trust in the health system that these fundamental principles of respect and non-interference with each person's bodily integrity will be honoured.

As set out in case law—with the consideration of a long-distance bus driver and the information provided to him on options for the repair of his ruptured Achilles tendon—patient autonomy means that patients should be placed in a position with sufficient information to be able to decide between two alternatives. This judgment also noted the High Court case *Wallace v Kam* [2013], in which the High Court said the duty 'to inform the patient of material risks of physical injury in proposed treatment is founded on the underlying common law right of the patient to choose whether or not to undergo a proposed treatment'. It is necessary to be given adequate information, given 'the policy underlying the imposition of that component of the duty is to equip the patient with information relevant to the choice that is the patient's to make.' (*ACT v Gillan; Gillan v ACT* [2018], at paragraph 35, citing *KL v Farnsworth* [2002], and *Wallace v Kam* [2013] at paragraph 8).

The components of informed decision making are additionally supported and reinforced in administrative regulations, such as in guidelines available to employees in health services. Organisations are keen to offer health care services in a professional way, and to minimise the potential liability to the institution of any employees acting without due regard to the importance of clients' autonomy.

Ensuring documentation of robust informed decision making is a safety and quality governance policy issue. The regulation has been explicitly explained and developed on a foundation of legal and ethical principles. In Queensland, the Clinical Excellence Division of the Patient Safety and Quality Improvement Service has produced guidelines for the public health system clinicians, which reflect the 'often complex ethical, legal, policy and practical framework of contemporary health care in which public health services are delivered'. The guide is for the multidisciplinary and team environment, which may include medical practitioners, dentists, nurses and other allied health practitioners (State of Queensland, 2017, p. 3).

The Queensland guidelines set out the elements of consent, stating that:

All health practitioners must obtain consent from an appropriate decision-maker before touching (examining) or providing health care to adult and child patients[6] except in a limited number of circumstances where that is not possible.

(State of Queensland, 2017)

Footnote 6 reads: 'This includes persons who are offenders (persons incarcerated in prison).' The guidelines state:

Failure to obtain a patient's consent to health care may result in a criminal charge of assault or civil action for battery. In addition, failure to disclose material risks to a patient may give rise to civil action for negligence[5]. In either case, disciplinary action by Queensland Health may be pursued.

The footnote 5 is a reference to another state's policy, which had already summarized the relevant law, showing that it is acceptable and preferable in many matters of regulation and administration for a sector to benefit and learn from the reasoned approach taken in other jurisdictions (State of Queensland, 2017, p. 9, citing Department of Health Western Australia, 2011).

The Government of Western Australia makes generic consent forms available on their website. The minimum requirement is that 'details relevant to consent are documented', regardless of whether the proposed treatment is declined or agreed to, and explicit consent must be documented in the patient's medical record (Government of Western Australia, Department of Health, 2016, p. 10).

You will remember that disciplinary action is an administrative regulatory action. A health service can decide that conduct has been unacceptable by the standards that they expect within the organisation, and discontinue the services of a contractor or the employment of an employee. In Chapter 2 you read about assessment of departure from acceptable standards. It is possible that even if a complaint is not proven in the criminal courts— such as for assault—it could still be proven in either:

- a civil action—such as for trespass or negligence
- an administrative complaint—such as unsatisfactory professional conduct (sometimes termed 'unsatisfactory professional performance').

Criminal cases are decided on the 'beyond reasonable doubt' standard of proof, and civil and administrative cases are decided on the 'balance of probabilities' standard of proof.

INTEGRATED LEARNING AND PRACTICE

Who documents consent?

In law, each person who contributes to therapeutic interactions bears a legal responsibility to ensure that their touching of another is lawful and consented to—and is supported by appropriately documented consent.

In ethics, each team member should reflect on their professional integrity to ensure records are accurate—and the autonomy of the individual—to satisfy themselves that documented consent is accurate and current.

Under regulation, policies guide team members and units in how to share the information and consent processes, and to document their part in the processes accurately. Generally, the most senior person is ultimately responsible for ensuring proper communication processes have been followed, and that consent is documented, and they must take the consent themselves if they perform the procedure.

REFLECTION POINT

Integration of standards

Read one of the guidelines on documentation of consent more fully, as a contemporary guideline that seeks to illustrate the integrated nature of ethics, law and regulation. On your first read through, note the content and fundamental aspects of informed decision making as they need to be implemented in a public service setting. Make a list of practical tips for implementing informed decision making in a health care setting.

On your next read through, make a note of which portions of the guide are about ethics, law, and regulation. You will then be able to summarise the contribution made by each towards effective informed decision making in a public setting.

Health service organisations can collectively define such obligations—for example, on a national level. Working with consumers and adopting patient-centred approaches are important to safety, quality and cost-effectiveness, as well as to technical clinical standards. The Australian Commission on Safety and Quality in Health Care (ACSQHC) highlights that partnerships with consumers are an important part of its clinical care standards, including:

- checking health information is understandable
- checking decision support tools are tailored appropriately.

In the *Australian Charter of Healthcare Rights*, a Charter developed and subsequently endorsed by Australian Health Ministers, two of the rights are:

- 'I have a right to be informed about services, treatment, options and costs in a clear and open way'
- 'I have a right to be included in decisions and choices about my care' (ACSQHC, 2018).

REFLECTION POINT

Changing the pitch

Look up the *Australian Charter of Healthcare Rights*. Read and rewrite the rights and practical application of the rights in the Charter in a different common language—you could try the language of tweet, the language of SMS, the language of tweens (you might need to consult with a tween to get it right for the current language) or any other language you prefer. Have fun with it, but also try to reflect the complex ideas behind the principles expressed.

The elements of informed decision making are universal, which means that they are useful for people of all ages and capacity. Similar elements were explored in the context of potential law reform during the 1980s, which challenged the appropriateness of far-reaching paternalism and routine decision making on others' behalf. The 1980s discussions serve as early reminders of the importance of the elements of informed decision making for all people, including minors and people with disability involving cognitive impairment (Weeramantry & Giantomasso, 1983, p. 2). At that time, Australians were beginning to consider whether our laws were in step with our international obligations, and academics were actively contributing to the discussion. Contemporary human rights documents of the era had set out obligations to uphold the dignity and wishes of individuals, regardless of their current capacity or stage of development (United Nations, 1966).

You will remember from Chapter 1 that Australia has signed the International *Convention on the Rights of Persons with Disabilities* (CRPD). The CRPD is a key human rights document that emphasises similar full and equal civic participation for persons living with disability, who are to be respected equally as individuals who may exercise choice and will to the best of their ability (United Nations, 2006). The universal applicability of the elements in upholding autonomy is now accepted.

REFLECTION POINT

Remembering international expressions of human rights

Visit the Department of Foreign Affairs and Trade website to source and read one of the international agreements, or to read a different convention that relates to autonomy and decision making in health care (there are a quite a few): <www.dfat.gov.au>. As you read, notice how the language can be firm in expressing strict standards, but that it is also aspirational at times. As member states accept the obligations under the agreements, they embark on a process of checking that they have met their firm requirements, as well as striving to achieve the remaining aspirations.

Check back to your reflections and notes from previous chapters to see if any of these aspirational goals matches your own earlier thoughts about goals and duties.

As highlighted in the following discussions, the analysis prompted by the elements of informed decision making takes into account the nature of each decision to be made. A judgment of competency of the decision maker is a relative concept, in this instance, relative to the scope and nature of each decision to be made.

REFLECTION POINT

Decisions and choices in the news

Keep an eye on current news and commentary for discussions and critiques of health care. When you read the pieces, note how the issue of autonomy is dealt with, and whether 'best interest' features in the discussion. Take some time to think about it, then return to the topic a few weeks later and see if you can add further reflections.

Also, reflect on why you notice and then read that article; could you possibly be missing out on reading about other issues?

The following discussions about competency and decision making demonstrate that ethics analysis can be similar to an analytical legal process. Both processes identify elements and then explore and test those elements in a given situation. Remember that ethics ultimately emphasises the optimal standard, which is usually aspirational and encourages us to aim beyond the minimum required standard.

Health care decisions and young persons

Children and young people are a large part of our population, and a large proportion of the health care clientele. They also present some of the more perplexing dilemmas about autonomy, as health care workers negotiate treatment with both the child and their parent or guardian.

Children in health care contexts bring into focus who is able to make health care decisions, and what type of decisions they are able to make. Under Australian law, adulthood is reached at age 18 years, and children are 17 years and under. Parents or other authorised persons are assumed to be able to lawfully decide a range of life and wellbeing matters on behalf of their children. This is because the state supports the parents/authorised persons as decision makers and—as you will read below—this authority is always limited, and is at the discretion of the state.

REFLECTION: EVERYDAY ETHICS

Think of a time when you had care and control of some children. Perhaps you are a parent, aunt, uncle or much older brother or sister—or perhaps you were babysitting. Throughout the course of the day, decisions needed to be made. What to do? What to eat? How to prepare for activities and pack up afterwards? How to negotiate disputes? How to deal with minor accidents and injuries? Think about how these decisions were made, and how much involvement the children had in them. You will probably find that this was different, depending on the age of the children.

Keep those everyday situations in mind as you think about children in health care contexts, remembering what children of different ages seem capable of in everyday contexts, and also distinguishing between when they are happy and when they are hurt, sick or upset. You may also find that you had a tendency towards maximising the children's autonomy, or of keeping control and acting paternalistically. Recognising your own bias in terms of autonomy and paternalism is useful for professional contexts in which you will deal with children and young people.

A parent's decision making for a child diminishes as the child's increasing capacity and autonomy is recognised. This is also part of common law—the law that is developed through judgments handed down by courts—as expressed in this landmark judgment:

> The common law can, and should, keep pace with the times ... the legal right of a parent to the custody of a child ends at the eighteenth birthday: and even up to then, it is a dwindling right which the courts will hesitate to enforce against the wishes of the child, and the more so the older he is. It starts with the right of control and ends with little more than advice.
>
> *(Lord Denning, in Hewer v Bryant [1970] 2 QB 357 at 369)*

The United Nations *Convention on the Rights of the Child* (CRC) supports due weight being given to children's views, 'in accordance with the age and maturity of the child', which member states strive to uphold (United Nations, 1989, Article 12).

Legislators recognise that the key principles in our laws and policy frameworks that relate to protection of children are consistent with those found in the CRC. Our laws and regulatory and policy frameworks support early intervention in situations of risk to a child, and participation of children and young people in decisions that are made about them, such as where they live (New South Wales Parliament, 2017), referring to the *Children and Young Persons (Care and Protection) Act 1998* (NSW).

The laws and policies for treatment and health care for children are consistent with this approach. In our health care system, the development of autonomy is encouraged.

For instance, children—particularly mature minors (usually children over 14 years)—can consent to minor procedures alone. There is a tendency to adopt a gradual increasing presumption of capacity and competency for medical and health care decisions, between the ages of 12 and 14 years. Below 12 years, children are presumed to lack capacity and be incompetent for such decision making, unless proven otherwise. Above the midpoints, children are encouraged to take more responsibility for health care decisions. However, they do need to demonstrate that they are competent to reach a sufficient understanding of the treatment or care that is proposed.

This requirement to demonstrate competency has a common law basis rather than a statute legislative basis. The case law that established this was from an era when Australian courts still looked to the British courts for their precedents, and the principle has been applied in many cases since then. The most compelling precedent is still *Gillick* (*Gillick v West Norfolk AHA* (1986)). Even when different states and territories have different and broadly framed legislative provisions, there is discretion available, and this case law guides the implementation of those standards. Note that if there were firm rules set in the legislation, then the statute law would be applied in its precise terms, as the clearly stated intention of parliament must be applied by the courts. (To read more on this, see a statutory interpretation text.)

So, the precise terms of the legislative provisions must be considered, if states have legislated on the issue. In South Australia, the *Consent to Medical Treatment and Palliative Care Act 1995* (SA) provides at section 6 that consent to medical and dental treatment by a person 16 years and over is valid and effective. Medical treatment may be administered with a parent or guardian's consent for a child (see section 12(a)).

Alternatively, a child's consent can be accepted below that age, if certain conditions are met. The treatment proposed must be considered to be in the best interests of the child's health and wellbeing, and the treating practitioner must be satisfied that the child has demonstrated that they are capable of forming an understanding of the process and possible consequences of the decision, as at section 12(b)(i). This is to uphold the basic elements of informed decision making if the child is to assume the decision making role.

These two conditions are found in many other general legislative provisions in other states, even if specific legislation on medical and dental treatment has not been made. In South Australia, an added protection is that a second doctor must agree with this assessment, and this agreement must be documented as a written opinion, as in section 12(b)(ii). Notice that in referring to statutes, it is important for fullest referencing to give the section of the Act you say contains the provision or standard you are summarising. This is like giving a page number of a book or article that you are referencing. Precision is essential if you are explaining a standard in detail.

Notice also the legal language precision here. If the section had set the relevant age at over 16 years, it would not apply to someone on the day they turned 16, but would apply to someone who was 16 years and one day old. There are also statutory interpretation rules about when each day starts and stops—so you know the exact time a new set of standards applies (Pearce & Geddes, 2014).

REFLECTION POINT

Legislation source

Check if there is law in your state or territory on a child's age of consent for medical treatment. To begin your search, either use your library, or go direct to your parliament website or to a clearing house site that has up-to-date information on the law, such as the Public Interest Advocacy Centre (PIAC). PIAC is an Australian association that has researched and represented children's interests in many aspects of the law, making information available on their website: <www.piac.asn.au>.

We recognise that a child's autonomy over their own life and body continually develops. It would therefore make ethical sense, as a child grows older, to gradually place increasing reliance on their expressed wishes. This may mean taking into account a child's assent (or agreement) or dissent (or disagreement), even if these would not otherwise be sufficient to meet the criteria of informed decision making. In practical terms, health carers facilitate the expressions of those preferences in a way that maximises autonomy.

Health care teams constantly discuss how to resolve child and family best interests, particularly when there are conflicts with developing autonomy, lack of compliance with treatment regimes, and family rejection of treatment advice (Harrison & Laxer, 2000).

REFLECTION POINT

Emerging competence

Read the *Children and Young Persons (Care and Protection) Act 1998* (NSW), and then compare it to the *Consent to Medical Treatment and Palliative Care Act 1995* (SA).

When you find out how a child or young person is defined, check whether that definition gives any broad limits on decisions that can or can't be made. Are there general principles of how to check on the informed nature of the decision? Look at the wording that provides that consent to medical and dental treatment by a child 16 years and over is valid and effective, or that dissent is expressed by a child 14 years and over.

Considering whether a child has demonstrated capacity to understand the choices to be made about a proposed procedure should be a constant assessment. Each time children return to a treatment or care setting, they will be a little older than last you saw them, and they may have developed sufficient capacity through maturity, cognitive development and experience to make an autonomous decision on issues that were previously decided for them by their parents.

Also, consider how information is presented at each stage of a young person's maturity, and if communication techniques can enhance the capacity for informed decision making so that the threshold is reached. Some research on children's consent capabilities has shown that children understand information more readily if it is presented in a personalised way. For instance, rag dolls can be used to demonstrate how blood would be taken (Berryman, 1978, p. 94). Other techniques could be used that do not assume that the child has developed abstract cognitive abilities. Children should be given ample opportunity to ask any questions they like, as this will encourage them to elicit relevant information for themselves (Nicholson, 1986, p. 144). Developing the child's capacity for decision making is a necessary process given the basic ethics responsibility to the autonomy of all persons, and respect for each person's integrity and dignity.

So how does this work in practice? Practical help and pragmatic guidelines are there to help you achieve that. For instance, the medical code of conduct you looked at earlier pays particular attention to the process of decision making for care and treatment for children and young people.

For children, the Good Medical Practice Code states (at 3.6):

> Caring for children and young people brings additional responsibilities for doctors. Good medical practice involves: Placing the interests and wellbeing of the child or young person first (3.6.1; Ensuring that you consider young people's capacity for decision-making and consent (3.6.2); Ensuring that, when communicating with a child or young person, you treat them with respect and listen to their views, encourage questions, and answer their questions to the best of your ability, provide information in a way that they can understand, recognise the role of parents or guardians and when appropriate, encourage the young person to involve their parents or guardians in decisions about their care (3.6.3); and Being alert to children and young people who may be at risk, and notifying appropriate authorities, as required by law (3.6.4).
>
> *(Medical Board of Australia, 2014, p. 9)*

The Good Medical Practice Code neatly captures the responsibility towards children, to consider their protection, and also to consider their evolving input into decisions which—at the start of their life—others make almost entirely on their behalf.

Considering limits to decision making is not only for the child. There are also limitations that society places on parents making decisions for their child. What these limits have in common is that the reasoning behind the limitation relies on the overriding responsibility to protect the child, given the child's vulnerability and dependence on others for safety, security and wellbeing.

For example, the responsibility that parents have to make decisions on behalf of their children is effectively taken away when the procedures at issue are regarded as non-therapeutic and too risky. For instance, legislation limits parents' capacity to consent to female circumcision and tattooing on behalf of their children (Dworkin, 1987, p. 193). Their power to make decisions on behalf of their children is also limited if it has been shown that they have acted against the child's best interest in the past.

Society effectively reserves the right to intervene to ensure that the best interests of each child are upheld (Shawndra, 2007). The authority of parents to give proxy consent for their children is, in essence, a mechanism that is only supported if it is used in the way the state has agreed it be used—to protect the wellbeing of children. So, the state reserves the right to intervene and the authority may be limited if the child's best interests were not being served. However, differences can emerge internationally in different state's administrative and legal systems, such as trends in research guidelines promoting greater involvement of children in research participation decisions, and legal trends for children restricting choices, and mandating the involvement of parents in certain decisions—such as for abortion in the USA in recent times. Intervention is generally more frequent for mature minors in mental health, personality disorders or life-threatening conditions, but it is not limited to these. Donna Dickenson argues that the agreement of the older child is needed for effective treatment participation, so forcing treatment is problematic in a practical sense and an ethical sense (Dickenson, 2001, p. 209). When children's decision making is restricted, their parents or others who are judged to be suitable resume their decision making role.

The gravity of the decisions that need to be made make a difference to whether a mature minor is deemed capable of making a competent decision. One example is explored in the following Reflection.

REFLECTION: EXPRESSED WISHES AND CAPACITY

In the UK in 1999, a 15-year-old girl known only as M became suddenly ill and required a heart transplant in order to survive. Her refusal of the transplant was overridden by a High Court judge, who deemed she was 'too overwhelmed' to make that informed decision. He approved the operation on grounds of best interests.

As a group exercise, discuss what you would do when faced with M's reported wish:

> It's hard to take it all in. I feel selfish. If I had the transplant I wouldn't be happy. If I were to die my family would be sad. Death is final—I know I can't change my mind. I don't want to die, but I would rather die than have the transplant, and have someone else's heart, I would rather die with 15 years of my own heart.

(Foster, 1999)

In the case of M, once the legal ruling was explained to her, M gave her consent. The presiding judge, Johnson J, said in judgment, 'M will live with the consequences of my decision, in a very striking sense ... There is the risk too that she will carry with her for the rest of her life resentment about what has been done to her' (*R v M* (1999), as cited in Forrester & Griffiths, 2001).

There is a subtle re-emergence of weak paternalism in acknowledging the special knowledge and experience that health carers have and, consequently, their great importance in helping to direct patients to sensible treatment options. Decision making entails a shared role—to work towards reasonable and achievable goals. It has probably always been the case, but now it is explicitly argued that the balance of decision making should shift back to the health care professional in different circumstances, depending on the urgency and gravity of decisions at hand.

The complexity of technological options for care may have also influenced this shift. The ethical justification for such paternalism is discussed in professional literature. For instance, in caring for children with cancer, a health care team wrote about how the balance in sharing of decisions between parents, clinicians, and (mature) children can vary depending on the likelihood of cure for the ill child and the range of reasonable options the clinician considers to be available. The team argued that the clinician could feel justified in strongly directing the family to one realistic course of action, based on his or her knowledge and experience. The child's preferences may be more practically important when two or more reasonable choices are available for their care. The child assumes greater decisional authority with maturity, and expected greater capacity for understanding complex issues (Whitney et al., 2006).

There are countless ethical and legal grey areas in the course of children's maturity towards full capacity for autonomous decision making. Discretion is needed as each situation is different, and ethics and law work together best to inform the decision maker and professionals who are assisting the decision maker. One quandary illustrates this. Imagine a minor who is pregnant. Legally, she has not yet exercised full competency over all decisions for her own health, yet by virtue of becoming pregnant, finds herself potentially assuming decision-making responsibilities for her child. In a paper written with legal academic John Devereux, we argued on both ethics and legal grounds that developing and supporting the minor is a high priority, as her competence is crucial to ethically rigorous decision-making processes for herself and her own child in the future (Berglund & Devereux, 2000, pp. 25–6).

Bear in mind that some circumstances may require the appropriate institutional response—for example, child to child harmful sexual behaviour when the behaviour has been coerced or non-consensual, and child protection issues (Australian Government, 2017, Recommendations).

INTEGRATED LEARNING AND PRACTICE

Developing autonomy and important decisions

1   As a tutorial exercise, map all the decisions you can think of that a pregnant 14-year-old girl might be faced with.

2   Write a list of ways to check if she will have the legal capacity to make the decisions herself, or with assistance.

3   Write a corresponding checklist of ethics concerns for each of those decisions.

People can feel coerced into agreeing, and this is particularly so for people with limited capacity, as they tend to be dependent on others. Children can feel unable to disagree with the suggestions of their parents or health care workers (Grisso & Vierling, 1978, p. 423). So extra care is needed to check who or what is influencing their decision, and that the young person is comfortable with the decision they are expressing.

REFLECTION

Family matters

If you are ready for something even more complicated, try the next exercise. Pay particular attention to the components of consent that you have now learnt about, as well as the overall objective of maximising autonomous decision making.

The exercise challenges you to consider the place of children in relation to their relatives who seek health care. In this case, a related child is present and available as an interpreter—a relatively common presentation in health care settings. However, should the child be accepted as an interpreter? What are the ethical risks in terms of the child and the relative? You will need to consider the decision-making elements for both the relative and child to solve the puzzle.

A child's place in others' medical decisions

An 84-year-old woman, Mrs M, comes to casualty at 10 am with her nine-year-old grandchild, Emi. They have arrived by taxi, and Emi has helped her grandmother to walk in and sit in the waiting area. Mrs M doesn't speak English, but Emi says that she can translate. Emi says her grandma hasn't felt well since last week, and is wheezing and has a pain in her chest. Emi's parents are at work and won't be home until 8.30 pm.

Professional interpreters who are part of medical consultations advise others to:

- interpret the content, sense and intent of what is said
- relay information in a neutral way, without withholding information or influencing decisions (Gietzelt & Jones, 2002, pp. 22–3).

Interpreters and translators recognise that their role is to provide language services. This includes services in interpreting and translating written, oral and sign language forms of language. The Australian Institute of Interpreters and Translators (AUSIT) Interpreter Code of Ethics provides the basis for professional conduct for nationally credentialed interpreters and translators, and many agencies and institutions require interpreters to abide by the code—even if they are not accredited members of AUSIT. Translators are expected to maintain the confidentiality of information, to be impartial, accurate and comprehensive in transferring messages between parties (AUSIT, 2012, pp. 3–5).

In principle, public hospital and health centres make interpreter services available to patients, in their preferred language. Commonly phone (or video conference) interpreter services are used, but some on-site services may also be available in community languages. For example, many health services are publicly committed to providing confidential and professional interpreter services to patients and their families or carer if they use a language other than English as their first and preferred language, or they are hearing impaired and use sign language to communicate.

One health district restates the state's public health service policy and standard procedures requirements for use of interpreters for multicultural health issues on their public website (New South Wales Government, 2017a). This ensures the principles are accessible to all, regardless of their status:

The need to understand and be understood is fundamental to safe and effective health care. Poor communication can result in misunderstandings which may be confusing, distressing and dangerous. Interpreters help health staff and patients (and the family and carers of patients) to communicate clearly.

… With the exception of emergencies, health staff are required to inform patients of all relevant information regarding their treatment and associated risks such as any side effects or adverse outcomes prior to commencing treatment or intervention. …

… It is mandatory that professional health care interpreters are used when seeking informed consent for surgery, treatments and/or research. It is essential that interpreters are present in the following situations:

- Admission
- Medical histories, assessment and treatment plans
- Medical instructions
- Pre and post operative instructions
- Psychiatric or psychological assessment and treatment
- Counselling
- Discharge procedures including instructions, medications and community resources
- Assessment and treatment regarding sexual assault, physical and emotional abuse
- Terminal illness/bereavement counselling
- Explanation of medication
- Mental Health Review Tribunals and magistrate hearings.

(New South Wales Government, 2017a)

These policies are supported by further linked policies on working with interpreters and general information and consent issues (New South Wales Government, Ministry of Health, 2005, 2006).

INTEGRATED LEARNING AND PRACTICE

Facilitating information flow

Look up the public website for information about interpreters. Follow the links to see how many departmental policy directives and guidelines you can find that explain the practical commitment made to fully informed decision making for people who are receiving health care services conducted in a language that they are not fluent in. These represent the institution regulatory standards.

Then, think of a time you or someone you knew needed health care in another country where the language and system was different to home: How was the communication managed?

So, what should you do in the real world when a readymade 'family' solution to interpreting is readily available? You may like to read further about this topic in the same article jointly written with John Devereux, which questions the ethical robustness of decisions made using a child as a link in the exchange of information between carers and patient. We also discussed the risk to the best interest of the child, who may feel an adult sense of responsibility and burden when placed in that position. On ethics and legal grounds, we argued that the child's input would rarely be acceptable (Berglund & Devereux, 2000).

Limitations in cognitive capacity

Declining capabilities are a routine part of a lifespan. At some stage, frequently in old age, we can all expect to diminish in our capacities and health. This is not a dramatic ethics dilemma in itself, but it does raise ethics issues in terms of decision making for care throughout that phase of life. Any of us can at some point—due to injury, sudden debilitating illness, or emotional or physical shock—be temporarily or permanently limited in our autonomy. At each of these times, we present health care workers with challenges as they go about the business of providing us with care. In the face of these challenges, health care workers remain committed to the integrity of their clients.

capacity
Legal capacity of competence, such as for informed decision making.

As a health care worker, you can probably sense when your clients have limited **capacity** for autonomy. They may seem slightly or grossly incapacitated—mentally, physically, or both. By virtue of their incapacity—temporary or permanent—it may be difficult for you to ascertain with precision what they want and, therefore, to know what course they wish to pursue in their health care. Nevertheless, the process remains centrally important.

Our society recognises that a person with diminished autonomy may not be able to make all the necessary decisions for their own care. The common objective is to act in a way that is to their benefit, and able to be judged by others to be acting in their 'best interest'. We rely on a parental obligation to children and a mechanism of guardianship for others with diminished capacity to make decisions in their interests if they cannot do so, after initially maximising their **mental capacity** and ability to make their own decisions.

mental capacity
Cognitive capability for specific thought process.

When a situation is urgent

In emergencies, paramedics and emergency department staff act to preserve life. It is assumed that this is an acceptable objective, and the workers are support by legislation given the common law doctrine of necessity, as you read in Chapter 3. Provided treatment is not contrary to the known and properly documented wishes of a patient, they can be treated in an emergency even when instructions are unable to be sought from the patient. Similarly, a child brought into emergency needing life-saving measures will be treated, and efforts to contact their parent or guardian will be made as quickly as is practical and possible. Treatment will not be delayed while that is done.

In the health care professions—where the autonomy of clients is a highly valued ethics principle and treatment decisions depend on patients being partners in treatment plans to the extent of their capacity—health care workers have additional protective obligations towards people with limited capacities. This is to ensure that appropriate substituted decision making is in place for decisions that a person is unable to make themselves.

Making practical arrangements when offering and delivering appropriate care to maximise the dignity of each client remains of central importance—particularly when caring for people with developing or diminished capacity. Identifying which decisions are able to be made competently is an important first step. Simple and routine decisions may still be able to be made autonomously by a person with limited capacity, even though complex or urgent decisions may need to be made with assistance.

An assessment of the client's capacity—that is, their ability to understand the care process or treatment on offer—is routinely made in health care, and particularly in aged care. A question about capacity is often asked by nurses, medical practitioners, relatives or other visitors. Each is monitoring whether the patient understands their situation and the options available. The assessment of capacity is routinely carried out, and is a vital skill for all health carers. One helpful list of issues to consider as a practical guide has been formulated by a team of clinicians and ethicists. You can pose these issues as questions, as you consider the circumstances of each patient:

- conducive environment and conducive frame of mind for decision making
- extent of cognitive function and stability over time
- adequate information available to the patient, which has been given and understood
- view of health professional
- additional factors relating to social situation and family (Finucane et al., 1993, p. 402).

These questions clearly go beyond a simple 'mini-mental examination' of the patient—which focuses on the patient's orientation to time and place, and their awareness of environment—to the environmental constraints on competence and decision making.

The general guideline is that it is rare for people to lack capacity for all the decisions they must make. The competency of any particular client should be assessed with respect to their current circumstances and the specific decision that faces them—consent is agreement to a specific proposition.

This routine assessment of capacity (or competence) is ethically critical. Without capacity, a person cannot give valid consent. If their capacity is limited, then there are corresponding limits to what a person can consider and consent to. Generally, the limits are that only minimally risky and minimally invasive procedures can be consented to without another decision maker being consulted, which is similar to the guidelines for children. That is because someone must be capable of making a decision before they can be judged to have made it.

PRACTICE EXAMPLE

Substitute decision making

Jayne Hewitt

Jayne has been a Registered Nurse for 30 years, working predominantly in critical care areas such as intensive care and coronary care.

Imagine that you are the senior nurse working in a residential aged care facility. Khalid, a resident you having been caring for over the years, and who has just turned 92, is suffering with declining cognitive function. You've noticed that over the course of the past few months he is increasingly forgetful, and frequently becomes disoriented. Khalid has two daughters and a son who visit him regularly, although there have been occasions when he is unable to recall their names.

During your morning shift you notice that Khalid is breathless and struggling to get out of bed. You undertake further assessment and note that Khalid is febrile and his heart rate is elevated. Concerned that he may be suffering with an infection, you ask for Khalid to be reviewed by his GP. Khalid is diagnosed with pneumonia, and the GP recommends that he be transferred to hospital for treatment with intravenous antibiotics. She asks that you make arrangements for Khalid's transfer as soon as possible, and leaves the facility.

You call Khalid's elder daughter, who is listed as the emergency contact, to update her on Khalid's condition and planned admission to hospital. There is no answer when you ring, so you contact Khalid's son. He tells you that as Khalid is suffering with dementia, and probably toward the end of his life—he should be provided with comfort measures in the care facility where he currently resides. The son tells you that he and his sister have discussed what should be done in these circumstances, and they all agreed that Khalid would not want active treatment. He says that he does not consent to Khalid's transfer.

1   Describe the ethical conflict that you find yourself in as the senior RN in this situation.

2   In seeking a solution, identify whether the law in your state or territory would permit Khalid's son to refuse admitting his father to hospital.

3   Are there any other people authorised to make this decision on Khalid's behalf?

4   Armed with this knowledge, what steps would you take?

You probably know from your own experience as a family member that practical safeguards can be implemented at a time when someone is unwell or has diminished capacity. If an elderly person seems unable to fully participate in all decision making at that time—in not understanding the decision to be made or the consequences of it—family members who may have accompanied them could be consulted about their prior expressed views. The carer may also have an indication about likely preferred options, given a person's past choices. This should be documented in the health care record notes, and the carer may be able to discuss previous decisions that have been made in a person's care. The person's expressed wishes should always be explored and noted.

REFLECTION POINT

Choices to be made by those close to you

Share examples of the process of decision making for an elderly relative or friend.

- What safeguards can you identify in the process of looking at treatment options and moving forward to decisions about that care?
- What process can you see to gauge their preferences?
- Are the recommended processes in place to further and protect autonomy for your own family and friends?

If capacity seems to have diminished to such an extent that a person is not likely to be able to make a decision, weigh up options and fully understand the process—such as the treatments being considered and the consequences of a decision—a different decision maker may be sought. A person may potentially need a substitute decision maker if they are:

- intellectually, physically, psychologically or sensorily disabled
- of advanced age
- mentally ill
- otherwise disabled.

A 'person responsible' can be identified to assist if substituted decision making is needed for a client, such as a guardian, a spouse or partner, a carer, or a close friend or relative. This search for a 'person responsible' is undertaken routinely because of the fundamental legal principle that some consent is needed. Any treatment could otherwise be seen as trespass. Family members and other suitable persons can become legally appointed decision makers, and are then called 'substitute decision makers'. As also explained in a comprehensive guide on guardianship provisions, discretion is needed—as much as possible—to preserve the person's freedom to manage their own personal, domestic and financial affairs to the extent of their capability (O'Neill & Peisah, 2011).

For instance, as you read in Chapter 4, some decisions, such as assistance in dying, cannot be made by a substitute decision maker (Victorian Government, 2017, pp. 180–2).

A person can make this decision about managing their personal affairs in nominating enduring guardians in advance of it being needed, including for medical and dental treatment. Then, when circumstances arise, as predicted, which prompt the enduring guardian's role to begin, a decision maker is already nominated to make certain types of decisions according to the instructions set out in the enduring guardian appointment. At the time enduring guardians are appointed, a person must be of 'full legal capacity'. Health professionals—usually their GPs, may be routinely asked to check a person who is nominating an enduring guardian. This is to ensure that their overall health and cognitive function is intact for that decision-making purpose (O'Neill & Peisah, 2011). Also, the GP will then be alerted to the arrangement if the substitute decision maker is needed in the future.

Guardians and substitute decision makers grapple with the concept of what decisions need to be made at a time when the person is unable to make that decision themselves, and what is in the best interests of the client if the client cannot make that decision.

The decision regarding what is in the client's best interests is also informed by the professional opinion of the health care worker. The best interests of the client are the primary interests of the client in maintaining and furthering their health and welfare. Even a close family member will differ from the client in many ways, and therefore cannot replicate the values and personal choices of the patient. The best that can be hoped for is that an informed decision—based on the best interests and broad life-choices of the patient—will be made on their behalf. There are limits to what enduring guardians and surrogate decision makers can decide, just as parents are limited in the decisions they can make that affect their children in significant ways. Guidelines and laws relating to surrogate, substitute or assisted decisions are constantly evolving.

While Australia does not yet have a uniform approach to capacity, it is an issue being contemplated by the Australian Law Reform Commission (ALRC). Principles drawn from various state policies are highlighted, such as assuming that a person has capacity unless proven otherwise, and remembering that capacity is specific to the decision to be made, and using substitute decision making as a last resort. The principle drawn from the UN *Convention on the Rights of Persons with Disabilities* is that assuming that a person lacks capacity because they have a particular diagnosis or condition is not justified (ALRC, 2013).

Under the principles of guardianship, decisions can be made on a person's behalf by a legally appointed decision maker or on an order of a recognised legal authority, such as a Guardianship Tribunal. The types of decisions that can be made will be limited by the function and power afforded to the guardian as substitute decision maker. The arrangement can be authorised under temporary or continuing orders, and all are subject to periodic review. The guardianship tribunal can appoint a suitable guardian. The tribunal can also hear and make a lifestyle or personal decision such as a medical or dental decision for someone who is incapable of doing so themselves. Normally, this option is only used if there is no alternative.

The guiding principle for all types of guardianship arrangements is that restriction of a person's freedom of decision making and action is a significant imposition, and only as much restriction as is needed in the circumstances should be imposed. Decisions should be made to promote the best interests of the person with the decision-making disability. Their wishes should still be sought and carried into effect, if possible (O'Neill & Peisah, 2011).

The process preserves the autonomy of the person. By involving the person as much as possible, they are facilitated to be ready to make certain decisions autonomously when that is appropriate. The substituting of each decision requires a different process, of checking that it is appropriate and acceptable, and that the freedom of the person is preserved into the future.

You will notice the language of important philosophers, such as Mill, in the guiding provisions. This is not surprising, as the balance that is to be arrived at is a considered restriction on a person's liberty.

INTEGRATED LEARNING AND PRACTICE

Why is assessing capacity and involving a person in decisions so important?

Under law, capacity underpins lawful decision making.

Ethics frameworks commonly emphasise enhancing capacity, as it is central to a person developing their autonomy and exercising some choice and control over what is happening in their life, including in a care setting. Allowing and furthering autonomy and a person's dignity is part of respecting a person.

Under regulations, international conventions and local policies provide guidance on fundamental human rights—including the right to be involved in decisions on all aspects of one's own life.

Caution is needed as the aged and frail can have difficulty disagreeing with the suggestions made by their practitioners, health care workers, family members, carers or guardians. As this includes you, you need to take care to set out a range of options for your client to consider, rather than place only one suggestion before them. Cognitively impaired adults are known to be particularly vulnerable to undue influence by others— such as their children or 'helpful' neighbour or friend, or formal or informal carer, or even their lawyer, doctor, accountant or religious adviser (O'Neill & Pesiah, 2011).

Try the next Reflection as a review of the issues of capacity, competency and decision making. As you consider the elements of consent, reflect further on autonomy and whether the words of wisdom that we have available from early philosophers can help you decide what you should do.

REFLECTION: DIMINISHING CAPACITY AND FREEDOM OF MOVEMENT

This reflection reviews the capacity and competency issues.

Enid and Martin both have advanced dementia. They live in an aged-care home in separate female and male wings. They are married, but there is no suitable accommodation for them to be cared for together. They are in secure wings. At times, they ask about each other, and Martin wonders when his wife will visit next. He mostly talks about Sarah, his first wife, whom he hasn't seen in 35 years. Enid is active and wanders, and is likely to forget where she is. Martin is mainly resting during the day, with limited mobility.

1   What, if anything, should staff say to Martin?

2   What issues about competence, veracity and choices permitted does this situation raise for Enid and Martin, their families and staff?

With declining capacity to make sensible decisions for one's own safety and welfare, others begin to step in and assume the day-to-day aspects of care, safety and comfort. Ensuring a safe environment for patients is difficult—particularly in contexts that are inherently dangerous if a person is prone to wander or fall.

Nursing professionals routinely face the ethically complex issue of how to ensure a patient remains in a safe environment, if the patient's own capacities for avoiding danger are impaired.

Ethics tools can help with this consideration, as a paper by Ann Gallagher demonstrates. Different restraint techniques, including psychological and technical (physical) options for stroke care patients were analysed with reference to Jonsen, Siegler and Winslade's model (Jonsen et al., 1998). Written from a practical nursing perspective, Gallagher reasoned for restraint only as a last resort, after consideration of alternatives and the impact of such a choice, given the medical indications, patient preferences, quality of life and contextual features that are part of the situation under consideration (Gallagher, 2011). Even this cautionary view would now be considered carefully, given international obligations. Using the least restrictive option available to ensure safety is supported under Conventions, such as the *Convention on the Rights of Persons with Disabilities* (United Nations, 2006). Restraint is very rarely justifiable.

A nurse was reprimanded and disqualified for 12 months when he inappropriately physically restrained a patient. He also put his arm around the patient's neck, appearing to cause airway restriction, and placed his finger in the patient's eye. He had been suspended pending the outcome of the hearing at Tribunal level (Nursing and Midwifery Board of Australia, 2017).

Care planning in advance

advance directive
A directive given by a patient in advance that represents their autonomous wishes and is intended by them to guide their treatment and care in the future.

Advance indication of the decisions that a patient has made that they would like to guide their future treatment and care is called an **advance directive**. Advance directives are increasingly being sought from patients whose condition makes it likely that they will lapse into a critical situation or be unable to express their wishes as their health situation changes. Their autonomy continues to be important, and what they would wish in particular clinical circumstances is taken into account.

However, as is the case with informed decision making, the patient's expression of choice needs to be specific. Advance directives can be difficult to accept because—although a patient may express what they would like to happen given a particular situation—the unpredictability of their symptoms means that the patient may not be able to grasp the true nature of what it would be like for them if that situation did come about. This means that the validity of carrying out their wishes can seem questionable to those evaluating the directives in the context of the emerging situation.

In an ideal situation, anticipating the end of life allows the patient and carers to be comfortable about the 'plan' ahead when the inevitable does occur. Ethics reflection can be helpful in exploring the path ahead for both patients and carers. Consider the compelling description of the collaborative application of Beauchamp and Childress's principles in a Californian intensive care unit, when a young woman became ill 10 months after her lung transplant—and subsequently died. You will remember the explanation of Beauchamp and Childress's principles of beneficence, non-maleficence, autonomy and justice in Chapter 1 and Chapter 4 (Beauchamp & Childress, 2001, pp. 83–7). The process of the young woman coming to terms with the imminent death, and the role of the clinical team in 'creating a warm and open environment' is described as a collaborative and ethically aware engagement, with frequent open discussion of quality of life and end of life issues, and limits to options in care. The patient herself made the decision of the timing to remove her intubation tube and stated her final wishes by writing letters to her family and fiancé (Stecher, 2011).

The practice of patients providing advance directives relies on the assumption that a competent patient is able to choose whether or not to undergo further treatment, including life-sustaining treatment. 'Living wills' mandate which treatments patients do or do not want, and are prepared ahead of time to be used if the patient becomes 'incompetent' (Devereux, 2002, pp. 322–3). Their practical use as the only expression of an autonomous care decision is limited, as routine decision-making power may be retained by many more people—that is, family—than was anticipated. When no specific patient advance directive has been given, clinical judgment and the 'guardian process' is routinely used. Such a decision that is made for others is based on the grounds of best interests, effectively upholding beneficence rather than the autonomy of the patient.

In Australia, individuals can refuse further active treatment if they are judged to have capacity—that is, they are competent—to make that decision, and so under common law right of inviolability, consent should be given before treatment or assessment is undertaken, as you read in Chapter 3.

Advance care planning provides for the ongoing autonomy of a person, including setting out the types of circumstances in which a person would not wish further active treatment to be initiated, and the type of care they would consent to receiving. A key part of advance care planning is in letting others know wishes, and also arranging a substitute decision maker who understands those wishes, who will then be informed when stepping in after a person is no longer able to express their wishes. These preferences can be written down or documented in advance care planning and advance care directives forms, which can then be taken into account in planning future care. The common law right stands even in states without specific forms. However, it is more straightforward for the decision maker— who needs to be comfortable implementing these wishes—if they have been properly documented, so using the forms are available in the relevant jurisdiction is a practical and useful way to document the wishes. Advance care planning is similar to telling someone what you would like to happen with your assets after you die, and formalising your wishes in a valid will. The directives forms are a transparent way of documenting competent informed preferences for existing or future health conditions—and making them known clearly to others. Just like consent forms, they document the process of decision making that has been undertaken.

The Australian Government supports projects on advance care planning in both acute care settings and palliative care, with support and training available for medical practitioners and nurses and other health care workers working in complex care environments (Australian Government, 2017). A National Framework for advance care directives has been supported by all Australian health ministers (Coalition of Australian Governments, 2011). The legislation in each jurisdiction is not the same, but the framework demonstrates a shared policy direction.

REFLECTION: ADVANCE CARE PLANNING

Look at the Advance Care Planning Australia website <http://advancecareplanning. org.au> and check the options for practical documentation in a different jurisdiction. (Advance Care Planning Australia is a national organisation funded by the Department of Health.)

Find the forms and process used in at least two other jurisdictions, and notice how the legislative arrangement in each jurisdiction impacts on the documentation process that is advised.

You may like to revisit the wishes exercise in Chapter 5 'Respect for a patient's journey' as you think further about what expressing wishes or values means for a patient.

Victoria, an instance of a state jurisdiction which has specific legislation, explicitly recognises advance care directives in the *Medical Treatment Planning Decisions Act 2016* (Vic). Under that legislation, which took effect on 12 March 2018, advance care directives have greater practical instructional force for circumstances and treatment preferences outlined by the person who made the directive. Directives can be expressed either as binding instructions, preferences, or values, as at section12. At section 6, the types of directives are defined as follows:

6 Types of directives

(1) For the purposes of this Act, an *instructional directive*—

    (a) is an express statement in an advance care directive of a person's medical treatment decision; and

    (b) takes effect as if the person who gave it has consented to, or refused the commencement or continuation of, medical treatment, as the case may be.

Examples

A statement that a person consents to a heart bypass operation in specified circumstances.

A statement that a person refuses cardiopulmonary resuscitation.

(2) For the purposes of this Act, a *values directive* is a statement in an advance care directive of a person's preferences and values as the basis on which the person would like any medical treatment decisions to be made on behalf of the person, including, but not limited to, a statement of medical treatment outcomes that the person regards as acceptable.

Examples

The following statements—

"If I am unable to recognise my family and friends, and cannot communicate, I do not want any medical treatment to prolong my life."

"If a time comes when I cannot make decisions about my medical treatment, I would like to receive any life prolonging medical treatments that are beneficial. This includes receiving a medical research procedure to see if the procedure has any benefit for me."

(3) For the purposes of subsections (1) and (2), an instructional directive or a values directive—

    (a) may be given in relation to—

        (i) medical treatment or a medical research procedure to be provided in a particular instance; or

        (ii) a course of medical treatment or medical research procedures to be provided over a period of time; and

    (b) may be given about—

        (i) one or more particular forms of medical treatment or medical research procedures; or

        (ii) generally about all medical treatment or medical research procedures; and

    (c) may be given so as to apply—

        (i) in all circumstances; or

        (ii) only in specified circumstances; or

        (iii) in all circumstances except in specified circumstances.

Note
See section 12.

(Medical Treatment Planning Decisions Act 2016 (Vic)]

When patients suffer a cardiac event, it is sometimes unexpected. However, it is mostly an expected part of the decline of an elderly or seriously ill patient, and marks the natural end of their last phase of life. Nevertheless, a choice must often be made about whether or not to resuscitate a patient. Many commentators have lamented that cardiopulmonary resuscitation (CPR) was being increasingly used in all hospital deaths—as people are not being allowed to die. Intervention could then be seen as prolonging suffering and doing harm in what often seem to be inevitable deaths. Legislation was thought to be needed to excuse health care workers from the obligation to resuscitate patients who are classified as 'Do Not Resuscitate' (DNR) (Lederberg, 1997). So, where a patient had rapidly diminishing lung or heart functions, care and comfort could be given instead of CPR (or other resuscitation techniques). Being ready to provide some care is ethically important. The imminent death of a patient does not excuse health care workers from offering help—but the goal of this help may not be saving life.

Advance care planning is an integrated regulatory tool that has been devised with assistance from law, ethics and policy to help with such complex decisions.

A health care professional's responsibility in informed decision making

Informed decision making and informed consent is really a process, not a discrete event. It is a process of information exchange and autonomous or facilitated decision making. The professional and health service remains responsible for having ensured that an informed decision has been made. A record or note of this must be kept.

A consent form documents:

- the patient's condition
- the proposed or required treatment
- the general nature and effect of the treatment
- the significant risks or side effects of the treatment
- reasonable alternatives and their risks
- the views of the patient
- how much the patient understands about the treatment
- whether the patient is able to consent.

There may be only a small space for writing these things down on the form. It is a shorthand document that points to a larger process. The health departments in each jurisdiction routinely provide an explanation of health care professionals' responsibilities in gaining patient consent, as well as a sample consent form. (For instance, New South Wales Ministry of Health, 2017b, New South Wales Ministry of Health, PD2005-406, Consent Form at 9.123.)

Health services can recommend that some types of decisions be obtained in writing, particularly if there is significant risk to the patient from a proposed process, such as:

- it requires sedation or anaesthesia
- there are known complications or significant risks
- the individual patient presents with a risk profile for the procedure or treatment
- there is some doubt about a patient's capacity to consent
- the type of health care offered is controversial (State of Queensland, Queensland Health, 2017, p. 10).

For all procedures—and even if written consent such as a signed consent form is not required—documentation can be made so that the notes reflect the discussion process. Queensland Health states:

> In the absence of a Queensland Health consent form, the details of the conversation between the patient and health practitioner is considered to be a part of the care given to the patient and as such can be recorded in the patient's clinical record.
>
> (State of Queensland, Queensland Health, 2017, p. 16)

The responsibility for information disclosure falls largely to the health care worker because, as the 'expert', the health care worker knows how to describe the process, and knows its risks and benefits (and their likelihood), as they are known to the profession. These risks should be communicated to the client so that a decision can be made about whether to go ahead with the treatment or management plan.

However, not all of the responsibility for information disclosure falls to the health care worker. Some information about the client's values, preferences or wishes also needs to be voiced, as this may make a difference to the type or range of treatment offered. Ideally, this information should be voiced by the client.

Informed decision-making guidelines and regulations protect and promote client autonomy. Informed consent has only been given if clients have given permission for examinations or procedures with the optimal amount of information available to them. It is a health care quality issue that is being given increasing attention in health care contexts and in the training of health practitioners and health care workers.

Of course, a balance needs to be struck between informing a client and overwhelming them. If there is too much information, the client may not understand or attend to any more details on the proposed procedure or treatment processes.

The challenge is to be able to communicate essential information, and provide opportunities for requests for further information, and ensure that each client understands and remembers crucial pieces of information so that their decisions are informed. If a minor risk or effects of small likelihood do not concern them in the slightest, then listening to all of the effects may be more of a burden than a help in their informed decision.

On the other hand, if the ethical significance of a process is important to them, or involves a question of religious significance to them, then much more information may be needed, and they may wish to also consult with others before reaching a decision. The ethical consequences, the social and personal significance, and the relevance of information are increasingly part of routine information disclosure in health care work.

The key point is that you should try to look through the everyday nature of what you are doing when you provide a service. To people who are receiving that service for the first time, it is not 'everyday'. You need to take the time to consider what it is that you do, in an everyday sense, and then try to explain it to others and discuss what it means for them. After all, it is in the everyday that health professionals work.

For you, as health care workers, a 'simple' operation is as straightforward as buying a sandwich or having a haircut. The challenge you face is to unpack the process and the things you take for granted about it. The process, risks and benefits must be documented in minute detail so that they can be communicated and discussed with the health client. This facilitates an informed consideration of health care choices.

Summary

In this chapter, you have spent time exploring the development, enhancement and respect for all patients' decision-making capabilities. You will have gained a working understanding that this is one way that autonomy is upheld in everyday health care practice. By looking at decision making as a whole of life theme, you have been encouraged to consider how autonomy could be enhanced in all situations and for all patients, no matter their age or circumstance. Guardianship principles have been explored, and special attention has been given to applying the principles of respect for engagement and participation in decision making in disability and aged care. You have been able to consider the principles derived from law, ethics and regulation in advance care directives.

STUDY QUESTIONS

1   Make yourself some flash cards for a memory test of concepts and definitions. Write each word about capacity and decision making on one side of a card, and then write the matching definition on the other. Check through previous chapters for any additional words you should make a card for. You can either test yourself by turning a card over to reveal the answer, or work in pairs by holding a card up for a friend to suggest the definition.

2   International human rights conventions are reflected in practical legal, regulatory and ethics standards for capacity and decision making. Discuss in 500 words.

SAMPLE ESSAY QUESTION

1   Law, ethics and regulation are applied in a comprehensive way when treatment and care decisions are made to protect the client's part in that decision-making process, in a way that is consistent with their stage of development and capacity.
    Illustrate this proposition, with reference to examples drawn from law, ethics and regulation.

REFERENCES

Australian Commission on Safety and Quality in Health Care [ACSQH]. (2018). *Australian Charter of Healthcare Rights*. Retrieved from www.safetyandquality.gov.au

Australian Government, Department of Health. (2017). Palliative Care: Advance care planning. Canberra: Department of Helth. Retrieved from www.health.gov.au

Australian Government, Royal Commission into Institutional Responses to Child Sexual Abuse. (2017). Final Report—recommendations. Retrieved from www.childabuseroyalcommission.gov.au

Australian Health Practitioner Regulation Agency [AHPRA]. (2016). Case 2016.0778, decision dated 30/12/16, *Panel decisions*. Medical, Qld. Retrieved from www.ahpra.gov.au

Australian Health Practitioner Regulation Agency [AHPRA]. (2017). Case 2017.0789, decision dated 29/3/17. *Panel decisions*. Medical, Tasmania. Retrieved from www.ahpra.gov.au

Australian Institute of Interpreters and Translators [AUSIT]. (2012). *AUSIT code of ethics and code of conduct*. Retrieved from www.ausit.org

Australian Law Reform Commission [ALRC]. (2013). *Equality, capacity and disability in Commonwealth laws*. IP44. Retrieved from www.alrc.gov.au

Beauchamp, T.L., & Childress, J.F. (2001). *Principles of biomedical ethics* (5th edn). New York: Oxford University Press.

Berglund, C., & Devereux, J. (2000). Consent to medical treatment: Children making medical decisions for others. *Australian Journal of Forensic Sciences*, 32, 25–36.

Berryman, J. (1978). Discussing the ethics of research on young children. In J. van Eys (Ed.), *Research on children: Medical imperatives, ethical quandaries, and legal constraints*. Baltimore: University Park Press.

Coalition of Australian Governments, COAG Health Council. (2011). *National Framework for advance care directives*. Australian Health Ministers' Advisory Council. Retrieved from http://coaghealthcouncil.gov.au

Department of Health Western Australia. (2011). *Consent to Treatment Policy for the Western Australian Health System* (3rd edn). Perth: WA Department of Health.

Devereux, J. (2002). *Medical law* (2nd edn). Sydney: Cavendish.

Dickenson, D.L. (2001). Consent in children. In M. Parker & D. Dickenson, *The Cambridge medical ethics workbook: case studies commentaries and activities* (pp. 209–13). Cambridge: Cambridge University Press.

Dworkin, G. (1987). Law and medical experimentation of embryos, children and others with limited capacity. *Monash University Law Review*, *13*, 189–206.

Finucane, P., Myser, C., & Ticehurst, S. (1993). 'Is she fit to sign, doctor?': Practical ethical issues in assessing the competence of elderly patients. *Medical Journal of Australia*, *159*, 400–3.

Forrester, K., & Griffiths, D. (2001). *Essentials of law for health professionals*. Sydney: Harcourt.

Foster, P. (1999, 17 July). Girl, 15, forced to have new heart. *Sydney Morning Herald*, 19.

Gallagher, A. (2011). Ethical issues in patient restraint. *Nursing Times*, *107*(9), 18–20.

Gietzelt, D., & Jones, G. (2002). What language? In C. Berglund & D. Saltman (Eds), *Communication for health care*. Melbourne: Oxford University Press.

Government of Western Australia, Department of Health WA. (2016). *Health consent to treatment policy*. Perth: Department of Health. Retrieved from www.health.wa.gov.au

Grisso, T., & Vierling, L. (1978). Minors' consent to treatment: A developmental perspective. *Professional Psychology*, *9*, 412–27.

Harrison, C., & Laxer, R.M. (2000). A bioethics program in pediatric rheumatology. *The Journal of Rheumatology*, *27*(7), 1780–2.

Jonsen, A.R., Siegler, M., & Winslade, W.J. (1998). *Clinical ethics: A practical approach to ethical decisions in clinical medicine* (4th edn). New York: McGraw Hill.

Lederberg, M.S. (1997). The psychological repercussions of New York State's do-not-resuscitate law. In A. Surbone & M. Zwitter, Communication with the cancer patient: Information and truth (pp. 223–36). *Annals of the New York Academy of Sciences*, *809*.

Medical Board of Australia. (2014). *Good medical practice: A code of conduct for doctors in Australia*, March. Retrieved from http://medicalboard.gov.au

Mill, J.S. (1975). On liberty. In *Three Essays* (pp. 92–114). London: Oxford University Press.

Museen der Stadt Nürnberg. (2013). *Memorium Nuremberg Trials, Nürnberger Prozesse*. Retrieved from www.museen.nuernberg.de

National Health and Medical Research Council [NHMRC]. (2004a). *General guidelines for medical practitioners on providing information to patients*. Retrieved from www.nhmrc.gov.au

National Health and Medical Research Council [NHMRC]. (2004b). *Communicating with patients: Advice for medical practitioners*. Retrieved from www.nhmrc.gov.au

New South Wales Government, Ministry of Health. (2005). *Patient information and consent to medical treatment*. PD2005_406. Retrieved from www.health.nsw.gov.au

New South Wales Government, Ministry of Health. (2006). *Interpreters—Standard procedures for working with health care interpreters*. PD2006_053, 2006. Retrieved from www.health.nsw.gov.au

New South Wales Government, Ministry of Health. (2017a). *Multicultural health*. Retrieved from www.health.nsw.gov.au

New South Wales Government, Ministry of Health. (2017b). Health Records and Information, Chapter 9. In *Patient matters: Manual for area health services and public hospitals*. Retrieved from www.health.nsw.gov.au

New South Wales Parliament. Legislative Council. (2017). General Purpose Standing Committee No. 2, *Report no. 46*. Sydney.

Nicholson, R.H. (1986). *Medical research with children: Ethics, law, and practice*. Oxford: Oxford University Press.

Nursing and Midwifery Board of Australia. (2017, 19 May). *Nurse disqualified for 12 months for professional misconduct*. State Administrative Tribunal File VR: 54/2016. Retrieved from www.nursingmidwiferyboard.gov.au

O'Neill, N., & Peisah, C. (2011). *Capacity and the law* (2nd edn). Sydney University Law Book 2. Sydney: Sydney University. Retrieved from www.austlii.edu.au

Pearce, D.C., & Geddes, R.S. (2014). *Statutory interpretation in Australia* (8th edn). Australia: Lexis Nexis.

Shawndra, S. (2007). State intervention in the family: Child protective proceedings and termination of parental rights. *Columbia Journal of Law and Social Problems*, *40*(4), 485–93.

State of Queensland, Queensland Health. (2017). *Guide to informed decision-making in health care*. Brisbane: Patient Safety and Quality Improvement Service. Retrieved from www.health.qld.gov.au

Stecher, J. (2011). Ethics at the end of life in transplant recipients. *Progress in transplantation*, *21*(1), 83–7.

United Nations. (1966). *International Covenant on Civil and Political Rights*. Entry into force 23 March 1976. New York: United Nations. Retrieved from www.ohchr.org

United Nations. (1989). *The United Nations Convention on the Rights of the Child*. Adopted by the General Assembly of the United Nations on 20 November 1989. Geneva: United Nations. Retrieved from www.ohchr.org

United Nations General Assembly. (2006). *Convention on the Rights of Persons with Disabilities and its Optional Protocol*. Annexed to resolution 61/106. Adopted by consensus 13 December 2006. Ratified 2008. Retrieved from un.org

Victorian Government, Ministerial Advisory Panel on Voluntary Assisted Dying. (2017). *Final report*. Melbourne: Victorian Government. Retrieved from www.health.vic.gov.au

Weeramantry, C.G., & Giantomasso, D.F. (1983). *Consent to the medical treatment of minors and intellectually handicapped persons*. Melbourne: Faculty of Law, Monash University.

Whitney, S.N., Ethier, A.M., Frugé, E., Berg, S., McCullough, L.B., & Hockenberry, M. (2006). Decision-making in pediatric oncology: Who should take the lead? The decisional priority in pediatric oncology model. *Journal of Clinical Oncology*, *24*(1), 160–5.

LEGISLATION

Children and Young Persons (Care and Protection) Act 1998 (NSW)

Consent to Medical Treatment and Palliative Care Act 1995 (SA)

Medical Treatment Planning Decisions Act 2016 (Vic)

CASES

ACT v Gillan; Gillan v ACT [2018] ACTSC 223.

Gillick v West Norfolk AHA (1986) AC 112.

Hewer v Bryant [1970] 2 QB 357.

KL v Farnsworth [2002] NSWSC 382.

R v M, Unreported, Royal Courts of Justice, Family Division, United Kingdom, 15 July 1999.

US v Karl Brandt Nuremberg Code. In the *Trials of War Criminals before the Nuremberg Military Tribunals under Control Council Law*, 1949, no. 10, vol. 2, Washington DC: US Government Printing Office.

Wallace v Kam [2013] HCA 19.

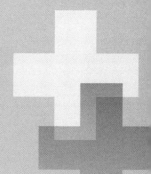

CHAPTER 9

Timeless quandaries at the beginning and end of life

LEARNING OBJECTIVES

- To explore dramatic issues at the beginning of life.
- To consider the contribution of classic philosophy to contemporary discussions.
- To consider evolving legal positions on status and interests in human tissue.
- To appreciate the practical limitations for clients and health professionals in different jurisdictions.
- To recognise the opportunity for renewed discussion when laws and guidelines are suggested or changed.

KEY TERMS

person   potentiality

personhood

CASE EXAMPLE

Snippets of information

From these notices, brainstorm as many potentially significant issues as you can that remind you of classic beginning of life quandaries.

Notice: 10/2/44: Mr and Mrs Frank Mallory are delighted to announce the birth of their first child, Judith Maree, born 1 January 1944, 5lb 3oz. Mother and baby now well. Thanks to the doctors and nurses in the special care nursery at St Luke's Hospital.

Notice: 17/5/65: Frank and Jean Mallory are delighted to announce the engagement of their only child Judith Maree to Martin Christopher Francis, the third son of Beverley Francis and John Francis (deceased). Both families wish the happy couple well in their future together.

Notice: 10/10/65: Martin and Judith Francis are delighted to announce the birth of their first child, Crystal Jennifer, born 4 October 1965, 7lb 4 oz. Mother and daughter well.

Notice: 15/9/77: Judith and Martin are delighted to announce the much awaited birth of their second child, Jimmy Christopher Francis, born 13 September 1977. Many thanks to the wonderful staff at the New Beginnings IVF program, and the team at the Royal Hospital.

Reproduction and beginning of life

Dramatic issues at the beginning of life highlight timeless quandaries and classic philosophical positions. The classic debates are reflected in contemporary commentary. In this chapter you will see how ethical professional choices that can be made vary between countries, given the limitations provided by the guidelines and laws of each jurisdiction. That doesn't mean that the ethics debate isn't raging in every country. Rather, it means that what can and can't be carried out currently is different in each country, and that a window for full ethics debate is opened when changes to these guidelines or laws are suggested. Some of the contemporary ethics debates are explained in this chapter, as well as the legal, regulatory and ethics forums in which they are held. We will make a start by looking through a 'legal lens' at the debate about morally significant elements of life.

At what point do we give life moral and ethical significance? Human beings essentially start as clusters of cells and, before that, as separate yet potentially significant elements of human life (single cells). The moral and ethical significance of life has been debated since the beginning of early philosophical thought.

person
Live human being, or live human being in development, with essential and recognised qualities of intrinsic capacity or function.

The thirteenth-century philosopher St Thomas Aquinas spent considerable time studying the Greek philosopher Aristotle, who had debated form and matter. Aquinas's position was that the human soul was integral to the **person**. He believed that the soul determined what made an individual a distinct human being, different from all others (Collinson, 1987, p. 34).

Modern philosophers continue the tradition of that debate. There is debate among some philosophers over whether life itself is an absolute good—the view that life is itself an absolute good can encompass the notion that even the mere potential for life is significant—or whether there is a particular point in development at which time human life takes on a moral significance (Noonan, 1973).

More controversially, other philosophers argue that the right to life depends on the desire for life (Tooley, 1973). This may mean that only beings that are conscious, self-conscious and desiring have a right not to be killed. Such philosophers even suggest that—depending on when this consciousness begins and whether memory is associated with it—all people, at least up to the age of four, are without a moral right to life, as are those who, by virtue of some degeneration, lose consciousness or their capacity to be desiring beings. Other philosophers have suggested that the indicators of the moral significance of life are brain development and an interest in human life (Lockwood, 1985).

Solving this ethical problem is crucial in relation to processes that intervene in natural human reproduction. In-vitro fertilisation (IVF) is one such process. It involves the external fertilisation of cells, and then implantation of the cellswhich are then implanted into the uterus. In order to refine this process, research was needed on human ova and sperm. The risk of damaging cells, and of 'wasting' cells, was ever present. Debate was needed on the moral value of mature male or female reproductive cells on their own—sperm and eggs, known as *gametes*—with potential to fuse with each other to form a new organism—fertilised eggs, known as *zygotes*. Debate was also needed on the moral value of zygotes and of early embryos. Dame Mary Warnock, who chaired the British Government's Committee of Inquiry into Human Fertilisation and Embryology, has written a seminal article on this early debate, which occurred in the mid to late 1980s, at the time when the United Kingdom was pioneering IVF (Warnock, 1987). The Warnock committee reached a compromise on the issue of when **personhood**, and therefore moral significance, can be said to come into being, settling on 14 days after fertilisation. You might have a different view of when to begin attaching moral significance to life.

personhood
Quality of being a person.

Dame Warnock's book *Making Babies* is an excellent essay-style summary of the history of reproductive technology and the choices allowed within that technology. Warnock argues that it is a privilege, rather than a right, to have access to as many opportunities as science now affords us in making babies (Warnock, 2002).

Heated debates have occurred about the rapid pace and ultimate worth of modern technological reproduction, also with a gender politics perspective Le Moncheck, 1996). Feminist ethics emerged as a forceful tool of analysis in examining what society is offering women in terms of medically assisted reproduction (see, for instance, Dickenson, 2017).

In the early days of IVF, ethics classes discussed issues such as the creation and storage of embryos, as well as their disposal. Rules to 'flush' unused embryos at the end of five years prompted questions about why so many embryos were being created, and the position of the embryos as potential children if their potential parents changed their minds about their creation. For example, couples who:

- plan to have a child but then decide otherwise
- fail to establish successful pregnancy and give up
- separate, and now have different plans for the embryos.

Consider the dilemma in the following Reflection.

REFLECTION: CHOICES AND LIMBO

In 1992 in the USA, a court case was heard to decide if a divorced woman could use cryopreserved embryos that she and her former husband had created and lodged with a clinic. Her former husband (the potential father) did not want this to happen.

One newspaper headline at the time read 'Frozen Embryos in Legal Limbo' (*New York Times*, 1992). The case prompted debate on right to procreation, and the right to avoid procreation. The right to life of the embryos was not established, as the embryos—essentially a cluster of cells—were classified as having a legal status somewhere between property and persons. The decision over whether or not they should develop to their full potential was thought to lie with the donors. This Tennessee case applied best interests principles and ordered the discarding of the embryos (*Davis v Davis* (1992)).

1   Do you agree with this position?

2   If the donors disagree, should another 'guardian' make a decision on behalf of the cluster of cells?

3   Does the fertilisation make a difference to your reaction to the significance of the stored cells?

Consider the development of law that is evident in a subsequent case. In this case, the parties used the term 'pre-embryo' to refer to a fertilised egg prior to implantation. After five months of dating, a man and a woman created eight cryopreserved pre-embryos for possible future use, because the woman was diagnosed with non-Hodgkin's lymphoma. She had been advised that the chemotherapy she needed was likely to make her infertile. Both attended and signed the consent forms. They broke up two months later. Years later, the sperm donor sought to exercise his choice in when and if the pre-embryos were implanted, and worried about them being implanted if he was not to be involved as a father. The preliminary hearings concentrated on contract law—whether or not a contract had been signed. If no contract had been signed, then the matter would be decided on the balancing of interests in the different courses of action.

The comprehensive article in the *New Yorker* at the time of the hearings includes comment on the legal discussions in the hearings (Schwarz, 2015). The parties happened to both be working in health care: the male as a nurse, the female as a doctor. The appeal court granted custody of the embryos to the woman, based on it being her only opportunity to have a child with her own eggs, so outweighing the man's interests in not having the embryos used. The dissenting judge disagreed, on the basis that there was no oral enforceable contract in place.

Since then, contracts such as Embryonic Disposition Agreements have commonly been used in the USA, as an indication of private 'contractual' agreements to guide future decisions in relation to the embryos, and so disputes could be tested in the courts under contract law (Leventis Lourgos & Miller Rubin, 2015). The case under discussion *Szafranski v Dunston*

(2015) also demonstrates that when judges disagree, they write dissenting judgments, but the majority judgment forms the decision for the parties.

INTEGRATED LEARNING AND PRACTICE

Don't judges just decide what is fair using their own wisdom?

Judges use their wisdom to apply the society's standards to the circumstances of the case. The law provides the framework for the possible logic that can be applied by the judges in considering the claims made by parties—partly by statute and partly by common law or case precedent.

Ethics can inform the arguments, such as when best interests reasoning is applied, as a fair consideration in the absence of clear contractual agreements.

The court processes and rules provide guidance to all parties in bringing their issues before a court to resolve. The possibility of appeal is available to both parties, so that a matter is reconsidered and the process is conducted fairly.

Beginning with legal status

When ownership or interest is considered in legal forums, the fundamental assumption in law has been that human tissue belongs to no one, and is 'res nullius'. There is some acknowledgment that in some circumstances—such as disputes over failure to store tissue with reasonable care—damage in the loss of reproductive tissue can be dealt with in ways that make it very similar to property. In *Yearworth and others v North Bristol NHS Trust* (2009), reproductive material stored during cancer treatment was the subject of dispute. Five men and the estate of a sixth man successfully claimed that negligent damage could be considered, as their samples were similar enough to property to be considered in the tort law of negligence, with the harm including their psychiatric injury or mental distress when the sperm they owned had not been properly stored (*Yearworth and others v North Bristol NHS Trust* (2009), cited in Dickenson, 2017, p. 2). Other aspects of the body may also be protected given accepted ways of demonstrating respect.

In UK legislation such as the *Human Tissue Act 1961* (UK), a balance is sought between the possible use of the body after death—such as the ability of medical practitioners and institutions to remove tissue for examination or further research—and traditions of respecting the wish of relatives, and leaving a body in peace, so as to uphold dignity and respect, particularly under some religious beliefs. The Royal Liverpool Children's Inquiry was critical of the removal of hearts and other organs and tissue from the bodies of children who had died at the Alder Hey Children's Hospital. The organs and tissue were removed after post-mortem examination—and sometimes without post-mortem reports being completed—and stored in a tissue library for possible further histological examination, or for use in medical education and research, for many years, all without the consent of the families (House of Commons, 2011, p. 359). This led to the enactment of the *Human Tissue Act 2004* (UK).

From an ethical perspective, the dead can still be thought of as being part of a cultural and moral community—meaning that they might not have rights, but they may have interests, as a person still has significance in the community and has not entirely ceased to be a member (Brecher, 2002, p. 113, as cited in Sperling, 2008, p. 83).

The labour expended on tissue may be protected, as held in the classic Australian case *Doodeward v Spence* [1908] and the English case *R v Kelly* (1998). The product of preservation—that is, embalming—is owned, but this stems from the work of embalming in preserving the body rather than the body and tissue itself (*Doodeward v Spence* [1908]). In *R v Kelly* (1998), in a case of an alleged theft of tissue from an anatomy school, whether there was a 'theft' depended on the classification of the tissue, given the tissue had been worked on.

It has been suggested that this concept has its foundations in the philosopher John Locke's writings, which shows the extensive influence of the early philosophers on the way we deal with complex issues in our society. Locke argued that property is derived from nature, and is transformed into property if we claim some interest in it by virtue of our work on it, the labour being unquestionably the property of man (Locke, 1946, p. 15).

From a legal and feminist perspective, Donna Dickenson has noted that so far, the law has not yet considered the labour perspective for the woman's labour in the extraction of eggs, which is arguably far greater than a man's in the collection of sperm (Dickenson 2017, p. 3).

Despite the basic assumption that human tissue in itself is not property, the controversy surrounding that assumption in legal contests is noted, and this means that the controversy in the storage of biological materials, tissues and specimens in 'biobanks' and then their use, is recognised. Academic discussion of biobanking highlights that if, hypothetically, human tissue could be treated as property, then the law of gifts in the equity law field may be helpful in considering the tissue that is used (Stewart et al., 2014), so the decision makers could draw on a field of law other than contract law to help solve difficult situations.

In some jurisdictions it is possible to retrieve sperm from a recently deceased partner, and then seek to use the sperm, provided the partner is thought to have given implied consent (Conway, 2016, p. 173). Sometimes the retrieval is possible in one jurisdiction (such as England), but the use of it is only permissible by travelling to another jurisdiction (such as some northern European states), given the regulations on how to interpret and give effect to the implied consent for use.

REFLECTION: TRAGEDY AND FURTHER CHOICES

An interesting yet tragic combination of ethics issues has been debated in various countries when married men die from sudden illness or traumatic injury, and their wives have sought to obtain semen from them before they die so that they can store the semen in an IVF facility and use the semen to conceive a child at a later date.

See if you can list the ethics issues raised by the following scenario.

In 1995, Mary's husband became suddenly ill from meningitis, and died aged 30 years. Mary said they planned to have children, and asked doctors to extract and store his semen, which they did. Later, Mary was denied permission to use the semen in the UK but subsequently won a High Court case to take the semen to Europe and use it there, in an agreeable IVF facility. There, she conceived a first child in 1998, and a second, four years later, in 2002. Initially, the birth certificate did not list a father's name. This scenario is based on a media article by Schlink (2002): 'New baby from dead husband'. You might be able to find other contemporary examples.

Think about choices and how they are made and expressed, and the process of reproductive assistance involved.

In some jurisdictions, use of sperm posthumously has only been held to be possible if there is implied consent, and when sperm has been retrieved prior to death. A separate court order is needed for each step of retrieval of sperm, and for use of the sperm. Australian federal government guidelines require clearly expressed and witnessed consent—but it does not need to be written consent. In the revised *Ethical Guidelines on the Use of Assisted Reproductive Technology in Clinical Practice and Research* (2017), considering options for use—including posthumous use—is part of the consent process before gametes are collected or embryos are created.

Similar consent applies to the storage of gametes; clinics are required to:

- ensure the supported decision-making process was in place
- consider what consent was indicated if one person was unable to provide further instructions (Australian Government, National Health and Medical Research Council, 2017).

However, different laws in states and territories must also be applied, so the practices set out in the guidelines apply unless prohibited by law.

In one case before Justice Hulme of the New South Wales Supreme Court, a woman won the right to take possession of her dead husband's sperm, which was cryopreserved at an IVF laboratory, having claimed it was incidental to her rights as an administrator of the deceased's estate. The couple had not yet signed the fertility treatment consent forms. A duty judge had initially considered that the circumstances were favourable under the provisions of the *Human Tissue Act 1983* (NSW), and ordered that sperm could be extracted after Mr Edwards had been fatally injured in a workplace accident—but also that it could not be released without further court order.

The Supreme Court then considered the release of the sperm as a succession issue of possession. The sperm had been lawfully removed under the duty judge's orders, and skill was applied to it to prepare and store it. Justice Hulme found the sperm was capable of being property. The work had been carried out on behalf of Ms Edwards, so the facility did not have sole interest in it. Considering possession issues alone, rather than use, the court found the interest in the 'property' was in the widow's partly because no one else in the world was claiming an interest in it. The sperm could not be used in New South Wales as the *Assisted Reproductive Technology Act 2007* (NSW) required written consent from the provider for its specified use. It was noted that Ms Edwards would likely seek assisted reproductive treatment in another state, and that if no specific legislation existed then current Federal Guidelines applied. (Jocelyn Edwards: re the estate of the late Mark Edwards [2011], at paragraphs 13, 20, 82, 88, 91, 110–15).

Posthumous sperm retrieval is ethically complex. In one case, a clinical ethics consultant recommended against sperm retrieval from a man who had been depressed after a separation three months earlier, and was brought to emergency suffering a self-inflicted gunshot wound. He was an only child, and his parents requested sperm retrieval so they might possibly have a grandchild. In another case, the ethics consultant recommended sperm retrieval for a previously healthy man who deteriorated rapidly with pneumonia and suffered multiple organ failure. He and his wife had been trying to have children for two years, and had seen fertility consultants. Even though his views on his wife possibly raising children as a sole parent had not been discussed, he had talked about his wish to have children and continue his family's name. All of the health care team believed that his wife's request to continue to try to have children was partly based on his expressed wishes, amounting to implied consent (Orr & Siegler, 2002).

REFLECTION POINT

Reasoned decisions

Thinking further about consent and implied consent and wishes, read the full paper by Orr and Siegler (2002): Is posthumous semen retrieval ethically permissible? *Journal of Medical Ethics*, *28*(5), 299–303, which you can find at <http://jme.bmj.com>.

See if you can analyse the process of ethical reasoning that was followed by clinical ethics consultants. Try to summarise the considerations in a way that helps explain the ethics reasoning framework you think was used. You might like to look back at Chapter 4 before trying this exercise.

In a Supreme Court case heard in Queensland in June 2018, a woman was granted permission to use the stored sperm of her partner who had died suddenly. His sperm had been retrieved after his death (*Re Cresswell* [2018]). This landmark case contains a detailed summary and application of the principles from previous legal cases, providing a clear application of the principle of precedent as well.

The judgment sets out key issues, such as:

- authority to remove the sperm (given in the specific legislation and jurisdiction)
- work done on the sperm so as to make it 'property'
- whether more than one party had made a claim for possession and use of the sperm.

The family of the deceased man supported the application that was made by his partner.

INTEGRATED LEARNING AND PRACTICE

Why not just let the law decide the complex issues in reproductive rights?

The acceptable standards are so difficult to agree on, which shows us that reproductive rights is an unresolved contemporary issue that needs the combined intellectual force of many fields in order to negotiate ways forward in each community setting: science, medicine, law, social sciences, philosophy, ethics, public policy and government. There is not necessarily a right answer, but discussion is part of working towards an acceptable solution. A comprehensive and inclusive public policy approach is relied on to shape and inform the ongoing debate. This is a complex area in a legal, ethical and regulatory sense, so all forms of analysis essential to reasoning and setting standards are needed.

There are arguably aspects of property in the way we deal with human tissue—a person's expressed wish (or a relative's wish) is considered, before transferring the use of human tissue after death—for instance, in organ donation. While it may not be a possession, we uphold an interest to 'exclude' others without our permission, a concept arguably closely aligned with the ethics principle of autonomy (self-rule). As yet, our 'rights' in our own tissue remains a collection of interests that may be elevated to institutional rights by the society we live in. You might like to read ahead to the organ donation discussion in Chapter 10.

First delivery

PRACTICE EXAMPLE

Narelle Biedermann

Narelle has been a Registered Nurse for 25 years and has worked predominantly for the Australian Defence Force as both a uniformed Nursing Officer and civilian Registered Nurse.

Mike is a medical student who has just delivered his first baby as part of his obstetrics/gynaecology rotation. The first baby is a highlight for any medical student, so Mike was rather excited about the experience and felt honoured to have been part of it. He posts a photo of him holding the newborn with the caption 'Meet Baby Jonah Harrison Markson, my first delivery!' on Instagram and Twitter, and states that he had the permission of the parents to share this joyous occasion with all of his Twitter followers.

1   Assume Mike didn't gain permission. Outline all the ways in which he breached confidentiality.

2   Because Mike said he got permission from the parents of the newborn, could he still be seen as breaching confidentiality?

(Adapted from Birks, M., Davis, J., Chapman, Y. (2015). Professional and Therapeutic Communication. Melbourne: Oxford University Press, 209)

Frontiers of science and ethical dilemmas

IVF and related technologies have led to a myriad of ethics dilemmas because of the availability of viable and reproducible human cells. Embryonic stem cell research has captured the world's attention, as it involves complex and provocative ethics issues. Stem cells can develop into any type of cell. They are embryonic, not only in coming from an embryo, but also in terms of their undifferentiated form. The technology now exists to harvest embryonic stem cells from embryos, then implant them into other tissues to research their development into all manner of human cells. The proposition is that the cell regeneration could aid in the management of diabetes, Alzheimer's and Parkinson's conditions—and possibly aid with spinal cord injuries through generating fresh fully functioning cells for affected organs and tissues.

However, a consequence of stem cell retrieval is that the embryo would not survive. So, the debate has been about the intentional production of embryonic material, and about the use of those created for another purpose. The concepts of personhood are central to the debate. If you acknowledge the 'personhood' of an early cluster of cells, then a person's interests and rights would be expected to be respected; the potential for developing into a person can be treated as equivalent to attaining personhood. Even if rudimentary rights are afforded, the intentional cell creation and destruction would then be objectionable.

Before embryonic tissue can be used for research, there is a consent process that often involves couples who have had IVF therapy. It is these people who have a reason to seek reproductive assistance, and therefore it is their embryos that have been created and stored, and are most readily available for such requests. In this context, the embryo or embryonic tissue is regarded as a part of the fertility patient—that is, the potential mother and father—and their consent is needed before the embryonic tissue can be used for other than treatment purposes. You will remember a detailed discussion on informed decision making in Chapter 8 'Lifelong practice in decision making' and a discussion of consent to participation in research in Chapter 7 'The limits of care', and you will also remember that the rigour of decision making is open to ethical scrutiny.

There is some research on that process of consent to suggest that couples that have agreed to donate surplus IVF embryos for research were generally concerned later about the social status of embryos that had not been selected to become a baby. In terms of the research request, they tended to view the donated embryonic tissue as an 'entity' rather than as a person or potential child. Their consent had been given at the start of the IVF treatment cycle, when they were mainly preoccupied with their treatment rather than the research request—and their main focus was on being able to have a baby. They didn't subsequently know if any of their embryos had actually been used in research. A number of interviewees were ambivalent, when 'good', 'viable' embryos had become 'spare' and neither implanted nor frozen for later use. Then, after the embryos became 'surplus' to the couple's own treatment needs, the prospect of them having been used for research generated strong emotions (Haimes & Taylor, 2009).

It remains a sensitive issue, and jurisdictions differ on how permissible research is decided and conducted. Regulations are in place so that only transparent and accountable and approved processes are conducted. In Australia, research can only be undertaken with a licence from the NHMRC Embryo Research Licensing Committee, with licences that are currently issued listed for public viewing on the website, along with the regulations that apply (NHMRC, 2018).

We can learn from history, in terms of the debates that have taken place and the decisions that have been made, given the reasoning that was applied in a particular historical context. Much of the debate so far has been on the nature of the cell and the embryo, and their ethical significance.

In the USA in late 2001, there was extensive media coverage of the presidential decision on stem cell research, and the ethics and religious advice on the issue. President Bush decided on a compromise: to allow federal funding for research on embryonic stem cell lines already created out of 'spare' embryos no longer planned to be used for IVF, but not to allow further stem cell lines to be intentionally produced for that purpose (Hall, 2001). It was a compromise that did not satisfy those objecting on religious grounds against any use of human life for other ends, nor did it satisfy the scientists and researchers seeking full research flexibility. The Catholic Church always opposed IVF, as it increased the risk of disrespect for each individual life **potentiality**.

potentiality
Capacity to develop in a certain way, given the opportunity and suitable development options.

Subsequently, the President's Council on Bioethics issued a white paper on alternative ways of sourcing embryonic stem cells—specifically human pluripotent cells, a type of self-replicating cell—without the intended production, use and destruction of such cells. The suggested options included:

- deriving cells from dead embryos
- using a biopsy to extract single cells
- manipulating somatic cells to alter their potential development as human embryos.

The emphasis was on finding alternatives to creating embryonic cell lines from viable embryos, which would then be discarded (The President's Council on Bioethics, 2005). On the scientific front, the US National Academy of Sciences issued guidelines to encourage embryonic stem cell research, with careful surveillance and oversight (Johnstone, 2005).

The guidelines are amended from time to time, as the science develops and as the monitoring processes evolve. The National Institutes of Health actively oversee human stem cell research in the US. The monitoring systems are particularly scrupulous because of the caution surrounding this area of science. Of course, the debate on allowable research directions was far from over and further heated debates have been evident, particularly towards the election of a new president. President Obama removed the restrictions on federal funding of research involving new stem cell lines from embryos left over from, for instance, IVF treatment (Robertson, 2010).

In 2010, the Presidential Commission for the Study of Bioethical Issues was formed to advise the US president on emerging issues in science, and on ethically responsible practices in research, health care and technological innovation, including in its charter the examination of issues relating to the 'creation of stem cells by novel means' (Secretary of Health and Human Services, 2010). The tone is of encouragement for exploration of use of synthetic or adult stem cells as an alternative to embryonic stem cells.

We can learn from the debates and discussion of others when forming our preliminary views on a matter. Try the following Reflection as part of your early personal reflection on this topic.

REFLECTION: IN THE NEWS

Either individually or as a group, source an article on one aspect of the use of human stem cells or reproductive technology. You can look for your article in newspapers, editorial reviews or professional journals.

Identify the words that have an 'ethics' feel in your article, list them, and find definitions for them.

Try to identify how the words were used in forming an argument or position on the topic.

These words can facilitate your own process of reflection on a topic. You may find yourself in general agreement or disagreement with an argument. Try to identify why you feel that way. Using your own words, rather than technical philosophical terms is fine—your own thoughts are the starting point for further ethics reflection.

The UK allowed human embryos to be knowingly created for research purposes, including cloning techniques and stem cell research by licensed researchers. It was permitted up to 14 days after fertilisation, as in IVF research, when the primitive streak appears (Plomer, 2002, p. 133). Extensions to the originally allowed uses for fertilisation were added to allow specifically for therapeutic cloning for the development of treatments for 'serious diseases' (*Human Fertilisation (Research Purposes) Regulations 2001* (UK)), but also noting that these regulations are now revoked, and the *Human Fertilisation and Embryology Act 2008* (UK) applies. These guidelines relied on deeming an early embryo of less than 14 days old to lack 'qualities' and to have 'potentiality', but not actual capacities (for thought, action, communication and sentience) and so to have limited moral status. There was criticism that this was objectionable, and that the resulting embryo research was therefore immoral (Deckers, 2005). The UK stem cell bank stores cell lines derived from adult, fetal and embryonic tissues and makes these available to researchers with international monitoring and oversight by the Medical Research Council (Stacey & Hunt, 2006). UK law has continued to develop, and a new *Human Fertilisation and Embryology Act 2008* (UK) and many new regulations apply, including *The Human Fertilisation and Embryology (Mitochondrial Donation) Regulations 2015* (UK). Research on genetic defects has burgeoned under these provisions.

Given increasing hypothetical scientific benefits of extending the research work as embryos become older, one leading genetics researcher publicly voiced her concern to the press about science creating embryos for research in 'factories' or allowing embryos to be kept alive for longer than two weeks. She was prompted to comment after new research was published on removing individual genes from embryos. She explained her personal discomfort: 'I can't put my finger on why but it feels like it cheapens something about human life' (Moody, 2017, p. 23). It is part of her professional responsibility to speak up and prompt further reflection and debate when, given her skill and experience in the scientific field, she was able to identify a complex quandary that needed to be discussed further.

Other countries have had similar rigorous debates, and alternative cell methods, such as harvesting specified adult stem cells, have been supported. These are differentiated, and specific in function to a specific type of tissue. Then, less than 20 years ago, it was thought possible, though more difficult, to culture cells from one part of the body and transplant them to other damaged sections, such as from a thigh muscle to a heart (Robotham, 2002). Research into this area has burgeoned, with success in rejuvenating various muscles and even with building tissue on a scaffold for a trachea using a person's own cells, which has the advantage of the body recognising and accepting rather than rejecting the reintroduction of the tissue. No anti-rejection therapies are needed, and the ethical debate on harvesting stem cells was sidestepped (Epstein & Parmacek, 2005). In a way, the ethics debates prompted the exploration of alternative methods of therapy. There are now multiple options in stem cell research for researchers, with the community actively providing funding and constraint when considering research directions to concentrate on. If the debate hadn't been so heated on the ethics issues of personhood, potentiality and sanctity of life, then it may have taken longer before the adult stem cell field was actively supported.

There is continuing community assessment of the acceptability of the product of the research, as well as its process. For instance, the European Court of Justice was asked by Greenpeace in Germany to consider if it was acceptable to profit from some stem cell research if the commercialisation violated public order or morality. The decision was much anticipated, as it would potentially impact on the feasibility of embryonic stem cell research in the UK and Europe. The Court's ruling, in 2011, was that it was not acceptable to patent research that has involved the destruction of a human embryo (Naik, 2011). Such decisions have the potential to reshape the direction of research endeavours, if it is not feasible for companies to invest in an area in which there is no commercial gain. As you will now realise, the commercial decision they must make in this case is made in a context of community discussion and debates of ethical significance.

REFLECTION: CREATION FOR OTHERS

The manipulation of life and of people's lives is at the heart of the personhood debate. The following example provides a useful opportunity for reflection on the creation of and respect for human life.

A story reported in the global media in 1991 captured attention and focused debate on what the limits are for a family trying to help their dying child. A *Time* magazine article recounted how a couple had conceived a child in the hope that she would provide compatible bone marrow for a transplant to save an elder sibling who was suffering from a form of leukaemia (Morrow, 1991). The ethics of conceiving a child for that

+ continued

purpose and, more generally, of using family members as live donors, were touched on in the media and actively debated by health care workers and ethicists.

The case of the two sisters is particularly challenging because it forces us to consider the sanctity of life. The younger child would not have been conceived if her older sister's life had not been threatened. Is it acceptable to use or manipulate life in that way? How important is the obligation to care for each child? How far should each child's autonomy, and the family's autonomy, extend? As part of your reflection, make a list of the benefits and drawbacks of this bone-marrow transplant. Make separate lists for each child, their family, and the community.

Once you have your lists, try to decide whether the pluses outweigh the minuses. The crucial item on your list that makes you decide in favour or against the procedure is likely to shed light on which fundamental principles are important to you, and what ethical framework you prefer to use. Is your decision guided by any of the legal obligations from Chapter 3?

On occasions, questions of best interests are decided by the courts. A process similar to the ethics analysis of gauging risks and determining limits to autonomy is used. In an Australian case, a 10-year-old child was able to donate bone marrow to his aunt, who had leukaemia, after the Family Court ruled that this was in his best interests. The risks to him were judged to be minimal, and the psychological benefits were weighed against these risks (*Re GWW and CMW* (1997)). (Notice the use of initials in the case citation. It is common in cases involving minors to deidentify the report of the decision in the interests of privacy and confidentiality for the child.)

Psychological benefit can include the exercise of one's own autonomy. In this case, the Family Court assumed the role of guardian, as it does when there is a conflict of opinion over the best interests of a child. The crucial factor in a guardian's appraisal of the medical situation facing their charge is the value judgment involved in weighing the risks against the benefits.

As you think further about ethical frameworks, you could try to work out whether you are, for instance, more comfortable with deontological or utilitarian theories (see Chapter 4 for a discussion of these and other theories). You may remember that the deontologist is an absolutist. The deontologist decides which fundamental obligation is the most important—such as right to life, or right to freedom—and whether a proposed action violates that rule (or 'deon'). On the other hand, a utilitarian weighs up the outcome of any action or situation, and then decides whether it is permissible and what action should be undertaken. A utilitarian takes care to choose the action that is likely to yield the greatest good for the greatest number. The fundamental concern of each utilitarian is reflected in what they use as a measure of 'good'—for example, happiness or health.

It is worth spending time working out which of the philosophical stances you agree with. This will help to determine your reaction to the dilemmas posed by the specific genetics issues that follow in this chapter, and in thinking back to the abortion issues in Chapter 3.

Genetics and safeguards

An international genetic project has studied the genetic composition of the human race. Called the Human Genome Project, its aim was to describe, or map, the human genetic structure to determine which genes are responsible for certain physical and behavioural characteristics. All human chromosomes carry DNA (deoxyribonucleic acid), and the human genome project analysed and sequenced this DNA. An international group, the Human Genome Organisation, coordinated the project's funding and scientific efforts, and the project was declared 'completed' in 2001, after which attention turned to mapping, variation and identifying applications for personalised medicine (Jasny & Zahn, 2011). The long-term aim is to improve the health of all individuals, but minority groups began asking whether this project would result in benefits for them. Many others were asking whether it was dangerous to understand exactly what we are made of too well, as that brings with it the possibility that someone or some group will control other people or all humans.

UNESCO cautioned against the misuse of the burgeoning knowledge in the *Universal Declaration on the Human Genome and Human Rights*, urging respect for dignity and rights regardless of genetic characteristics. As stated in Article 2b of the Declaration, 'That dignity makes it imperative not to reduce individuals to their genetic characteristics and to respect their uniqueness and diversity.' Also at Article 4: 'The human genome in its natural state shall not give rise to financial gains.' (UNESCO, 1997). This Declaration and the *International Declaration on Human Genetic Data* (2003) were republished together in 2017, underlining their contemporary importance for the international community (UNESCO, 2017).

REFLECTION: UNESCO DECLARATIONS

As an exercise, source the *Universal Declaration on the Human Genome and Human Rights* (1997) and *International Declaration on Human Genetic Data* (2003). Both are available on the UNESCO website: <http://unesdoc.unesco.org>.

Read through the Declarations, and summarise the concerns addressed in each of the sections or 'articles'. You will notice that they generally point to the danger of a loss of freedom and dignity, and encourage member states to establish forums for further discussion of the issues, such as ethics committees. Try to identify the specific concerns, and gain an overall sense of the main concerns by reading the Declarations in their entirety, including the preamble.

Compare your list of concerns with a colleague who has also read the Declarations.

You will remember from Chapter 1 that international human rights documents are partly aspirational, in that they set ideals. Nevertheless they do have some legal force, as countries that agree to be signatories state that they will endeavour to uphold those principles, and then enact legislation to reflect their commitment.

The ongoing debate over ownership of genetic material or any work on it is highlighted in many legal and regulatory forums.

+ continued

An individual's genetic material can be the subject of study, and can lead to very valuable patents that are used in genetic testing processes, which are sold commercially. So far, the approach has been to deny an individual's specific property rights to their genetic material, on the grounds that such individual ownership would limit advances in research. In *Moore v Regents of University of California (1990)*, a patient's T-cells were used to create a cell line to be used in research, and perhaps later for commercial activities. The patient was found not to have 'owned' the cells, and so did not have any further rights in the cell line that was created. This case is used as a demonstration that property rights are at best tenuous, and need to be argued rather than assumed. The law in this area remains unclear (*Moore v Regents of University of California (1990)*, as cited in Dickenson, 2017, p. 3).

An Australian Parliament Senate Inquiry into 'the impacts of gene patents on healthcare, medical research and the health and wellbeing of Australians' was prompted by a private company attempting to enforce its patent rights over the BRCA1 and BRCA2 genes. If the company had pursued this claim successfully, it would have become the sole tester or license provider for testing for the genes that indicate a predisposition to developing breast or ovarian cancer. The Inquiry noted that the community was concerned about potential commercial exploitation of the test. The inquiry recommended the possible amendment of the *Patents Act 1990* (Cth), and the development of policy to guide the use of government mechanisms to intervene to restrict the rights of patent holders, or to 'acquire a patent for the purposes of promoting human health' (Parliament of Australia, Senate, 2010).

As more is understood about genes, the issue of predictive genetic testing, availability of genetic information, and the possibility of discrimination or inequitable treatment in a social sense is vigorously debated. The industry standard adopted by the Financial Services Council—the council of life insurance companies in Australia—is that private health insurance is not affected by results of genetic tests—however, life insurance products may be. Individuals are required to disclose to an insurer any risk-related information that is known to them, such as personal medical or genetic test information. This is because in the insurance contracts legislation, it is a matter relevant to the insurer's decision (New South Wales Government, Health Centre for Genetics Education, 2017).

You could look back to the general ethics and regulatory discussion on privacy protections in earlier chapters, especially Chapter 6. The *Privacy Act 1988* (Cth) does not absolutely prevent a health service provider using or disclosing a person's genetic information. Under guidelines that took effect from March 2014, if consent is not able to be obtained, and use or disclosure is necessary to lessen or reduce a threat to a genetic relative, and this belief of serious threat to the life, health or safety of the genetic relative is reasonable, then the information can be used and disclosed, as long as the section 95AA guidelines have been followed (*Privacy Act 1988* (Cth), s 95AA—Use and disclosure of genetic information to a patient's genetic relatives under Section 95AA of the *Privacy Act 1988* (Cth)—Guidelines for health in the private sector, 12 March 2014.)

The sensitivity of genetic information for individuals, genetic relatives and the community is recognised in the *National Statement on Ethical Conduct in Human Research* (2007/2018), which addresses human genetics as a distinct area of research with particular ethics considerations for researchers and human research ethics committees. Under one of the principles, when consent is sought for collection of genetic information for research, individuals should also be informed if the third-party disclosure legal requirements to employers, insurers, or financial or education bodies could be relevant, given the information to be generated in the research (National Health and Medical Research Council, Australian Research Council and Universities Australia, 2007/2018, Chapter 3, 3.3.23, p. 50). So, considerable regulation applies and guidance is available when genetic information is collected in a controlled environment, such as a health or research setting.

Perhaps you know someone who has considered having a genetic test done—either a test on themselves, or perhaps on a child or foetus in utero. It is a complex issue, with personal and social implications. If you do know someone who thought about having genetic testing, what were some of their hopes and fears? How did that person make their decision on whether or not to proceed?

REFLECTION: GENETIC PREDICTION

In the UK about 15 years ago, a simple genetic test kit became available in health-related lifestyle shops. For about £100 (roughly $180), nine genetically determined metabolism processes could be analysed for your body. The focus was on diet and lifestyle. In the USA, a combined genetic-based test of predisposition to osteoporosis, heart disease and immune deficiency became available through primary care practices, and it became available worldwide via the internet.

Commercial genetic testing is the subject of guidelines. However, these guidelines vary in different countries, and consumers then decide if they want what the technology claims to offer them. Whether to let the free market and consumers decide if they want the tests—and so 'regulate' their use that way—is itself a matter of ethics debate (Levitt, 2001). A range of genetic tests is directly available to consumers—and professionals would generally prefer that they were only offered within a professional context (Lovett & Liang, 2011).

1　In a small group, consider whether you are happy to have genetic tests available and, if so, whether they should be available:
   - in a shop setting
   - in a health-practice setting
   - via the internet.

+ continued

2   List your reasons for your support, or your objections, in order from least to most strongly held views.

3   Write an advertisement for one of the services you hypothetically support, and include some of the information a prospective customer may need to know.

Once an individual decides to undergo genetic testing, the information about the risks they face—or risks they may carry in terms of genetically inheritable conditions—raises perplexing future decisions. The individual then has to decide:

• should they tell others, or not?
• should they change lifestyle or further risk factors, or not?

The decision to have a test is generally accompanied by counselling, because of the complexity of consequences that may follow for themselves, their family and their future family members.

David Suzuki has written extensively on the ethics of the genetic manipulation of plant, animal and human life. His 'genethic' principles are, in summary:

• to understand, in detail, the nature of genes
• to be cautious in claiming to understand the complicated interplay of genes in behaviour and 'defects'
• to accept variation as a natural and desirable phenomenon
• to maintain individual autonomy over genetic decisions that affect us as individuals
• to preserve the distinction between genetic species (Suzuki & Knudston, 1989, pp. 345–6).

The next Reflection can be worked through either in groups or alone. It is a fictitious scenario about genetic manipulation (and genetic testing) that asks you to consider the ethical importance of the genetic process, and to nominate who or what groups might have ethical concerns about the process.

Suzuki's 'genethic' principles can be used as a discussion base for the Reflection. You could decide whether the principles should apply and, if so, what they would mean for the new colony proposed in the exercise. Alternatively, other principles, such as those of Beauchamp and Childress—beneficence, non-maleficence, autonomy and justice—could be used to examine the issues (Beauchamp & Childress, 2013). The ethical dimension of genetic manipulation is partly about control over individuals and species, and partly a scientific debate about what is most beneficial, in the long term, for the reproduction and survival of a species. You might also like to read ahead to review the models of justice in Chapter 10.

REFLECTION: SOCIAL GENETIC PLANNING

You might like to look at the discussions of resources and justice in Chapter 10 before trying this exercise.

Imagine it is the year 2100. A new multinational colony has been established in space. Its job is to investigate the further use of space, as Earth has become overcrowded and the climate is becoming unliveable. The results of the human genome project have enabled researchers to identify a gene that predisposes people to obesity. Obesity related complaints would be undesirable in the new colony, as people would need to stay for 10 years because of the travel time. Too many ill people would drain the resources of the colony and the project would have to be abandoned. The administrators propose either limiting work permits to those who are cleared of the defective gene, or rectifying the genes of those with the obesity gene before they can gain work permits.

- What do you advise should be done?
- Is it a national or international problem?
- Should the new colony go ahead?
- Should Suzuki's 'genethic' principles apply?
- What would be allowed under your country's guidelines for gene therapy?

1 Using the following justice models—justice as fairness, comparative justice, and distributive justice—advise how a genetic testing service could be distributed. You could come up with different advice for each model, or combine the models in producing your advice.

2 Determine what is a good that the community on the new colony agrees with, and how that good should be distributed. Your good could be either genetic testing for the gene, or the genetic manipulation of defective genes.

Apart from examining, understanding and 'rectifying' genes, the replication of entire genetic structures is possible. This scientific advance, termed *cloning*, captured the world's attention over 20 years ago (Kuhse, H. 1997). Since 1997, with the creation of Dolly—a sheep cloned from another sheep—the ethics of the creation and recreation of exact copies of individual humans has been discussed and debated. Dolly was created 'by transferring the nucleus from an udder cell into an egg whose DNA had been removed' (Pennisi & Williams, 1997). Many countries around the world were prompted to inquire into the process and the reasons for it, and to ask what the ethical limits of such a process were. Should cloning be allowed at all? Should cloning be extended to humans?

In the USA, President Clinton was very quick to promote public and government debate on the ethics of the process in relation to both animals and humans.

The US Senate Committee formed to consider the issue of cloning expressed a number of concerns about the issues raised by cloning, such as the essence of personhood, the control over life, and the risk and harm resulting from the hundreds of failed attempts that preceded the successful creation of the perfect Dolly. They publicly stated that experimentation on humans would not be allowed.

The progress of Dolly has been closely followed, as has the progress and sudden health failures of other cloned animals. Dolly developed premature arthritis in 2002 and progressive lung disease in 2003, which led to her being put down (Smith, 2002). Other cloned animals frequently suffer from heart failure and rapidly ageing constitutions. Despite occasional sensational claims that humans have been cloned, the risk of creating many unviable and desperately malformed embryos and babies in the process—not to mention the hidden uncertainties for the resulting live babies—acts as a strong deterrent to human cloning.

There are scandals in all research fields, but coverage is immense when the subject is cloning. The accuracy of cloned human embryonic stem cell research results, as reported by an eminent Korean researcher, was called into question, leading to considerable media coverage. Researchers in the field then immediately reassessed how many of the earlier reported results they could rely on from that previously leading laboratory (Chong & Normile, 2006). It was subsequently decided that much of the earlier reported research had been fraudulent, and issues such as better independent monitoring of research were canvassed in subsequent ethics commentary (Saunders & Savulescu, 2008).

Genetics institutes are working to minimise the impact that disabling conditions have on the lives of individuals. Further debate is needed on what should be considered a disability, and what is simply a part of the normal distribution and variation of characteristics in humans. The potential to develop a disability is also different to the actual development of disability, giving rise to these ethics issues:

- Should those with the potential to develop a disability be thought of differently?
- Should those with the potential to develop a disability be tested?
- Should such testing and information only be limited to what is socially and medically agreed to as being serious and disabling?

Early diagnosis of potential genetic disease is itself an ethics issue. It involves assessment of family responsibility for genetic predispositions and family ownership of genetic information, as well as individual autonomy and choice in investigating and controlling one's own health. Family members may well disagree among themselves about whether genetic disease is a collective problem or the responsibility of the individual. The balance between the responsibility of the individual for their own health, and the responsibility of the family—or of society—for the health of larger social units may vary between cultures. In a position statement on genetic testing, Kare Berg, writing from a Norwegian perspective, has outlined the importance of family responsibility in serious disease predisposition (Berg, 1996). The balance between family and individual responsibility is not the same in all cultures.

In China, the policy position that required couples to follow their doctor's advice to limit the number of children born with genetic aberrations worried physicians and ethicists in other countries. These physicians and ethicists felt prompted to comment on policy or rules in the Chinese jurisdiction, noting broader fundamental issues that they could comment upon as members of the international community. The concern was partly in relation to the use of genetic information and reproductive technologies, and then applying them to concepts of normality and disability, and partly in limiting the parents' autonomy (MacLeod & Clarke, 1998).

You could change the exercise about obesity testing in a hypothetical space colony of the future to include any number of potentially testable characteristics in any social situation. Genes predispose us to variations in appearance—such as height, weight, hair colour and complexion—as well as to internal physical variations, especially in our internal organs (and their effective function), and structural variations in essential organs such as heart vessels and lung capacity.

The debates that occur constantly in relation to the ethics of genetics are a prime example of the often-dizzying possibilities that science and health care present us with. The possibility of changing the very nature of the human race is increasingly real.

Every now and then, the community calls for a halt to such developments, and asks for reflection on their ethics and legality. The overall aim is to prevent us from losing control of our future to technology. The community seeks to agree on particular objectives for technology so that it can be harnessed, through agreed means, for those agreed aims. In setting these objectives and means, we can take into account the concerns of both:

- deontologists—in relation to the process of change
- consequentialists—in relation to acceptable outcomes.

REFLECTION: COMPLEX URGENT DECISION MAKING

As a review of this section, get together with some colleagues and try one of these exercises.

Exercise 1

There seem to be increasing reports of conjoined twins. Tragically, in many instances, vital organs are shared and parents face the impossible decision of watching both children slowly deteriorate in health, or agreeing to operate to separate them, knowing that at least one may die as a result. The religious background of the parents, the willingness of doctors to intervene, and the capacity of legal systems to make best interests decisions varies between countries.

- Think of a recent example the birth of conjoined twins, and research what happened.
- What were the views of those involved?
- What happened in the end? What was the reasoning that contributed to the decision?

You might like to consider the issues of personhood closely as you unravel this dilemma, or look back at the ethics reasoning choices in Chapter 4.

Exercise 2

In the Netherlands, early guidelines for withholding or withdrawing intensive care from newborns who are 'non-viable' (or dying) have been supported by paediatricians. In contrast to the approach in other countries of 'saving' babies born at progressively earlier weeks of pregnancy, the Dutch guidelines were justified on the grounds of:

- consequent suffering for the newborn from any active treatment process
- futility of treatment, when a beneficial outcome is highly unlikely
- quality of life, with significant impacts on expected life choices.

+ continued

The Dutch argument was that 'saving' babies results in tremendous morbidity—meaning ongoing disability and health issues—because of poor health outcomes for pre-term infants below 26 weeks of a normal 42-week gestation (Dutch Pediatric Association, 1992). (Note that Chapter 4 included a discussion on euthanasia law and end-of-life practices in the Netherlands as an example of a contemporary ethics debate.)

Given that limited information on the complications of a premature birth is routinely presented to an expectant mother—and that many premature infants are delivered in an emergency admission—there may be little time to prepare the parents for decisions that involve the treatment of their newborn. This presents an ethical difficulty for their optimal involvement in decisions about the infant's treatment—particularly in the earliest decisions of implementing intensive treatment (Schroeder, 2008).

Thinking about two prospective parents in this situation, look back to the decision-making components in Chapter 8 and consider what makes a decision and, especially, what makes an informed decision.

- Which of those decision-making components is readily achievable as the parents prepare to make decisions on behalf of their newborn?
- Can you guess which parent often becomes the primary decision maker in this situation? Why?
- Identify which parent is most likely to satisfy more of the decision-making components for an ethically robust decision-making process during an emergency admission.

Maximising the information available—in readiness for any such decision time—depends on both parents having had access to the professional advice and information throughout the pregnancy. It also depends on the couple sharing the information each had received separately during the preparation leading up to the birth. This would maximise their autonomy and increase the quality of their direct input into best interests decisions for their newborn.

Summary

This chapter has highlighted the contribution of philosophical reasoning to contemporary discussions on dramatic issues at the beginning of life. This learning will prompt you to remember ethics issues you learned about earlier in this book. Medical and surgical termination of pregnancy was discussed in Chapter 3, with a focus on how jurisdiction makes a difference to the options available; the philosophical debates behind the options were also discussed. Voluntary euthanasia was discussed in Chapter 4, with a focus on the ethics discussions that had informed the available legislative and regulatory options, as well as those under current community discussion and consideration. By now, you should be able to anticipate that regulations vary between jurisdictions. The exercises in this chapter gave you the opportunity to practise finding the relevant regulations and guidelines that apply in your own settings.

You have learnt that community—as well as professional discussion—is evident when statutes or regulations on a sensitive topic are contemplated. You have also learnt that when a legal case is heard on a matter that raises fundamental issues about the beginning of life, the judge's reasoning can reflect fundamental ethical and philosophical concerns.

STUDY QUESTIONS

Note: These questions also recap some issues that were covered in Chapter 3.

1   Define a 'person'. In your definition, include your opinion on when personhood or a claim to life begins. Support your position with references to law, ethics or philosophy.
2   Choose one aspect of reproductive health. Discuss a potential legal, regulatory and ethics issue for a health practitioner or health care worker working in this health field.

SAMPLE ESSAY QUESTIONS

1   Analyse the contemporary regulation of the availability of emergency contraception, as made available by a professional association, society or board.
2   Comment on the ethical and legal issues that have informed the contemporary regulation of emergency contraception.
3   The ownership of human tissue is a legal as well as an ethical issue. Illustrate the complex arguments that are considered, with detailed references to case law reasons for decision.

REFERENCES

Australian Government, National Health and Medical Research Council [NHMRC]. (2017). *Ethical guidelines on the use of assisted reproductive technology in clinical practice and research*. Canberra: NHMRC.

Australian Government, National Health and Medical Research Council [NHMRC]. (2018). *Database of licences authorising the use of excess ART embryos*. Canberra: NHMRC. Retrieved from www.nhmrc.gov.au

Beauchamp, T.L., & Childress, J.F. (2013). *Principles of biomedical ethics* (7th edn). London: Oxford University Press.

Berg, K. (1996). Ethical aspects of early diagnosis of genetic diseases. *World Health, 5*, 20–1.

Brecher, B. (2002). Our obligation to the dead. *Journal of Applied Philosophy, 19*(2), 109–19.

Chong, S., & Normile, D. (2006). How young Korean researchers helped unearth a scandal. *Science, 311*(5757), 22–5.

Collinson, D. (1987). *Fifty major philosophers: A reference guide*. New York: Routledge.

Conway, H. (2016). *The law and the dead.* Abingdon and New York: Routledge.

Deckers, J. (2005). Why current UK legislation on embryo research is immoral: How the argument from lack of qualities and the argument for potentiality have been applied and why they should be rejected. *Bioethics, 19*(3), 251–71.

Dickenson, D. (2017). *Property in the body: Feminist perspectives* (2nd edn). Cambridge: Cambridge University Press.

Dutch Pediatric Association. (1992). To treat or not to treat? Limits for life-sustaining treatment in neonatology [in Dutch]. Utrecht, Netherlands, cited in F.J. Walther (2005), Withholding treatment, withdrawing treatment, and palliative care in the neonatal intensive care unit. *Early Human Development, 81*(12), 965–72.

Epstein, J.A., & Parmacek, M.S. (2005). Recent advances in cardiac development with therapeutic implications for adult cardiovascular disease. *Circulation, 112*, 592–7.

Haimes, E., & Taylor, K. (2009). Fresh embryo donation for human embryonic stem cell (HESC) research: The experiences and values of IVF couples asked to be embryo donor. *Human Reproduction, 24*(9), 2142–50.

Hall, M. (2001, 10 August). Bush OKs limited stem-cell funding. *USA Today*, 2001, 1.

House of Commons. (2001). *The Royal Liverpool Children's Inquiry Report.* London: The Stationery Office.

Jasny, B.R., & Zahn, L.M. (2011). A celebration of the genome, Part IV essay: Genome sequencing anniversary. *Science, 331*, 1024–7.

Johnston, J. (2005). Stem cell protocols: The NAS Guidelines are a useful start. *Hastings Center Report, 35*(6), 16–17.

Kuhse, H. (1997, 12 June). Caution, not panic, on cloning. *The Australian*, 11.

Le Moncheck, L. (1996). Philosophy, gender politics, and in vitro fertilization: A feminist ethics of reproductive healthcare. *Journal of Clinical Ethics, 7*(2), 160–81.

Leventis Lourgos, A., & Miller Rubin, B. (2015, 12 June). Court gives frozen embryos to Chicago woman over ex-boyfriend's objection. *Chicago Tribune*. Retrieved from https://www.chicagotribune.com/

Levitt, M. (2001). Let the consumer decide? The regulation of commercial genetic testing. *Journal of Medical Ethics, 27*(6), 398–404.

Locke, J. (1946). *The second treatise of civil government: a letter concerning toleration*, J.W. Gough (Ed.). Oxford: Basil Blackwell. (Original work published 1689).

Lockwood, M. (1985). When does a life begin. In M. Lockwood (Ed.), *Moral dilemmas in modern medicine* (pp. 9–31). London: Oxford University Press.

Lovett, K.M., & Liang, B.A. (2011). Direct-to-consumer cardiac screening and suspect risk evaluation. *Journal of the American Medical Association, 305*(24), 2567–8.

MacLeod, P., & Clarke, F.F. (1998). Forget cloning and pay attention to China. *Canadian Medical Association Journal, 159*(2), 153–5.

Moody, O. (2017, 23 September). Pioneer warns of embryo factories. *The Times*, 23.

Morrow, L. (1991, 17 June). When one body can save another. *Time*, 46–50.

Naik, G. (2011, 19 October). Patent ruling sets back EU stem-cell scientists. *The Wall Street Journal*. Retrieved from http://online.wsj.com

National Health and Medical Research Council, Australian Research Council, & Universities Australia. (2007). *National statement on ethical conduct in human research*. (Updated May 2015 and July 2018). Canberra: NHMRC. Retrieved from www.nhmrc.gov.au

New South Wales Government, Health Centre for Genetics Education. (2017). *Life insurance products and genetic testing in Australia*. Fact Sheet 20. (Updated 21 March 2017). Retrieved from www.genetics.edu.au

[*New York Times*]. (1992, 3 June). Frozen embryos in legal limbo, *New York Times* article reprinted in *Sydney Morning Herald*, 15.

Noonan, J.T. (1973). An almost absolute value in history. In J. Feinberg (Ed.), *The problem of abortion* (pp. 10–17). Belmont: Wadsworth.

Orr, R.D., & Siegler, M. (2002). Is posthumous semen retrieval ethically permissible? *Journal of Medical Ethics, 28*(5), 299–303.

Parliament of Australia, Senate. *Gene Patents*, 26 November 2010, p. 5, & *Recommendations*. Retrieved from http://aph.gov.au

Pennisi, E., & Williams, N. (1997). Will Dolly send in the clones? *Science, 275*, 1415.

Plomer, A. (2002). Beyond the HFE Act 1990: The regulation of stem cell research in the UK. *Medical Law Review, 10*, 132–64.

Robertson, J.A. (2010). Embryo stem cell research: ten years of controversy. *Journal of Law, Medicine & Ethics, 38*(2), 191–203.

Robotham, J. (2002, 9 May). Thigh gives heart a leg-up and offers alternative to stem cells. *Sydney Morning Herald*, 3.

Saunders, R., & Savulescu, J. (2008). Research ethics and lessons from Hwanggate: What can we learn from the Korean cloning fraud? *Journal of Medical Ethics, 34*(3), 214–21.

Schlink, L. (2002, 10 February). New baby from dead husband. *Sunday Telegraph*, 46.

Schroeder, S. (2008). Ethical issues for parents of extremely premature infants. *Journal of Paediatrics and Child Health, 44*(5), 302–4.

Schwarz, M. (2015, 28 April). Who owns pre-embryos? *The New Yorker*. Retrieved from www.newyorker.com

Smith, D. (2002). Cloning study points to early end for Dolly. *Sydney Morning Herald*, 6.

Sperling, D. (2008). *Posthumous interests: Legal and ethical perspectives*. Cambridge: Cambridge University Press.

Stacey, G., & Hunt, C.J. (2006). The UK Stem Cell Bank: A UK government-funded, international resource center for stem cell research. *Regenerative Medicine, 1*(1), 139–42.

Stewart, C., Lipworth, W., Aparicio, L., Fleming J., Kerridge, I. (2014). The problems of biobanking and the law of gifts. In I. Goold, K. Greasley, J. Herring & L. Skene (Eds), *Persons, parts and property: How should we regulate human tissue in the 21st century?* (Chapter 3, pp. 25–38). Oxford and Portland, Oregon: Hart Publishing.

Suzuki, D., & Knudtson, P. (1989). *Genethics: The ethics of engineering life*. Sydney: Allen & Unwin.

Swain, M.S., & Marusyk, R.W. (1990). An alternative to property rights in human tissue. *Hastings Center Report, 20*, 12–15.

The President's Council on Bioethics. (2005). *Alternative sources of pluripotent stem cells*. Washington, DC: The President's Council on Bioethics.

The Secretary of Health and Human Services, Presidential Commission for the Study of Bioethical Issues. (2010). *Charter*. Washington DC: Presidential Commission for the Study of Bioethical Issues.

Tooley, M. (1973). Abortion and infanticide. In J. Feinberg (Ed.), *The problem of abortion* (pp. 51–91). Belmont: Wadsworth.

United Nations Educational, Scientific and Cultural Organization [UNESCO]. (1997). *Universal Declaration on the Human Genome and Human Rights*. Paris: UNESCO.

United Nations Educational, Scientific and Cultural Organization [UNESCO]. (2003). *International Declaration on Human Genetic Data*. Paris: UNESCO.

United Nations Educational, Scientific and Cultural Organization [UNESCO]. (2017). *Universal Declaration on the Human Genome and Human Rights (1997) and the International Declaration on Human Genetic Data (2003)*. Paris: UNESCO. Retrieved from http://unescdoc.unesco.org

Warnock, M. (1987). Do human cells have rights? *Bioethics*, *1*(1), 1–14.

Warnock, M. (2002). *Making babies: Is there a right to have children?* Oxford: Oxford University Press.

LEGISLATION

Assisted Reproductive Technology Act 2007 (NSW)

Human Fertilisation (Research Purposes) Regulations 2001 (UK)

Human Fertilisation and Embryology Act 2008 (UK)

The Human Fertilisation and Embryology (Mitochondrial Donation) Regulations 2015 (UK)

Human Tissue Act 1983 (NSW)

Human Tissue Act 1961 (UK)

Human Tissue Act 2004 (UK)

Patents Act 1990 (Cth)

Privacy Act 1988 (Cth)

Privacy Act 1988 (Cth), s 95AA—*Use and disclosure of genetic information to a patient's genetic relatives under Section 95AA of the Privacy Act 1988* (Cth)—*Guidelines for health practitioners in the private sector, 12 March 2014.*

CASES

Davis v Davis (1992) 842 S.W.2d588 (Tenn. 1992)

Doodeward v Spence [1908] 6 CLR 406

Jocelyn Edwards: re the estate of the late Mark Edwards [2011] NSWSC 478

Moore v Regents of University of California 793 P 2d 479 (Cal 1990)

Re GWW and CMW, Federal Law Court, unreported, 21 January 1997

R v Kelly (1998) 3 All ER 741

Re Cresswell [2018] QSC 142

Szafranski v Dunston, Nos 1–12-2975, 1–14-1539, June 12, 2015 (Appellate Court of Illinois)

Yearworth and others v North Bristol NHS Trust (2009) EWCA Civ 37; [2010] QB 1

CHAPTER 10

Regulation and availability of health and community services

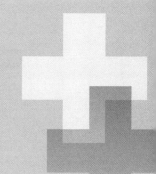

LEARNING OBJECTIVES

- To understand how law and regulation shapes the funding of health care.
- To appreciate ethics tools as part of planning service availability.
- To be able to illustrate how law and regulation protects the availability of the health care system.
- To identify ethics reasoning in the classic funding and distribution models.
- To be able to describe current health care funding models.
- To appreciate how administrative budgets are set to manage health priorities.
- To recognise ethics reasoning in discussions on public availability of health and community services.

KEY TERMS

claim	health
comparative justice	interest
cost–benefit analysis	justice as fairness
cost-effectiveness analysis	need
distributive justice	right
entitlement	utility

CASE EXAMPLE

Seeking a safe haven

Three people from the same family have just made an application seeking asylum in Australia. They ask your advice on what health and community services are available for them in your jurisdiction.

Gather your ideas as you work your way through this chapter, so that you can provide relevant information and perhaps some advice.

1   If you were to advocate for the family, what information would you provide, and what advice would you give, if any?
2   Alternatively, if you were to represent your local health service, what would you advise?
3   How would you explain the limits to available services to them?

Funding and billing of health services

The government (or the executive) and delegated authorities provide regulations to keep a society safe and orderly. Regulation is often set within schedules to the legislation, or separately tabled and agreed to by parliament. Alternatively, the authority to create regulatory standards and apply regulations can be sourced from broad powers set out in statutes. You read about the regulation of health services standards and of health practitioners and health care workers in Chapter 2.

Aspects of regulation and administration shape a patient's care. These include:

- funding for health
- deciding the level of publicly available services
- setting the public rebates for services available through Medicare
- setting budgets for service areas
- facilitating delivery of clinically appropriate services to those with entitlement to receive them.

Our society understands that a basic level of regulation and administration is essential to safeguard the public from too great a risk in accessing unapproved services, and to support the fair and efficient use of public resources—thus safeguarding the ongoing availability of decent and fair health service into the future. Ethics issues are highlighted in the discussion of these standards. Some of the classic ethics commentary on these issues is sourced from international discussions about health service provision.

Providing health care services is costly. The health care spending of many countries is periodically reported by the Organisation for Economic Co-operation and Development (OECD) as a proportion of gross domestic product (GDP). The USA spends an estimated 17.2 per cent of GDP, which is very high compared to Australia at 9.6 per cent of GDP, and the UK at 9.7 per cent of GDP. The European countries of Netherlands and France spend 10.5 per cent and 11 per cent of GDP respectively (OECD, 2017).

Economists routinely note that recession reduces spending growth in the short term, but spending then continues to rise with the increased routine use of medical technologies in health care (Smith et al., 2009). There is some evidence to suggest that survival rates from serious illnesses, such as cancer, are better in higher-spending countries, when viewed over time (Evans & Pritchard, 2000). Theoretically, that puts the USA in the lead. Even so, some critics argue that there is great inequity in the US system, despite the higher proportion of GDP available, and there is constant review of how to distribute care better. The proportion of funds available for health care in any given country is unlikely to change dramatically.

Australia has Medicare, a Commonwealth system. Medicare subsidises:

- medical consultations
- diagnostic imaging
- pathology services
- optometrist services
- prescription medicines
- free public health care in public hospitals (to a decent minimum level)
- dental and some other allied health services (in some circumstances).

Medicare pays health service providers with money collected by the Commonwealth through levies and taxes. A provider can receive payments of predetermined amounts for each service that attracts a Medicare benefit. Medicare is set up so that medical care is available when needed (and to a reasonable level) without personal financial considerations unreasonably restricting that care. All citizens and entitled visa holders can register to be Medicare card holders, thus demonstrating they are entitled to receive Commonwealth services. There is more discussion about entitlement to receive services later in this chapter.

The Commonwealth legislative basis for Medicare was noted in Chapter 1. The services that are subsidised by Medicare are regularly published as a list in the Medicare Benefits Schedule, and a maximum 'gap' that a patient can be asked to pay for out-of-hospital services is also set in that schedule (Australian Government, 2017). This list is read with the legislative provisions, and the authority supporting some payments is found in the legislation. The legislative scheme includes the following Acts and Regulations:

- *Health Insurance Act 1973* (Cth)
- *National Health Act 1953* (Cth)
- *Health Insurance Regulations 1975* (Cth)
- *Health Insurance (Diagnostic Imaging Services Table) Regulations 2017* (Cth)
- *Health Insurance (General Medical Services Table) Regulations 2017* (Cth)
- *Health Insurance (Pathology Services Table) Regulations 2017* (Cth).

In further legislation underpinning the Medicare program, the *Human Services Amendment Act 2011* (Cth) provides for a Chief Executive Medicare, with certain investigative powers—in, for instance, sections 41G and 43A.

The routine services for which patients' costs are covered by the public purse are tightly defined under the Medicare Benefits Schedule. What is included changes from time to time, as new treatment options become available. The rebates that are publicly funded are also altered from time to time so that areas of need are balanced with areas of demand—this ensures equitable distribution of the limited available public funds. Budgetary considerations are part of this assessment.

Entitlements can be further restricted if a larger than expected outlay is encountered for a particular service item number. For instance, in relation to a rebate for a particular psychiatric condition, the following proviso was added: 'it is not sufficient for the patient's illness to fall within the diagnostic criteria. It must be evident that a significant level of impairment exists which interferes with the patient's quality of life'. Implemented at the same time was a restriction on the availability of benefits for the removal of broadly classified skin lesions. This change was due to a '30 per cent increase in Medicare outlays above that anticipated' (Commonwealth Department of Health and Family Services, 1997, pp. 3, 7). The federal Cabinet has at times considered matters of potentially large budgetary impacts for pharmaceuticals that are to be funded or subsidised by the Commonwealth taxpayer. The government holds the decision-making power, even though it is routinely advised by its agencies, and some of its decisions have attracted critical comment for political interference in an independent process if it is done to protect a Budget surplus (Medicines Australia, 2011).

The resources are limited and must be used carefully. The Commonwealth legislation and regulation stipulates that professional services must be clinically relevant and part of the appropriate treatment of the patient in order for the benefit to be payable—that is, the services must be generally accepted in the medical profession as necessary. If a service is not clinically relevant or necessary or appropriate, the benefit should not be claimed by the service provider or patient. Professional integrity and ongoing reflection on whether each service is clinically appropriate and relevant for each patient is crucial to the fair operation and viability of the scheme.

Medicare fraud is a crime, as well as likely amounting to professional misconduct as a serious significant departure from acceptable standards in each health profession. To seek a benefit or payment when it is not warranted would be misleading and deceptive conduct in a legal sense, as well as being unethical professional conduct. Improper issuing of an account can result in charges under the *Health Insurance Act 1973* (Cth), at sections 128A or 128B, and the funds can be recovered from the practitioner under section 129AC. The following excerpts from sections 128A and 128B highlight the strict liability of a breach of the provisions on making false statements, and how the legislation is applied. Understanding the schedules and regulations and then making correct statements about the type of clinically relevant services that are provided is essential.

128A False statements relating to medicare benefits etc.

(1) A person shall not make, or authorise the making of, a statement (whether oral or in writing) that is:

(a) false or misleading in a material particular; and

(b) capable of being used in connection with a claim for a benefit or payment under this Act.

Penalty: 20 penalty units.

(2) Where:

  (a) a person makes a statement (whether oral or in writing) that is false or misleading in a material particular;

  (b) the statement is capable of being used in connection with a claim for a benefit or payment under this Act;

  (c) the material particular in respect of which the statement is false or misleading is substantially based upon a statement made, either orally or in writing, to the person or to an agent of the person by another person who is an employee or agent of the first-mentioned person; and

  (d) the last-mentioned statement is false or misleading in a material particular;

    that other person commits an offence punishable on conviction by a fine not exceeding 20 penalty units.

(2A) An offence under subsection (1) or (2) is an offence of strict liability.

Note: For strict liability, see section 6.1 of the *Criminal Code*.

(3) In subsection(2), a reference to an employee of a person shall, in a case where that person is a corporation, be read as a reference to:

  (a) a director, secretary, manager or employee of the corporation;

  (b) a receiver and manager of any part of the undertaking of the corporation appointed under a power contained in any instrument; or

  (c) a liquidator of the corporation appointed in a voluntary winding up.

(4) A prosecution for an offence under this section may be commenced at any time within 3 years after the commission of the offence.

(5) It is a defence if a person charged with an offence under this section in relation to a statement made by the person did not know, and could not reasonably be expected to have known, that the statement was:

  (a) false or misleading in a material particular; or

  (b) capable of being used in connection with a claim for a benefit or payment under this Act.

(6) In this section, a reference to making a statement includes a reference to issuing or presenting a document, and a reference to a statement shall be construed accordingly.

128B Knowingly making false statements relating to medicare benefits etc.

(1) A person shall not make, or authorise the making of, a statement (whether oral or in writing) if the person knows that the statement is:

  (a) false or misleading in a material particular; and

  (b) capable of being used in connection with a claim for a benefit or payment under this Act.

Penalty: Imprisonment for 5 years or 100 penalty units, or both.

(2) Where:

  (a) a person makes a statement (whether oral or in writing) that is false or misleading in a material particular;

(b) the statement is capable of being used in connection with a claim for a benefit or payment under this Act;

(c) the material particular in respect of which the statement is false or misleading is substantially based upon a statement made, either orally or in writing, to the person or to an agent of the person by another person who is an employee or agent of the first-mentioned person;

(d) that other person knew that the last-mentioned statement was false or misleading in a material particular; and

(e) that other person knew, or had reasonable grounds to suspect, that the last-mentioned statement would be used in the preparation of a statement of the kind referred to in paragraph (b);

that other person commits an offence punishable on conviction by imprisonment for a period not exceeding 5 years or a fine not exceeding 100 penalty units, or both.

(3) In subsection(2), a reference to an employee of a person shall, in a case where that person is a corporation, be read as a reference to:

(a) a director, secretary, manager or employee of the corporation;

(b) a receiver and manager of any part of the undertaking of the corporation appointed under a power contained in any instrument; or

(c) a liquidator of the corporation appointed in a voluntary winding up.

(5) In this section, a reference to making a statement includes a reference to issuing or presenting a document, and a reference to a statement shall be construed accordingly

Some health care practitioners choose to charge only the Medicare rebate, which is around 75 to 85 per cent of the scheduled fee for any particular service (depending on the provider and where the service is received). These providers are termed 'bulk-billers': their service is largely paid for by Commonwealth Medicare funds. Providers can enter bulk-billing agreements with the government, ensuring that no money changes hands between the patient and provider. The number of providers prepared to bulk-bill has fallen dramatically over the last few years, but there are some federal government schemes for GPs who bulk-bill patients in certain groups who face vulnerable circumstances, and safety net provisions for individuals who have high prescription medicines and medical care costs. Providers can choose to bulk-bill some patients who are Medicare card holders and who are also pensioners, who have a Pensioner Concession Card, and other people who hold a Health Care Card because they receive allowances to assist with transition from income support to paid work such as Newstart, Carer, Widow, or Sickness Allowance.

The federal government regularly updates the allowances details on the Department of Health and Ageing website: <http://www.health.gov.au>. Providers can now more routinely organise to issue an account to Medicare for the public portion of a service on behalf of patients, with patients only then needing to pay any gap direct to the health care provider when they attend for a service. Compliance audits of a provider's records can be undertaken by the Commonwealth Department of Human Services to check that documents substantiating the clinically appropriate and relevant service, and that the appropriate documentation to issue the account is held—a practical example of accountability.

Fair distribution and models of justice

Being a health professional or health care worker and providing care has a professional, community, institutional and societal context. What you do makes an impact on the health of individuals and communities. Every now and then, it is important to consider what you are offering to the community through your work, and to think about your responsibilities on a macro scale rather than a micro scale.

INTEGRATED LEARNING AND PRACTICE

What is the good that health care should aim to achieve?

Any response to this question will depend on your ethically informed value judgment of what is a good. Your answer will also depend on whether you think people have a right to receive that good, and this will be informed by ethics and legal issues about whether someone is within a community that then shares that 'health care'. (Remember that when we talk about justice the word *good* is a thing or concept—not an adjective.)

Many people would think about 'health' or 'life' or 'quality of life' or 'health care' or 'treatment' as a 'good' in health care. Aiming to make the 'good' available may be expressed pragmatically, and with value judgments such as 'when needed' or 'when available' or 'when reasonable' or 'shared equally'.

Thinking about how the way services are delivered shows us what sort of distribution is in action. If your health care institution has a queue system, or waiting times before a booking can be made, some ordering of patients is happening behind the scenes, before you, as a health practitioner or health care worker, even see them.

Before you can decide what is reasonable, you need to know how large the pool of resources is, including the source of funding that fuels the system, and what and who else requires resources from the pool. The legal and regulatory framework will provide a clue, as it defines how funding is drawn in to the pool, and who is entitled to access benefits. The question of who decides on how to prioritise resources is also a crucial justice question. Again, ethics can help here, by providing choices of distribution models that are compatible with certain ethics frameworks.

Your own idea of when you are available to work makes a difference to the type of work that you will do. Is 2 a.m. within your idea of proper availability of services? If it is, do you work that shift because your view is that that service should be available? Examining your own individual commitment to the type and availability of services that will be provided becomes part of the system. After all, a system is made up of many people like you who have chosen to become health care professionals. Ethics can help with these difficult questions, by examining the good that is aimed for and the models of justice that guide the distribution of that good.

Doing good is the basic premise of being beneficent—of caring. To 'do good' requires understanding what 'good' is, and then acting to the extent of your responsibility to that good. It is an active obligation. In simple terms, questions of individual client care, and doing good for them, come under the concept or principle of beneficence. The community obligation that is part of beneficence is also related to the principle of justice, in that it is about questions of the distribution of—and access to—health care.

Each profession has its own definition of 'a good'. For example, depending on the profession, a good might be:

- the preservation of life—for an obstetrician or midwife
- an 'easy death'—for a palliative care specialist
- 'quality of life'—for a rehabilitation team.

Getting consensus on what a good is—within a profession, or group of professions in the one system—is the first step in deciding reasonable beneficence responsibilities. Since that good must then be distributed, this consensus is important in deciding responsibilities concerning justice. The definition arrived at is an ideal, so while the good might not be achieved all the time, the ethical position is to continue to aim for it, thus maximising the possibility of doing good and minimising the possibility of doing harm.

Applying the concept of good, whether it is an absolute or decent minimum, is an illustration of the breadth of responsibilities that health care professionals undertake to do good. Many codes of ethics mention acting in the patient's or client's best interests, and furthering the health of the community. A professional's responsibility is not only to treat each client, but also to ensure that others have the opportunity to be similarly treated. In other words, the individual treatment that a professional gives to their client should not compromise the availability of such treatment to others.

All health care workers are part of the team that goes about distributing health resources on behalf of the community. At some point, it would be useful to reflect on the model of distribution that is applied where you work. Taking time to think about how the organisation is set up will inform your reflection on any difficulties you face in securing resources, or in making your idea of a health service a reality for your clients.

The way resources, or 'goods', are distributed is a justice concern. You will remember the definition of the principles of beneficence, non-maleficence, autonomy (or respect for persons) and justice from Chapter 1. The idea of justice has many underlying assumptions. Generally speaking, it is about the fair distribution of burden and benefit. How you think about justice depends on your values and what you think health care should achieve.

If you are to remain responsible by world standards, you may also need to check now and then that your approach to caring is consistent with the expectations expressed in international documents about human rights. Those expectations can appear to be quite stringent, and you should remember to check the definition of the 'good' as well as the way it would be distributed.

health
State of physical, mental and social wellbeing.

The World Health Organization (WHO) has defined **health** as 'a state of complete physical, mental, and social wellbeing and not merely the absence of disease or infirmity'. WHO's health goal for your clients and potential clients—which is essentially the good we should all be striving for—is expressed in the preamble to WHO's constitution: 'The enjoyment of the highest attainable standard of health is one of the fundamental rights of every human being without distinction of race, religion, political belief, economic or social condition'. At the start of the twenty-first century these objectives were viewed as ambitious, but they are used as a guiding mandate to tackle issues such as the preventable transmission of human immunodeficiency virus (HIV), malaria and tuberculosis and, more recently, to contain and track potentially pandemic influenza, as well as to seek attainable improvements in basic living conditions and health care access for all people (World Health Organization, 1976, p. 1).

REFLECTION: DEVELOPMENT OF A SERVICE

Pick a good that your profession offers, and trace its development and availability, as well as any regulations that promote or restrict its availability. This will make you revisit what your profession sees as a good, and how the potential for achieving that good is balanced against, on the one hand, possible harms, and on the other hand, the need to gather and deploy the resources necessary and available in society to aid its development and accessibility.

As you find out about your good, think about what it means for your commitment as a health care professional to the principles of caring, doing no harm, respecting autonomy and fair distribution. You may find that the relative emphasis you place on each of these will change as you gather your factual material or understand some of the practical regulations a little more. You should feel confident in your developing understanding of regulation and the process of ethics analysis, particularly in thinking about trained and skilled professionals ready to provide care in health care contexts, responding to consumer requests and needs.

There are a number of philosophical choices to be made under the principle of justice, in deciding just how to distribute what is available. So the question is this: given the current pool of resources, how can we distribute what we have in an ethical manner? All health care workers struggle to provide 'a good', however they define it, in a context of competing claims on resources and seemingly diminishing pools of those resources.

The reality of modern health care is competing **claims** for goods in a finite system.

The three justice models discussed most often are:

- justice as fairness
- comparative justice
- distributive justice.

The models derive from the philosophical writings of three well-known philosophers and, as the discussion progresses, you will notice that each model has different ethical theories or frameworks supporting it. All these theories and frameworks are about what a society might regard as a fair distribution of limited resources that are in demand by the members of that society.

The philosopher John Rawls writes about the concept of **justice as fairness**, which is a concept of absolute equality and fairness. The model has been applied, by others, to health, and is the justice model that is closest to the WHO definition of health (Beauchamp & Childress,

claim
Implicit or explicit demand to receive a good, as one's due.

justice as fairness
Justice model of equality, in which goods are distributed with the aim that community members are restored to equivalent levels.

1994, p. 340). Disparate treatment based on the financial circumstances, race or other distinguishing features of those to whom services are being provided is unacceptable under the justice-as-fairness model. The justice-as-fairness model cuts across lines created by nations or regions: nationality or place of residence do not determine rights to health care. Under this model of justice, differential treatment is justified only to compensate for disadvantages suffered by some people. The aim is that all people should end up roughly equal.

Think about what limits your clients in achieving health. Should the health-care agenda include the removal of barriers to health?

Indigenous education models are now incorporating culture and community into a holistic approach to health. This is one example of services that aim to alleviate historically accrued disadvantages and barriers, as well as putting in place physical health measures in the pursuit of health. Culturally appropriate and quality services are supported, which have been developed collaboratively in response to needs of the Aboriginal community. The approach that is supported by Aboriginal communities is evident in submission documents and resources that have been developed within communities, including leading advocacy organisations such as the Victorian Aboriginal Child Care Agency (VACCA); see <www.vacca.org>. The essential aspect of collaboration is reflected in key government planning documents (Victorian Government, 2008).

comparative justice
Justice model of need, in which goods are distributed on the basis of demonstrated most need, compared with the demonstrated needs of other community members.

need
Demonstrated interest in receiving a good.

Comparative justice, as its name suggests, involves assessing the relative importance of people's interests in receiving the health resource. This is a compromise between justice as fairness, in which the ideal is providing treatment based on nothing else but **need**, and acknowledging the limited pool of resources from which to provide that treatment. The triage system of health care delivery is an example of the comparative justice model in action: need assessment is carried out and treatment is given accordingly. Minor complaints wait longer, and more serious cases are rushed to the head of the queue.

A type of triage system exists in our emergency/casualty departments. It also exists in our waiting lists for public hospital care. The following extract from policy guidelines on prioritising patients on elective waiting lists for surgery is an example of the assessment of need that is the key to the triage system. Emergency admissions are excluded from this, as they are assumed to take place immediately.

A referring doctor completes the recommendation for admission form, obtains the patient's consent, and assigns a clinical priority category. Categories 1, 2 and 3 are deemed 'ready for care'; Category 4 is deemed 'not yet ready':

> Category 1—'Admission desirable within 30 days for a condition that has the potential to deteriorate quickly to the point that it may become an emergency.'
> Category 2—'Admission within 90 days desirable for a condition which is not likely to deteriorate quickly or become an emergency.'
> Category 3—'Admission within 365 days acceptable for a condition which is unlikely to deteriorate quickly and which has little potential to become an emergency.'
> Category 4—'Patients who are either clinically not yet ready for admission (staged) and those who have deferred admission for personal reasons (deferred).'
> *(New South Wales Government, 2012)*

Note also that even on the day of surgery, operating time can be reallocated if more urgent cases present to the hospital. Less urgent cases can be asked to return another day.

The modern application of distributive justice often takes comparative justice one step further. It allocates resources not just on need, but on what our society regards as an appropriate distribution of benefits and burdens. **Distributive justice** is really just the broad societal consensus on how to allocate rights, duties, and burdens among community members (Dickens, 1994, p. 315). The important point is that the burden is distributed according to the ability of sections of society to cope with it, and the benefit is given to sections of society that need or deserve it. This means that need is not the only deciding factor.

There is also some sort of social assessment of worth and deservedness going on here. If Rawls's model is applied in this assessment, then 'distribution' is interpreted as 'justice as fairness' or 'equality'. In distributive justice, any social difference can be the discriminating feature that decides whether or not a service will be provided, or at what level it will be supplied. For example, resources could go to the wealthy, if we judge they deserve it, and less to minority groups. Or the wealthy could be asked to bear more cost burden for the same care. The distinctions made between different social groups highlight the contemporary political and social divisions of the society that applies this justice model. You might like to revisit some of the ethics theories in Chapter 4 to help you decide how best to make a societal judgment on who deserves what treatment.

distributive justice
Justice model of need and entitlement, in which goods are distributed based on demonstrated and comparative interest and entitlement to receive community benefits and the expectation or capacity to bear burden.

Ethics reflection on economic tools as part of planning

There are tools that have traditionally been used to decide if a service is worth offering, and if society can afford to make it available, by focusing on the likely benefit of the service, and then compare the benefit with the likely demand for the service, and the drain on available resources that offering the resource or service would cause.

Two of these tools are **cost-effectiveness analysis**, and **cost–benefit analysis**. Cost-effectiveness analysis compares alternative ways of achieving a specific set of objectives or outcomes. Cost-effectiveness analysis is being increasingly used to decide program rationing in large health systems, such as in the US system. Cost-benefit analysis compares the cost of a program with the expected benefits in dollars. The quantification of outcomes makes it controversial in health. It is hard to quantify improvement in health or lifestyle or life years in a financial sense. In public policy and economics, clearly defining the population is part of the analysis of the social and financial costs and benefits for that group of persons (Svensson, 2010, p. 275).

cost-effectiveness analysis
A comparative assessment of costs in achieving an agreed objective or beneficial outcome.

cost–benefit analysis
A calculation of the cost of delivering a service with demonstrated and calculated financial benefits.

REFLECTION: PREVENTIVE TESTING BUDGETS

The following discussion focuses on the decisions involved in funding and making a service available.

A famous ethics paper by Ubel and colleagues reported on a study that posed the following scenario to experts in medical ethics and medical decision making (Ubel et al., 1996, p. 1176). Consider their scenario. What do you think should happen?

The federal government has set up a program to test for colon cancer in people enrolled in Medicaid, a government program that offers health insurance to low-income people and their families. The test allows doctors to find colon cancer at an early stage. So far, the federal government has offered the test to people at high risk for colon cancer, and this has prevented many of them from dying of colon cancer. Now the government wants to offer the test to the rest of the people receiving Medicaid, all of whom are at equally low risk for colon cancer.

A group of doctors was formed to help the government decide which of two tests to offer the low-risk people:

• Test 1 is inexpensive but does not always detect cancers in their early stages.

• Test 2 is more expensive but is better at detecting early cancers.

The decision is complicated by budget limitations: the government only has a certain amount of money available to pay for the screening tests. After evaluating the costs and benefits of each test, the doctors have reached the following conclusions. The budget is just large enough to offer Test 1 to all the low-risk people. With this approach, everyone can receive the test, and 1000 deaths from colon cancer will be prevented. The budget is just large enough to offer Test 2 to half the low-risk people. With this approach, half the people can receive the test and half cannot, and 1100 deaths from colon cancer will be prevented.

The ethicists and decision makers who thought about this problem were told that if the second scenario were to be followed—offering Test 2 to half the low-risk people—the persons selected for screening would be randomly selected on the basis of their social-security numbers. The ethicists who responded to the survey were uneasy about the assumption underpinning cost-effectiveness analysis. The assumption was: 'it is best to maximize the total benefit per dollar spent, even if this is achieved by offering a health care intervention to only a portion of a population that might benefit from it'. They rejected the more effective test, in favour of making a test equally available to all potential recipients. In doing so they implicitly challenged the utilitarian basis of cost-effectiveness analysis—that is, achieving the greatest good for the greatest number.

One critic of this hypothetical pointed out that it did not consider the possibility of moving money across from other budgets to be able to deliver a better test to all the low-income Medicaid recipients (McCombs, 1996). This alternative is similar to rearranging budgets and budget priorities on a large scale, which you will try your hand at in an exercise later in this chapter.

The controversy associated with tools such as cost–benefit analysis and cost-effectiveness analysis is the way it requires decision makers to make value judgments about who—or which groups of people—should receive treatments. Its controversial nature is also because the decision of worth is made before the actual consumer or patient enters the treatment context. The decision is made at a different time—for example, when setting up the service—or is made hypothetically—for example, for the type of situation that any given patient might, one day be in.

An early experiment in limiting the costs of public health service programs was conducted in the US state of Oregon. The community was involved in the planning. Before decisions were made about how many of certain types of services should be offered to public patients, the community was asked to rate how successful these services were in adding quality life-years. The Oregon experiment in consultative rationing has been discussed at length elsewhere. The controversial aspects of the Oregon program have also been debated, such as:

- making health-outcome or quality life-years the focus
- considering the worth of the expected life-span
- making assumptions about the worth of health-care programs.

Two key figures in the Oregon experiment were Kitzhaber and Kemmy. This is how they describe their personal experience of the budget dilemma they faced:

> In the interim spring of 1986, a variety of factors combined to produce a budget shortfall of $35 million, and the E-Board took steps to bring the budget back into balance—among them, a decision to drop over 4300 Oregonians from state medical coverage.
>
> ... Not many months later, however, some of those human consequences began showing up in my emergency room—people who had delayed seeking timely treatment because they now had no way to pay for it.

Despite the controversy surrounding it—you will remember the controversial aspects of generalising quality of life considerations to a group of people from Chapter 5—the Oregon program was one of the first social programs to acknowledge the limitations that health budgets pose to the goal of achieving health for all.

However, the application of an economic tool is not the end of the matter, as how the reasoning is approached and whether the end result is acceptable can be the focus of ethics reflection. Each definition that is used in an analysis is also open to discussion and considered reflection. The definition of good that is chosen for the assessment in the next Reflection is a broad concept of 'good'—detecting cancer in the greatest number of people in a certain population (or subsection) of a population. This is the common approach of utilitarian analysis. A 'good' is defined, and the process of achieving that 'good' for the greatest number of a defined group is then designed with the primary objective being the desired purpose or outcome. The issue is: what testing process is most useful—or delivers maximum **utility**—for the express purpose of detecting cancer? So utility is a concept of usefulness, applied in a previously defined notion of benefit or good. Under utilitarianism,

utility
Quality of usefulness for a desired purpose or outcome.

defining the good and utility aimed at is essential. It is then maximised according to the overall aim of delivery to the greatest number of the recognised community or portion of the community that is agreed to be in potential need of such delivery. The effect on those who miss out is acknowledged, but that is deemed to be an acceptable part of the process of working towards the greater utilitarian outcome.

Balancing budgets around the world

While Medicare is federally budgeted and provides for certain services, state governments have their own budgets to run hospitals, including inpatient, outpatient and emergency services. State governments also provide numerous community and public health services, with a strong emphasis on health promotion and preventive health, and keeping people healthier, fitter—and out of hospitals. Medicare Agreements between states and the Commonwealth cover many services and pharmaceuticals used in the state-run public hospitals.

Medicare is not meant to be used to fund health services in instances when compensation for an injury may be claimed, or when medical bills will be the responsibility of the person who caused the injury. Exceptions are provided for emergency treatment, even if the injury stems from motor vehicle or work accidents in which compensation or insurance claims may be routinely sought. This applies to state service provision as well. Ambulance officers arriving on the scene of an accident need not worry about who will pay for the service. For instance, in New South Wales there is a bulk-billing arrangement in place for the authority—the State Insurance Regulatory Authority—under the *State Insurance and Care Governance Act 2015* (NSW), to make payments for conveying injured persons by ambulance, making it possible to institute essential care and transport patients to hospital immediately, for instance, in New South Wales, *Motor Accident Injuries Act 2017* (NSW), section 10.9. Emergency departments in hospitals receive the casualties with the same expectations.

Both state and federal government budgets are routinely publicly available. When tabled in Parliament, they provide an insight into what the current government's key objectives are in delivering health care, and how money is spent to achieve those objectives. Debating a budget for a service makes little sense unless the good that is trying to be achieved is also discussed.

INTEGRATED LEARNING AND PRACTICE

Isn't a budget just for economists and accountants to sort out?

Here are a few reasons to get involved in budgetary matters. The law can shape a budget by making some aspects of care a societal requirement rather than discretionary spending. Ethics reasoning can help to resolve difficult choices between competing claims, and maintain a fair system for the community. Policy opportunities are plentiful in a budget, as money on a line item can mean that a theoretical objective can become a practical reality. Of course, budgets work best when designed in partnership with economists and accountants.

The following Reflection exercise illustrates the breadth of one state government's health department budget. This exercise demonstrates the difficult budget decisions that must be made when resources become even more limited than usual, or when primary objectives change. Inevitably, some services lose money as that money is shifted to other services, or is cut from the budget entirely. This is a macro exercise: it steps away from individual treatment decisions and asks you to think about what resources the system—or large service units—has at their disposal. Once budget cuts or rearrangements are instituted, those running the services have to:

- examine the objectives of the service
- agree on how best to distribute what they have
- decide whether they can still provide the 'good' that they believe they are there to provide.

REFLECTION: BUDGETS AND PRIORITY DECISIONS

This exercise uses a budget for the provision of health infrastructure and services in the state public health sector.

TABLE 10.1 HEALTH PROGRAM BUDGET

New South Wales Department of Health, total budget 2018–2019	
Area	$ million
Acute and sub-acute health services	21 300
Outcome: Improved service in hospitals 'boosting and improving acute hospital services (such as emergency care and elective surgery), sub-acute patient services (such as rehabilitation and palliative care) and ambulance services'	
Mental health	2100
Outcome: Mentally healthy communities 'improving admitted and community-based mental health services'	
Community health services	1600
Outcome: Healthy resilient communities 'strategies to reduce childhood obesity and improve oral health, immunisation rates and health screening', 'expand drug and alcohol services', and increased post-natal visits (pp. 4–9)	
Health and medical research	115
Outcome: World-class research and innovation including grants, fellowships and scholarships, 'clinical trials initiatives and research ethics and governance improvement initiatives, including faster ethics approval (45 days) and research governance approval (15 days) in newly introduced outcome indicators (pp. 4–10)	

+ continued

New South Wales Department of Health, total budget 2018–2019	
Area	$ million
Independent advisory bodies	29
Outcome: Continuously improving health care, the Health Care Complaints Commission, 'protecting public health and safety by processing, assessing and resolving health care complaints', and the Mental Health Commission of New South Wales, 'working with government and the community to secure better mental health and wellbeing for everyone'	

(New South Wales Government, 2018, pp. 4-1–4-11)

Examine the budget and consider the ministerial directive that priorities should change slightly. Think about how to achieve these changes in priority without allocating additional money. You can move money, but you cannot add more. Before you start, adopt the role of stakeholder. Stakeholder roles can include:

- health professionals—for example, doctors, nurses and others
- consumers of health services/clients—for example, patient advocates, particular client groups
- planners—for example, chief executive officers, government representatives
- general community—for example, local councils, parents' groups.

You may be able to think of other stakeholders.

The hypothetical ministerial directive for this exercise is that, in the coming year, the focus should be on health promotion, integrated preventative services, home-based aged care, disability services and palliative care, and procedures should ideally be carried out in local day-surgery settings rather than in large metropolitan hospitals with pre-operation and post-operation overnight stays.

A budget rearrangement can be combined with the additional scenario of a forthcoming pay increase for nurses, and a pay decrease for visiting medical officers (a similar exercise is found in an early ethics text) (Mitchell & Lovat, 1991, p. 136), or a proposed increase in staffing and a better staff–patient ratio in community health service settings, but keeping pay levels steady.

If you consider staffing and staff ratios, you might like to check the legislative requirements in any such as nurse to patient ratios, such as those found in Victoria in the *Safe Patient Care (Nurse to Patient and Midwife to Patient Ratios) Act 2015* (Vic), or the staff ratios policies within institutions.

This exercise prompts you to find out the objectives of each program, the good each is aiming for, and to consider them before budgets are rearranged. The detailed objectives can be found in the parliamentary papers (New South Wales Government, 2018, pp. 4-1-11; Health Cluster at Chapter 4).

Some health care workers are very uncomfortable about justice decisions being made that affect their treatment decisions about individual clients, but others are less so. It could be argued that the duty to care for the individual client is paramount, and therefore should not be subject to broad budgetary discussions. On the other hand, with a limited resource, health professionals' obligations are also to other potential clients whom they have not yet met, but who might walk through the door and need treatment in the near future. That is why professional codes of ethics emphasise duty to society as well as duty to the individual client, as read in Chapter 1, and as you found when you analysed a professional code of conduct or code of ethics using Beauchamp and Childress's principles. The modern business of health care forces you to consider others as well as those whose health needs are right in front of you.

In the UK, basic universal health care is available. Limited resources, rationing and managed care—and therefore limitations on the funds available to specific regions—have been a reality for over 20 years. GPs play a central role in fund holding and managing and integrating care with other services providers, such as NHS staff in community and social care services. British GPs are contracted to:

- manage essential services
- provide services during core hours
- manage their listed patients and temporary residents who are ill and expected to recover, or who are suffering from chronic disease or terminal conditions.

This behaviour is prescribed under a regulation, *The National Health Service (General Medical Services Contracts) Regulations 2004* (Addicott & Ham, 2014, p. 10). Patients 'join' a practice as a patient, and they do not have the flexibility of attending multiple practices for their primary care. Early in the NHS initiative, GPs became the 'commissioners' of services for their local populations (Mannion, 2011). Of course, not all GPs wanted this funding responsibility, as the time and financial responsibility involved was considerable.

Throughout the system refinements, there has been an early and ongoing concern that the UK system harboured inequality (*Lancet*, 1997). General practices are sharing their expertise and pooling their resources (Addicott & Ham, 2014, p. 23). How a system is funded and structured can challenge the way individual health care professionals relate to clients, as has also been debated elsewhere.

When District Health Boards in New Zealand began to organise the public funding and provision of health, public health and disability services, and district budget holding was trialled, there was a concern that the health professional needed to have good, coordinated information available to protect the clients and their interests in an increasingly competitive environment (New Zealand Medical Association, 1994, p. 13). The Association of Salaried Medical Professionals in New Zealand stressed the importance of the 'internal morality' of professionals, who strive to provide the best health care they can under different budget constraints and externally imposed limits, and through times of changing structures and systems (Powell, 2005). Parliamentary papers reported on subsequent reform processes and by the health department (New Zealand Parliament, 2009; <http://health.govt.nz>). The District Health Boards in New Zealand now own and fund the public hospitals in their area.

Private insurance is also part of our Australian two-tiered system. Considering the coverage in private care highlights the funding and billing issues in a defined pool of resources that is to be shared among the community members who have joined and contribute to the health care fund.

You may remember Monica's journey in Chapter 5, and you could look back to that story to think further about the gap between what is covered by a private (or public) health fund, and what is leftover for the patient to pay—in addition to their private health fund premiums.

In the USA, a managed care system is quite common, as many patients are insured with managed care providers. Defining entitlement is clearly a requirement before any care is received. Managed funds share money from the funding pot of the insurance provider, and very low income earners are granted access to public monies if they become entitled by satisfying certain residential and income requirements. Different models of managed care can place the rationing decision with one primary provider—usually medical or nursing staff—who then coordinates their own service provision with the services of other professionals. A number of models that help determine who should exercise that rationing decision have been proposed. In all these models, the value of the personal provider–client relationship remains extremely important (Urbina et al., 1997). Professionals strive for the best possible care for all clients under their ambit and care. To reflect from the patient's perspective, each person may be wondering:

- am I in the community that is provided for by that specific funding?
- can I expect that my request for the funding of my care will be seen as an equitable and affordable use of the funds?

Try the following Reflection which prompts you to think about personal need and entitlement in the context of the specific community that a person belongs to.

REFLECTION: PUBLIC PURSE AND DWINDLING PERSONAL ASSETS

Imagine that your uncle is quite ill and may need long-term nursing care. He lives in a small town in the USA. Most of his money is tied up in his house, which he shares with his wife. His children have grown up and left home. The couople worry about how the nursing care is to be paid for. One of your cousins secretly worries that there will be little left to care for their stepmother in her old age, much less any inheritance for the children or grandchildren.

All of your uncle's joint cash savings have been used up in his convalescence from a fall injury and a worsening heart condition. He is still quite weak and unable to care for himself. His wife is also elderly and has health problems, so is unable to care for him at home by herself. Your uncle wants to return home, and worries about the nursing home fees, which will slowly whittle away the nest egg of stocks he had hoped to pass on to his children. He worries that even the house may have to be sold if he is in a nursing home for much longer, as the bills keep coming in.

The difficulty is that the US national insurance Medicare can cover hospital costs for seniors, but not long-term care costs, and the state government cover for the poor and permanently disabled can only apply once assets and income are both reduced.

What would you suggest be done ethically? Also consider legal and regulatory responsibilities. What sort of official declarations of financial need could you honestly document? Many administrative forms, like tax returns, involve a statement of honest belief of the accuracy of answers given to public authorities.

A gatekeeper in managed fund arrangements is effectively positioned between the provider and the patient, and the question of community and equitable entitlement questions will be answered before care commences.

Hospitals can be nominated as care providers by insurers, and they negotiate contracts for reimbursement for care provided. These contract negotiations can be heated and difficult, as hospitals seek to ensure they have sufficient funds to cover anticipated care costs properly. The large US government-funded plan for very low income earners (Medicare—which is not to be confused with the Australian universal scheme of the same name), once provided a buffer for hospitals as contracted care providers, but a context of falling Medicare rates, tighter margins with insurance contracts, and a continuing backlash against managed care developed (Benko & Bellandi, 2001).

The US largely private health insurance system was the forerunner in practices being nominated as providers of 'capitation contracts' to provide care for certain insured people. The physician needed to balance both individual care and care costs—including those generated in a setting and those outsourced through referral. When asked about their practice in a managed care setting for a study in the USA (Pearson et al., 2002), many physicians expressed concerns about:

- the request for referral or use of outside care
- when to authorise treatments that would help, perhaps more 'socially' than medically
- patients' requests for specific treatments that may be expensive and that may require specific criteria to justify the expense under a managed care plan
- feeling pressured to provide services outside their own level of expertise
- wanting to give additional service, advice or supply of goods for free, but feeling obliged to limit expenses for the sake of the practice.

These comments remain relevant today, reflecting the tension in being a care provider and budget holder. The managed care or coordinated care system, however it is formulated for each community or group within a community, relies on 'trust' that pursuing the best possible care for each patient is the shared aim of the carer, the health service and the funder. Managed care members interviewed by researchers have spoken about how important it is to have trust in the doctor, and also trust in the hospital and, now, trust in the insurer, that best possible care will be made available (Dorr et al., 2002).

Working in managed care brings into sharp focus decisions like drug prescriptions, hospital admission, referrals and use of affiliated resources. The limited referral process—or more strictly controlled and budgeted referral process—can mean waiting lists and longer waiting times for patients to access those secondary services.

The 'budgets' that have to be balanced can be at area level or, in the US system, at insurance coverage level. The different style of practice implicit in this organisation of care delivery began to be taught routinely in resident training in the USA. The case discussions during rounds involved clinical issues, but also issues of referral that could lead to resource-use problems. Residents can expect use of expensive procedures and specialty referrals to be scrutinised (Gomez et al., 1997). This is clearly a different style of practice from that focused solely on maximal care of individuals using any or all available technology and resources.

Asch and Ubel have also described the way that, under the managed care system operating in the USA, doctors could feel forced to take responsibility for choosing the cheapest treatment that accords with the 'standard of care' set by the managed care policy. They described how the government 'caps' (or puts a limit on) the costs of particular services; this forced the physician to think beyond the individual client, appeal to the 'standard of care' (which, in most cases, is the most commonly used treatment rather than the best), and, finally, make do with less than the best, unless other options have failed (Ash & Ubel, 1997, p. 1670).

REFLECTION POINT

Primary care decisions

GPs in a budget-holding context in the UK are encouraged to prescribe generic drugs whenever possible rather than brand-name drugs. Those prescribing brand names consistently are 'visited' by representatives of the budget team for their area to try to encourage more cost-effective patterns of prescribing.

1   What should the GPs be asked to do? What should the GPs' response be?

2   Set out your reasons, and then explain them to a colleague or friend.

In a similar funding problem discussion, in Thailand, a set affordable contribution was sought from patients for each treatment, and then the local hospital covers all further treatment costs. There was controversy over the 30-baht health care scheme, when referral to tertiary care specialist or intensive treatment facilities for complex or chronic conditions was likely to be costly, and some local hospitals were reportedly reluctant to refer their patients for that further treatment (Lyall, 2002).

In Australia, various initiatives have been trialled that encourage coordination and care planning that goes beyond episodic service provision. The early trials focused on care management and budget coordination for high-service clients, such as elderly persons with dementia, who are unable to manage their own care in the current system. The focus was on complex and chronic conditions, which, by their nature, consume enormous amounts of the health budget—particularly chronic asthma, diabetes and heart conditions—as well as for people in Aboriginal communities with chronic disease issues (Commonwealth Department of Health and Ageing, 2000). For Australian veterans, widows or their dependants, care is provided by the Commonwealth Department of Veterans' Affairs. For those who have complex care needs, one or more chronic conditions and who are at risk of being admitted or readmitted to hospital, a form of coordinated care is in place—rather than managed care—in the Coordinated Veterans' Care (CVC) Program. Additional funds beyond that available under Medicare are provided so that a GP and nurse coordinator are able to coordinate ongoing care, and encourage participants to self-manage care coordination. Professional associations, including those for nurses, actively support their members participating and training for their roles in the CVC program (Australian Nursing & Midwifery Federation, 2017).

The aim of any system of care is to reduce error and inappropriate or wasted services, improving quality and effectiveness so that the maximum benefit can be achieved with the pool of resources available. Each professional will need to make practical ethical choices when they are working within a finite system.

Fidelity or loyalty

PRACTICE EXAMPLE

Jennifer Haines

Jennifer has been a Registered Nurse for 40 years and spent most of those years practising in critical care areas, ICU, CCU, Neurosurgery ICU and Emergency Department.

Fidelity is the obligation of an individual to be faithful to commitments made to themselves, and also to others.

In health care, nurses are expected to be faithful and loyal to the profession of nursing, and this includes loyalty to agreements and responsibilities accepted as part of the profession. But nurses can also be expected to be loyal employees of their employer—as required in industrial law. What happens when a nurse faces a clash of loyalties? Which comes first?

For example, if a nurse works in a ward or unit where there is chronic understaffing that is affecting the standards of patient care, what should the nurse do? To whom does the nurse owe their primary loyalty here? If the nurse chooses the employer, they may continue to work in a ward where they can see that patients are being hurt by not receiving the care that they should. If they choose their loyalty to their profession and its standards they may face disciplinary action by the employer.

Which would you choose: loyalty to the employer? Or loyalty to the profession?

Interests and entitlement

Once a system is in place, and is mandated by the institution in which you work, the real question for you as a professional health care worker is: what discretion do you have in applying that model? When professionals disagree violently with the model that seems to be operating, they may decide to protest. Our health care history is replete with examples of professionals protesting about the resources provided for them to get their job done, or about the way in which some types of treatment seem to be undertaken (or some clients treated) but not others. Patient groups too can voice dissatisfaction with how resources are shared, how some treatments are developed and others not, and how long it seems to take for their health care needs to be met. The concerns can demonstrate a clash between individual autonomy and a community concept of fair distribution, under justice.

In an everyday setting, we live with queues. We queue at the bus, we queue at a café, we queue at various offices, and so on. So, what if we jump the queue? Are we 'entitled' to, or not? Think about how you feel if people jump queues. Also, if you have ever jumped a queue, think about why you felt entitled you to do that. Was it your need? Or was it some other deservedness? You will probably find that the social agreement of waiting in line for a resource that everyone is waiting for is an accepted one, but that there are certain exceptions that people may feel justifies allowing others to go the head of the queue.

Justice has at its heart our everyday sense of ethics of what we should do, and how we should behave towards one another, in taking our share of community resources or ensuring others are able to benefit from their share of community resources. You could consider the issue from the patient's perspective by raising similar reflective questions. Remember: the answers could be quite different in a context that is different to the one that you are used to—such as in a developing country, or in a situation of crisis.

REFLECTION: EVER PRESENT QUESTIONS TO CONSIDER

Consider these reflective questions as you read further:

- What community am I in?
- Can my community help me with health care?
- What sort of health care is available to me?
- What do I owe my community in return as part of my duties of belonging?

right
Claim that is recognised as imposing obligations on others to fulfil it.

interest
That which is to one's advantage or benefit.

You may decide that acting beneficently is only required when someone has a **right** to whatever good you would be promoting. You would be correct, because there is a difference between rights and **interests**. That can be illustrated fairly easily, with an exercise that works best in a group. First, ask 'Who owns a car?' Many hands will probably go up. The rest of the group may have an interest in those cars, but they don't necessarily have a right to them ... or do they? The people with the goods—the cars—might be caring for others by giving their cars to people without them, but is that an obligation? Ask the people with the cars, 'Who would give their car to someone who doesn't have one?' Wait, and watch the hands disappear. So, what interests are reasonable? Perhaps if I told you that I want your car so that I can get to work more easily, or so I can get to university to study, you might feel swayed. Can I have it? I have shown you a good reason why I want it. I have asked, and made my autonomous decision clear. Do you have a duty to give the car to me?

Under our current societal structure, the answer to this question is 'probably not', and the same applies to whatever else I ask for, unless there is model of justice operating that obliges you to fulfil that wish or want. (You read about wishes and autonomy in earlier chapters.) If I were to take your car, I might be depriving your similar interest to get to work or to university. There is also the consideration that you have probably earned the car by buying it. However, all is not lost. Society does acknowledge my interest in coming to work, or university, and makes public transport available at a reasonable cost. There are some human rights agreements—for example, the United Nations *Convention on the Rights of the Child*—reflecting a commitment to education as a basic right, but only to the level of a decent minimum of primary school level, with encouragement for states to develop different forms of secondary education (United Nations, 1990). Studying or working is seen as a good, so my interest in pursuing that is reasonable, but getting there quickly or more conveniently may not be pursued to the exclusion of others' interests. There is a similar limit to obligations relating to beneficence in health care. Like access to education, it is thought that we only have a right to certain levels of care; beyond those levels our right becomes an interest only.

Thinking about an everyday ethics issue of what is owing (or due) to you, can help you to distinguish between rights and interests.

REFLECTION: EVERYDAY RIGHTS, INTERESTS AND DUTIES

Imagine that Sally is out shopping with her two primary school-aged children. They return to their car in the shopping centre car park to put their shopping in the car and head home. They are surprised to see, lying on the ground, neatly behind their car boot, two absolutely brand new $20 notes. No one else is in sight in the car park. They are really in a rush, hoping to be home within a few minutes to get ready for an activity that afternoon.

Well, two children, two notes, you think, and that $20 is a lot of money in the eyes of the two children. So what should Sally do? It clearly is an opportunity to think about whether the children should claim the money as their own. What would you allow them to do, or would you even keep the $40 as your own, being the adult?

Sally asked the children how they thought the person who had lost it would be feeling. They then thought about the options: keep it, look around for the person who might just have dropped it then keep it if they can't find them, or go and hand it in to the centre's lost property to see if the owner contacted the office. They agreed on the latter, with parental encouragement, but not enforcement, from Sally. She tried to impart the values of honesty during the process, along with the idea that doing what restores the money to the other person is really reward enough.

The money was handed in to an impressed manager, who flattered the children with praise for their action. There was also an offer by the manager that, in keeping with the centre policy, if it was not claimed by the rightful owner within a week, she would contact the children as the new owners. It was actually picked up that afternoon by an elderly shopper who had rung in, quite distressed about the loss. The children were called by the manager to pass on the grateful thanks of the owner of the money, who

+ continued

had then been able to do her shopping with that money. The owner had also expressed her renewed faith in the honesty of the young people of today.

Try to identify the values that were evident in the process. Try also to identify why an interest in keeping the money was not necessarily a right of 'finders-keepers'.

Now, try to analyse another everyday situation. After having a quick lunch at a café, you line up to pay your bill. It is very busy, and the crowd around the till is restless, with many people in a hurry to get back to work. The cashier seems flustered. When your turn to pay comes up, you give your table number. The cashier reaches for the details of what you ordered, as written on the waiter's order notebook, and asks you for $14.50. This is substantially less than what you have just eaten, having had an extra order of dessert and then coffee, which on your quick calculation hasn't been added to the bill. What should you do? Should you pay just what is asked, or disagree with what is asked and suggest paying more?

Try to examine the issues of rights, interests and duties from the perspectives of yourself as patron, the waiter, the cashier, and the café owners, before you make your decision.

You could also think back to the legal issues covered in Chapter 3. Consider whether there is a contractual duty as a consumer to pay the full amount of what you have ordered and had supplied to you. Consider your general professional responsibility to act in a way that upholds the reputation of the profession, which you read about in Chapter 2. What would be the expectation of the public for your conduct?

As you work your way through this chapter, return to this exercise to see if your reading helps you to further unravel the complex interplay of roles and duties.

As a general guiding rule, when there is strong agreement that service obligations are mandated, that service will be a right. When there appears to be considerable discretion about whether or not to provide the service, the service is meeting a strong interest (or claim)—not a right.

Raanon Gillon has noted the difference between institutional and moral rights: institutional rights are simply claims that have been justified. The institution can decide, collectively, to grant such things as free medical care, but equally it may take those things away. On the other hand, moral rights cannot be taken away. Gillon also notes that only some rights impose obligations on others to act in a particular way (Gillon, 1986, pp. 54–8.). This distinction between rights that impose obligations and those that don't is not new to the field of law, which tries to clarify which of our obligations are contractual, and therefore enforceable, and which are merely goodwill. Jurist and theorist, W.N. Hohfeld, outlined the difference between wishes, or liberties and 'claim-rights'. Claim-rights imply an obligation on others to satisfy those claims, but wishes, or liberties, do not (Devereux, 2002, pp. 450–2). Daniel Callahan, an eminent US ethicist, also notes that there are limits to our ability to satisfy health interests. He argues that before we talk in terms of health rights, we must re-examine the fundamental goals of medicine—paying particular attention to how realistic and affordable those goals are—and that countries must meet agreed-upon goals (Callahan, 1996).

The two-tiered nature of the Australian health care system reflects this division of health care into 'rights' and 'interests'. There is a publicly funded, government-provided sector and a privately funded, privately provided sector. While these are designed to operate in parallel, there is constant debate about what should be publicly available, and how much public provision should be available to those who can afford private care. In some countries, such as Australia and England, publicly funded care is available to all, regardless of income, with automatic cover for many aspects of basic, or decent, minimum health care but not for 'extras' like private rooms in hospital or patient choice of doctor. Patients who are not privately covered must pay for extras somehow. Thus, we could say that the minimum publicly covered care is considered a right within the community, but this does not extend to the 'extras'.

To complicate this further, some people in a community may not seem 'entitled' to access care at all, so have no **entitlement**. Usually, before people become your patients, they have been deemed to be 'eligible' to be treated in some way. So, in a clinic, they might be eligible to receive publicly funded care. In a private practice, they may be 'covered' by insurance or public funding, or both. Or they may be in a position to pay the full cost. Try to imagine a situation in which a person is not entitled to access subsidised health care (in a given community) and does not have the resources to pay the fee upfront before receiving care. This is the situation for people in the USA who are caught between government-subsidised health coverage for the very poor and employer-subsidised coverage for middle to upper income earners. Their interest is in being treated, but is it their right? Illegal immigrants are in an invidious position of not having joined a community officially, and not having access to that community's health care. Despite universal basic health coverage provided in many countries, the public system is for citizens and residents, and not necessarily for those with pending visa decisions or certain visas. Some visas restrict rights to work, and also restrict access to the Commonwealth-funded Medicare.

entitlement
Recognised need to create community obligation to fulfil interest or claim.

States can make separate decisions on behalf of their own community and, in practice, each jurisdiction decides the level of access to their health services that they will afford to those on temporary visas. For instance, in Victoria, special access arrangements and funding has been afforded to asylum seekers who have arrived into the country and are living in the community or are being held in community detention facilities pending an administrative decision on an application for a protection visa, so that they can access some services such as hospitals and community health services.

The community detention guidelines state:

> Community detention (residence determination) was introduced in June 2005 and is a form of immigration detention that enables people to reside in the community without needing to be escorted. Community detention does not give a person any lawful status in Australia, nor does it give them the rights and entitlements of a person living in the community on a visa (for example, the right to study or work).
>
> Community detention clients are informed of the conditions of their community detention arrangements upon entry into the program. Conditions include a mandatory requirement to report regularly to the Commonwealth Department of Immigration and Citizenship (DIAC) and/or their service provider, and reside at the address specified by the minister.

(State Government of Victoria, 2011)

The guidelines explain the position and ongoing discussion between the governments on the issue:

> Under current arrangements with the Commonwealth, Victorian public hospitals provide some health services to people in immigration detention under a full cost recovery model (including hospital care and ambulance transport). The Victorian Department of Health is currently in discussions with the Commonwealth to expand this arrangement to include people living in community detention.
>
> International Health and Medical Services (IHMS) has been contracted by DIAC to arrange and provide health services to people in immigration detention, including community detention. As such, IHMS has established a network of health service providers across the state to provide necessary health services. People living in community detention have access to this network of health service providers through IHMS. If a community detention client presents to any Victorian public health service to access the services listed below, DIAC will reimburse the Victorian state funded service provider on a fee-for-service basis.
>
> *(State Government of Victoria, 2011)*

The Victorian Government (2011) states in the *Guide to Asylum Seeker Access to Health and Community Services in Victoria*:

> Asylum seekers are eligible for most health and community services funded by the Victorian government, such as community health services and the Home and Community Care program, as eligibility for most services is not determined by visa or residency status. However asylum seekers without access to Medicare often have difficulty accessing services that ordinarily require a Medicare card. It is also important to note that no asylum seekers have access to a Health Care Card and so often face financial difficulties meeting out-of-pocket health expenses for items such as pharmaceuticals.

Asylum seekers in Victoria have special access arrangements for the following services:

- Public hospital services
- Ambulance services in emergency situations
- Community health and Home and Community Care Program services
- Dental services
- Catch-up immunisation
- Other Victorian government programs for which asylum seekers have special access.

The Guide then sets out the practical arrangements, such as the following for public hospital services:

> Medicare ineligible asylum seekers are to be provided full medical care (including emergency and elective) including pathology, diagnostic, pharmaceutical and other services in Victorian hospitals as either admitted patients or non-admitted patients. Medicare ineligible asylum seekers are not to be billed, except in situations where they receive the following services as non-admitted patients:
>
> - spectacles and hearing aids
> - surgical supplies

- prostheses
- aids, appliances and home modifications for the first 30 days post discharge until they are eligible for the Department of Human Services' Aids and Equipment Program ...
- pharmaceuticals:
  - Note: these should be billed at a level consistent with the Pharmaceutical Benefits Scheme statutory copayments.
  - Note: a co-payment for prescriptions to treat tuberculosis should not be charged.
  - Victorian hospitals may bill Medicare ineligible asylum seekers for pharmaceuticals supplied to admitted patients upon separation.

While this describes the minimum standard of health service provision, hospitals at their own discretion may choose to provide an extended level of service to Medicare ineligible asylum seekers where appropriate.

(State Government of Victoria, 2011)

This means that the State of Victoria has decided to extend health care entitlements, and to also allow hospital services to make a further discretionary decision if they deliver services that are not funded by either the Commonwealth or state governments. Local areas can exercise discretion if their budget allows.

CASE EXAMPLE

Current guidelines and regulation

Think back to the Case example 'Seeking a safe haven' on p. 308. Prepare to elaborate on the information you could provide—and perhaps even alter your advice—for the family seeking asylum in Australia.

Check if these guidelines, or one of the other regulations you read earlier in this chapter, are still the same or if they have been updated. Compare them to guidance in one other jurisdiction.

Note in your own words why checking current guidelines in your jurisdiction is important.

So, the right to access health care is not granted to all. It depends on membership of the community that holds the resources for distribution. Illegal immigrants are in a dubious position in every country that provides care on the basis of right of recognised citizens to access care. The international responsibilities to afford basic human rights to persons classed as refugees in their territory—including facilitation of access to welfare services, which includes access to welfare afforded by non-government organisations—as set out in the international conventions such as the United Nations *Convention and Protocol Relating to the Status of Refugees*, are implemented at the discretion of each country in a way they decide they can afford (United Nations, 1951, 1967). Classifying a person as a refugee is the first step in relying on these international obligations. Under the Convention, refugees should not be penalised for illegal entry or stay in a country.

Medical treatment after life-threatening injury is, under our current system, a near absolute right because life itself is threatened, and our concept of an interest to health holds our right to life to be fundamental. However, we may not have such an absolute right to receive counselling after injury because—although it could be argued to be essential to recovering a decent minimum of health—it may not be available in places that are convenient to the client, or at hours that suit them perfectly. It may even be left to state or regional bodies to decide how much of a right or interest counselling is. Distinctions between rights and interests can also be illustrated by considering prevention and innovative or costly treatment issues. Advice on diet to prevent heart disease is a good that is so fundamental to health that it is currently seen as a right in Western countries; publicly funded dietary advice begins in early childhood clinics and at primary school. In contrast, transplant of a diseased heart is not seen as a right; we know this because this treatment option is not made available to all. Looking into the future, a life-saving organ transplant may one day be seen as a 'right'— provided sufficient organs are available—but repeated organ transplants may not.

Availability and distribution of a human resource

From time to time you will notice interesting community debates on whether individuals should opt in or opt out of their organs being available for organ donation to others in the event that they die. Consent processes used to be routinely built into driver's licence registration because of the practical context of sudden accident and death in motor vehicles. Many countries use the renewal of a licence as an opportunity to invite a person to indicate a positive hypothetical decision that they would be prepared to have their organs donated. This then forms the basis of discussion with family members if they are called to a hospital and learn that a person has passed away or is close to passing away. An opt-in process emphasises the importance of an individual's autonomous preferences over their own body. Families can still then decline, and are more likely to do so if they do not know their loved one's wishes.

Australia has an opt-in system, with a national register for people wishing to donate organs to record their consent, the Australian Organ Donor Register, administered by the Department of Human Services. In a coordinated national approach, authorised medical personnel can check this register to see if a person has given consent, and which organs and tissues that person wished to donate, such as heart, lung, kidney, liver, pancreas, pancreas islet, intestines, eye tissue, bone, skin and heart tissue such as valves. As well as registering online, people can also register through Medicare. Families are asked to confirm this decision, so talking to next of kin and families is a crucial part of expressing this hypothetical wish and ensuring it is known to others (Australian Government, 2017). South Australia maintains a driver's licence consent process (Government of South Australia, 2017). Theoretically at least, and putting logistics of transport and timeliness to one side, if a national system is used, the availability of organs would be anticipated to be to everyone in need nationally, the Australian community, rather than to primarily those within a particular state.

In the UK, the British Medical Association (BMA) has supported a soft opt-out system for organ donation, 'with safeguards for organ donation, as we believe this is the best option for the UK to reduce the shortage of organs and save lives' (BMA, 2017). The BMA highlight the latest government developments on their website: that Wales already has an opt-out system, and people are treated as having given consent for donation for organs and tissues unless they register otherwise. Scotland has committed to similar legislation. At the end of 2017, the Prime Minister Theresa May announced an intention for England to adopt similar provisions. The BMA planned to continue its lobbying for an opt-out system in Northern Ireland (BMA, 2017). The media discussion that ensued in the UK noted that the current opt-in system had prospective donors registering and holding an NHS Organ Donor Card, and that an opt-out system would presume permission to use an adult's body for transplant purposes, with the 'soft' proviso that it would not go ahead if a family objected. A consultation process was planned through the Department of Health (BBC, 2017). Singapore, Israel and some European countries—including Croatia, Spain, Norway, Portugal, France, Sweden, Italy and Finland—have had an opt-out system for decades. It is recognised that appropriate transplantation facilities are also needed to translate organ donation into high rates of transplants in practice (Brennan, 2015).

If the consultation in England demonstrates stakeholder and community support, regulations would then effect this change—provided it is also supported by parliament—with debate and discussion at grassroots stakeholder and community representative levels, which are essential to clearly defining what is acceptable in the community. If an opt-out process is implemented, it would show that the community views each organ as a potential community resource that may be distributed as needed after it is no longer needed by the individual who has died. If an opt-out system is adopted in the UK, it arguably emphasises justice and resource distribution of the defined 'good' of community resource of organs over the principle of autonomy.

REFLECTION POINT

Defining the interests in organs further

Organ donation is closely related to the ownership of bodily tissue after death. The discussion in Chapter 9 'Timeless quandaries at the beginning and end of life' will be helpful if you would like to think further about the legal status of one's own organs. You could consider if it is a personal interest in autonomy that is in conflict with justice if no consent or preference is sought before distribution of organs, or if the dilemma illustrates a clash of public interests (such as you read about in the availability of personal information for research purposes).

We have grown used to looking back on earlier health care as characterised by paternalistic beneficence. We may look back on the 1980s as the decade of autonomy. In the 1990s, our enthusiasm for patient and client autonomy was tempered, and the financial realities of the modern times have brought into sharper focus the limited availability of resources for public funding. The new kind of beneficence imposed by the system—and then practised by health care professionals—is increasingly limiting the available client choices, as the health care professions and the surrounding regulatory system impose limits on client wishes according to which wishes they are comfortable with and are able to grant. In the modern health care context of stretched resources and fluctuating financial situations, justice concerns were predicted to dominate health care ethics in this century (Berglund, 1997). In the context of global financial uncertainty, that trend of budgeted and managed care is set to continue. The restrictions are posed either by the public purse-holder or the private fund manager, with similar effect—limitation on complete patient autonomy. Care is delivered and received in context that recognises health resources as a valuable asset to be conserved and used wisely.

REFLECTION: LOOKING BACK

Now is the time to look back to how you felt at the start of your learning on law, regulation and ethics. Write down how you feel now.

Your learning will continue to develop, and you will be extended as you face challenging and complex issues in your work, so keeping a reflective portfolio going is a handy way of capturing your thoughts as it allows you to look back to these thoughts at any time. Many people think about their learning and development journey periodically, particularly at times they feel the urge to stocktake, regroup and plan where and how they would like to offer their skills in the future.

As you continue to learn more about the integration of law, ethics and regulation in your daily life and work pursuits, remember that you will always have experienced guides with you on the journey. The philosophers, jurists, parliamentarians, scholars, policy makers and regulators, professional colleagues and researchers from previous generations will be available to you through their writings. You will see their voices reflected in contemporary discussions and debates. When you contribute to the discussions, your voice will also become part of the legacy of learning for others in the future.

Summary

This chapter has provided the opportunity to reflect on the way practical regulations actively support the delivery of health care and health and community services. With a focus on availability and restriction, and distribution of services, you will now understand that legal provisions support the regulation of availability of services. Examples of funding restrictions and priority-setting policies have given the opportunity to explore the classically debated funding and distribution models, and to learn that those models are informed by ethics reasoning. Some everyday examples have been used, from the perspective of a potential client or patient, such as considering refugees seeking information on available services, bringing into sharp focus the difficult topic of resource allocation and justice.

STUDY QUESTIONS

1 Define interests and rights.
2 Briefly describe the way a health care system is organised to enable providers to provide a health care service to potential clients. Explain briefly how law, regulation and ethics combine to establish and maintain the system for a particular community of potential clients.
3 Describe the three models of justice.
4 Choose one of the models of justice, and provide examples of its application in a health care service setting.

SAMPLE ESSAY QUESTION

1 Define rights and interests, and entitlement to health care. Set out the positions of the citizen, permanent resident, tourist and asylum seeker in seeking health care services in your jurisdiction.
2 Review the Glossary terms to revisit concepts that you have covered throughout the text.

GLOSSARY QUIZ

Choose glossary terms at random. See if you can define each term, and also explain what it means when it is applied in a specific legal, ethical or regulatory context that you have read about in the text.

REFERENCES

[ ] Editorial. (1997). Health Inequality: The UK's Biggest Issue. *Lancet*, *349*, 1185.

Addicott, R., & Ham, C. (2014). *Commissioning and funding general practice: Making the case for family care networks*. London: The King's Fund. Retrieved from http://kingsfund.org.uk

Asch, D.A., & Ubel, P.A. (1997). Rationing by Any Other Name. *New England Journal of Medicine*, *336*(23), 1668–71.

Australian Government, Department of Health. (2017). *Medicare Benefits Schedule Book Operating from 1 November 2017*. Retrieved from http://mbsonline.gov.au

Australian Government. (2017). *Organ and Tissue Authority: About donation, and myths and misconceptions*. Retrieved from http://donatelife.gov.au

Australian Nursing & Midwifery Federation. (2017). *Department of Veterans' Affairs Coordinated Veterans' care (CVC) Program*. Retrieved from http://anmf.org.au

BBC. (2017, 4 October). England to consider optout organ donation. *BBC News*. Retrieved from http:// bbc.com/news

Beauchamp, T.L., & Childress, J.F. (1994). *Principles of biomedical ethics* (4th edn). London: Oxford University Press.

Benko, L.B., & Bellandi, D. (2001). The rough and tumble of it. *Modern Healthcare*, *31*(12), 53–4.

Berglund, C.A. (1997). Bioethics: A balancing of concerns in context. *Australian Health Review*, *20*(1), 43–52.

Brennan, S. (2015, 25 November). New opt-out system in Wales aims to revolutionise organ donation. *The Guardian*. Retrieved from http://theguardian.com

British Medical Association [BMA]. (2017, 16 October). *Policy and research ethics: Organ donation*. Retrieved from http://bma.org.uk

Callahan, D. (1996). Achievable goals. *World Health*, *5*, 6–8.

Commonwealth Department of Health and Family Services. (1997). *Supplement to Medicare Benefits Schedule Book of 1 November 1996*, effective 1 May 1997. Canberra: AGPS.

Commonwealth Department of Health and Ageing, Acute and Co-ordinated Care Branch. (2000). *Primary care initiatives: Further co-ordinated care trials.* Retrieved from www.health.gov.au/hsdd/primcare/acoorcar/abtrials.htm

Devereux, J. (2002). *Medical law: Text, cases and materials* (2nd edn). Sydney: Cavendish.

Dickens, B.M. (1994). Legal approaches to health care ethics and the four principles. In R. Gillon (Ed.), *Principles of health care ethics*. Chichester: John Wiley & Sons.

Dorr-Goold, S., & Klipp, G. (2002). Managed care members talk about trust. *Social Science & Medicine*, *54*(6), 879–88.

Evans, B.T., & Pritchard, C. (2000). Cancer survival rates and GDP expenditure on health: A comparison of England and Wales and the USA, Denmark, Netherlands, Finland, France, Germany, Italy, Spain and Switzerland in the 1990s. *Public Health*, *114*(5), 336–9.

Gillon, R. (1986). *Philosophical medical ethics*. Chichester, United Kingdom: John Wiley & Sons.

Gomez, A.G., Grimm, C.T., Yee, E.F.T., & Skootsky, S.A. (1997). Preparing residents for managed care practice using an experience-based curriculum. *Academic Medicine*, *72*(11), 959–65.

Government of South Australia. (2017). *Planning ahead: Organ and tissue donation, provisions*. Retrieved from www.sa.gov.au

Kitzhaber, J., & Kemmy, A.M. (1995). On the Oregon Trail. *British Medical Bulletin*, *51*(4), 809.

Lyall, K. (2002, 24 April). 30-baht health care a fatal prescription. *The Australian*, 8.

Mannion, R. (2011). General practitioner-led commissioning in the NHS: Progress, prospects and pitfalls [Review]. *British Medical Journal*, *97*(1), 7–15.

McCombs, J.S. (1996). [Letter]. *New England Journal of Medicine*, *335*(19), 1465.

Medicines Australia. (2011, 16 June). *Parliament condemns Cabinet decision to block listing of new PBS medicines*. Retrieved from http://medicineaustralia.com.au

Mitchell, K.R., & Lovat, T.J. (1991). *Bioethics for medical and health professionals*. Wentworth Falls: Social Sciences Press.

New South Wales Government, Department of Health. (2012). *Waiting time and elective surgery policy*. PD 2012_011. Retrieved from www.health.nsw.gov.au

New South Wales Government. (2018). *Budget Paper 3. Budget Estimates 2018–19*. NSW Budget 2018–19.Retrieved from www.budget.nsw.gov.au

New Zealand Medical Association. (1994). *New Zealand Medical Association Newsletter*, *108*, 3.

New Zealand Parliament. (2009). New Zealand Health System Reforms, Parliamentary Library Research Paper. Retrieved from http://parliament.nz

Organization for Economic Cooperation and Development [OECD]. (2017). *OECD health data 2017: Health expenditure and financing*. Paris: OECD. Retrieved from www.oecd.org

Pearson, S.D., Sabin, J.E., & Hyams, T. (2002). Caring for patients within a budget: Physicians' tales from the front lines of managed care. *Journal of Clinical Ethics, 13*(2), 115–23.

Powell, L. (2005). Providing quality healthcare under funding constraints. *New Zealand Medical Journal, 118*(1215), U1471.

Smith, S., Newhouse, J.P., & Freeland, M.S. (2009). Income, insurance, and technology: Why does health spending outpace economic growth? *Health Affairs, 28*(5), 1276–84.

State Government of Victoria, Department of Health. (2011). *Guidelines for Victorian public health services on community detention*, as at September 2011. Retrieved from www2.health.vic.gov.au

State Government of Victoria, Department of Health. (2011). *Guide to asylum seeker access to health and community services in Victoria*, revised May 2011. Retrieved from www2.health.vic.gov.au

Svensson, M. (2010). Cost–benefit analysis. In R.C. Free (Ed.), *21st century economics: A reference handbook* (pp. 275–83). Thousand Oaks, California: SAGE.

Ubel, P.A., DeKay, M.L., Baron, J., & Asch, D.A. (1996). Cost-effectiveness analysis in a setting of budget constraints. *New England Journal of Medicine, 334*(18), 1174–7.

United Nations. (1951/1967). *United Nations Convention and Protocol Relating to the Status of Refugees.* Resolution 2198 (XXI) adopted by the United Nations General Assembly, adopted in 1951 and as amended by 1967 protocol. Retrieved from http://unhcr.org

United Nations. (1990). *Convention on the Rights of the Child.* Entry into force 2 September 1990. Retrieved from www.un.org

Urbina, C., Kaufman, A., & Derksen, D. (1997). The managed health care scenario: Challenges to future medical training. *Education for Health, 10*(1), 25–33.

Victorian Government, Aboriginal Affairs Victoria and Department of Planning and Community Development. (2008). Indigenous Family Violence Partnership Forum. *Strong Culture, Strong Peoples, Strong Families 10 year plan: Towards a safer future for Indigenous families and community.* Retrieved from http://dhs.voc.gov.au

World Health Organization. (1976). Preamble to the Constitution of World Health Organization. In *WHO Basic Documents* (26th edn). Geneva: World Health Organization.

LEGISLATION

Health Insurance Act 1973 (Cth)

Health Insurance (Diagnostic Imaging Services Table) Regulations 2017 (Cth)

Health Insurance (General Medical Services Table) Regulations 2017 (Cth)

Health Insurance (Pathology Services Table) Regulations 2017 (Cth)

Health Insurance Regulation Regulations 1975 (Cth)

Human Services Amendment Act 2011 (Cth)

Motor Accident Injuries Act 2017 (NSW)

National Health Act 1953 (Cth)

Safe Patient Care (Nurse to Patient and Midwife to Patient Ratios) Act 2015 (Vic)

State Insurance and Care Governance Act 2015 (NSW)

The National Health Service (General Medical Services Contracts) Regulations 2004 (UK)

GLOSSARY

Note: Numbers in brackets refer to chapters where these terms are defined.

Absolutism
An ethics theory in which a rule or rules are identified as fundamentally important, and of unvarying significance. (4)

Accountability
Process of being open to scrutiny for assessment of conduct of responsibilities. (3)

Administrative law
Principles and procedures of fair administration and administrative decision making for matters particularly affecting an individual's interests. (3)

Advance directive
A directive given by patient in advance that represents their autonomous wishes and is intended by them to guide their treatment and care in the future. (8)

Assault
Physical interference or causing fear of physical interference to a person. (1)

Autonomy
The principle of allowing and promoting self-rule, of people making decisions about their lives. (1)

Battery
An act of physical interference or force applied to a victim's body without consent. *Battery* is an old term. Many modern laws combine battery in the broader concept of assault, which includes the threat as well as actual force or touching. (1, 3)

Belief
Firmly held opinion or accepted understanding. (2)

Beneficence
The principle of doing good and providing care for others. (1)

Benefit
Positive effect or outcome. (7)

Best interests
That which is judged to be to the maximal benefit of a person or persons in maintaining or furthering their health and welfare. (7)

Bioethics
Reflective ethics process applied to the health care context and life sciences. (1)

Capacity
Legal capability or competence, such as for informed decision making. (8)

Casuistry
Ethics theory in which previous decisions are analysed in terms of values, and factual and cultural contexts, and used to guide future decisions. (4)

Character
Moral qualities of a person. (2)

Claim
Implicit or explicit demand to receive a good, as one's due. (10)

Client
Person investigating or receiving service. (2)

Code of conduct
Comprehensive listing of rules or principles to guide members of a group in their thought and action. (1)

Common law
Fair rules and principles set down in civil courts for the people to follow. (3)

Communitarianism
An ethics theory in which the relationship of a person to a specific community is identified, and the interests and needs of that community as a whole take priority over individual interests and needs. (2)

Community
Group of people defined by shared social engagement. (2)

Comparative justice
Justice model of need, in which goods are distributed on the basis of demonstrated most need, compared with the demonstrated needs of other community members. (10)

Competence
Ability to perform a specified task, and readiness to do so. (2)

Competencies
Skills that have been assessed and demonstrated by a person as able to be performed to an acceptable standard. (2)

Comprehension
Understanding, specific to issues under consideration. (8)

Compulsory
Required action for all, with enforcement provisions. (6)

Confidentiality
Limited distribution of another's personal information, due to respect for privacy. (6)

Conflict of interest
A situation in which two potentially opposing and incompatible interests exist. (6)

Consent
Agreement. (7)

Consequentialism
An ethics theory in which the consequences of actions are the focus, both on the actor and others affected by the action. (4)

Consultation
Active process of facilitating the expression of opinions, taking advice and cooperative deliberation. (2)

Contract law
Principles of legally enforceable agreements and procedure for testing breaches in a civil court. (3)

Conviction
Firmly held belief. (4)

Cost–benefit analysis
A calculation of the cost of delivering a service with demonstrated and calculated financial benefits. (10)

Cost–effectiveness analysis
A comparative assessment of costs in achieving an agreed objective or beneficial outcome. (10)

Criminal law
Jurisdiction's body of rules and principles on prohibited conduct and omissions and penalties for proven prohibited conduct. (3)

Cultural safety
Safety for a person given their culture, environment and personal experience. (2)

Culture
Social expectations and norms of a particular community or civilisation. (2)

Deon
Established morally fundamental rule. (2)

Deontology
An ethics theory in which the process and components of actual or proposed action is the focus, with reference to agreed values and rules. (2)

Descriptive ethics
An ethics tradition demonstrating or noting the stance adopted, and not necessarily the reason for the stance. (4)

Dignity
Quality of worthiness. (5)

Distributive justice
Justice model of need and entitlement, in which goods are distributed based on demonstrated and comparative interest and entitlement to receive community benefits and the expectation or capacity to bear burden. (10)

Doctrine
Tenet or lesson held out or taught as a true guiding rule. (4)

Doctrine of double effect
Ethics doctrine in which the intention of likely positive effects is considered to morally excuse certain foreseen negative effects. (4)

Duties
Obligations and specific tasks that you are bound to fulfil, or actions from which you are bound to refrain. (2)

Duty of care
An obligation to take reasonable care in dealings with a person, once there is an undertaking to provide care or advice, or contribute to such specific benefit for a specific person. (4)

Entitlement
Recognised need to create community obligation to fulfil interest or claim. (10)

Ethics
Reflective process of analysing and examining moral issues and problems. (1)

False imprisonment
Unlawful physical or psychological restraint of liberty, including detention. (1)

Fiduciary duties
Duties of good faith so that trust, confidence or influence over another person and their trust and confidence in the fiduciary relationship is not abused. (3)

Fit and proper person
A suitable person deserving of the trust of others to exercise certain privileges in an ethical manner. (2)

Goals
Ideals and objectives aimed towards. (2)

Good
A desirable end or object. (1)

Governance
Controlling, directing or regulating activities. (2)

Health
State of physical, mental and social wellbeing. (10)

Health care
The provision of care with the objective of maintaining, restoring, or improving health or comfort. (2)

Health care professionals
Those trained in recognised professions to be providers of health care. (2)

Health care worker
Person working in health service delivery who is not registered as a health practitioner. (1)

Health practitioner
Health care professional who is registered under the Health Practitioner Regulation National Law. (1)

Human rights
Basic rights, thought to be due to all human beings. (1)

Ideals
A standard or concept of excellence, which is aimed to be met. (1)

Impairment
Condition detrimentally impacting on competencies, competence, or capacity. (2)

Impropriety
Imprudence; stark and distasteful contravention to conventional standards. (2)

Information
Details specific to the issue under consideration. (8)

Informed consent
Agreement given based on information and understanding of the proposed process, significance of decision, and potential benefits or risks entailed. (8)

Informed decision making
Alternative term for 'informed consent', also encompassing the active participation of both parties in determining options to be potentially agreed to, and in identifying significant material risks and benefits to be explored. (8)

Insight
A reflective process of examining own behaviour and motivations, and recognising deficiencies. (2)

Integrity
Willingness to actively reflect upon and uphold the highest principles and standards of conduct consistent with roles, responsibilities and duties. (1)

Interest
That which is to one's advantage or benefit. (10)

Judiciary
Court system set up to adjudicate and resolve disputes between the state and a person, or between two persons. (3)

Jurisdiction
Scope of authority and power to set and enforce laws and regulatory schemes. (1)

Justice
The principle of fair allocation of community resources and burdens. (1)

Justice as fairness
Justice model of equality, in which goods are distributed with the aim that community members are restored to equivalent levels. (10)

Law
Body of formal and customary rules and principles, used to regulate interactions in a community. (1)

Legislation
Statutes and other rules in related instruments which are formally approved by a parliament. (1)

Libertarianism
An ethics theory that aims for the greatest good for the greatest number, with good defined by each person pursuing their own defined wishes and liberties. (2)

Liberty
Freedom of will, as expressed in choice of thought or action. (6)

Mandatory
Required action, contingent on being under certain command and corresponding enforceable obligations. (6)

Mandatory notification
Alert to relevant authorities. (2)

Medical ethics
Specific term for ethics in the medical and biomedical context. (1)

Mental capacity
Cognitive capability for specific thought process. (8)

Morals
Significant lessons prompting reflection to identify virtuous, right, or acceptable course of conduct. (1)

Need
Demonstrated interest in receiving a good. (10)

Non-maleficence
The principle of not harming others, and of minimising harm to them. (1)

Normative ethics
An ethics tradition in which moral positions that are held are demonstrated and reasons for the adoption of those positions are also explored. (4)

Norms
Accepted standards, which can be used to judge conduct. (1)

Obligation
Something one is bound to fulfil or perform. (2)

Paternalism
Decision-making framework in which care and control of another is undertaken. (5)

Patient
Person receiving care. (2)

Person
Live human being, or live human being in development, with essential and recognised qualities of intrinsic capacity or function. (9)

Personal morality
Significant lessons prompting reflection to identify a virtuous, right or acceptable course of conduct of an individual, largely affecting that individual. (7)

Personhood
Quality of being a person. (9)

Potentiality
Capacity to develop in a certain way, given the opportunity and suitable development conditions. (9)

Prima facie
Conclusion supported by first observation or apparent evidence. (3)

Principle
A fundamental proposition, from which specific goals or duties can be derived, or under which goals and duties can be described. (4)

Principlism
An ethics framework in which issues are understood and analysed with the assistance of broad descriptive principles. (2)

Privacy
State of secrecy or concealment. (6)

Private interest
Issues of importance and significance to an individual, defined on an individual basis to be in that person's best interest. (6)

Professional
Skilled person with high standards of skill and ethics, which they offer in the service of the community. (1)

Professional code of ethics
Expression of principles, rules, ideals, and values of specific professional group, creating responsibility to strive for states, ideals and goals, and to uphold certain rules, in each member professional's conduct. (1)

Professional misconduct
Unsatisfactory professional conduct that is so serious it could warrant suspension from practice or deregistration. (2)

Proportionism
An ethics theory in which rules and values can be used as guides, but their application takes into account the practical alternatives in a given situation, with allowance for human nature. (4)

Propriety
In keeping with prudent and supported conventional standards. (2)

Public health
Field of health care concerned with assessing and improving health and preventing illness or disease on a population basis. (6)

Public interest
Issues of importance and significance to the structure of a community, and to the general benefit of a significant group of a community's members. (6)

Regulation
Standards, rules, restrictions and procedures for social control and management in specific contexts. (1)

Reflection
A process of thought and analysis on past, present or future issues, applying deep and serious consideration. (2)

Relativism
An ethics theory in which divergent perspectives are canvassed, with a view to establishing courses of action that are acceptable to those perspectives in their given context. (4)

Religion
System of faith and belief according to recognised sacred teachings. (4)

Respect
Hold in high regard and esteem, and to refrain from interference with a respected person. (5)

Respect for persons
Principle of upholding autonomy, generally used for research participants. (4)

Responsibility
Obligation and duty to fulfil certain tasks or series of tasks. (1)

Right
Claim that is recognised as imposing obligations on others to fulfil it. (10)

Risk
Likelihood of negative effect or outcome; possibility of significant negative outcome. (7)

Rules
Derived and specific expression of fundamental principles or ideals that are agreed by a group to have force, in a moral obligation of members of the group to abide by them. (1)

Skill
Level of competence in a specific task or series of tasks. (1)

Slippery-slope argument
An argument that small 'slips' in standards will lead to larger 'downwards slides' and a

degradation of standards, so that any small slips should be vigorously guarded against. (4)

Social morality
Significant lessons prompting reflection to identify a virtuous, right, or acceptable course of conduct of individuals, with significant implications for the choices then available to others in society. (7)

Standards
Accepted benchmarks that are defined and available. (1)

Substitute decision maker
Person who makes decisions on behalf of another, acting as a proxy or surrogate. (5)

Tort law
Common law principles of wrongs committed against a person or the person's interests and the process of proving those wrongs in a civil court. (3)

Transparency
Being candid and open to scrutiny. (7)

Trust
Confidence in another person, or persons within an organisation, to act in an expected manner. (5)

Unsatisfactory professional conduct
Conduct that is judged by peers of good repute to be significantly below acceptable standards. (2)

Utilitarianism
An ethics theory in which the outcome of actual or proposed action is the focus, and the acceptable course of action is that in which the greatest good for the greatest number is achieved. (3)

Utility
Quality of usefulness for a desired purpose or outcome. (10)

Values
Concepts given worth or importance in life and interactions, making up a value system. (1)

Veracity
Truthfulness, accuracy, and completeness in information relied on by others. (5)

Virtue
Worth or quality of particular moral excellence. (1)

Voluntariness
To decide own course of action with free and unconstrained will. (8)

Wishes
Desired states, thoughts, or actions that would bring happiness if attained or realised. (5)

INDEX